A. JAMES PRINS
A LIFE IN LITERATURE

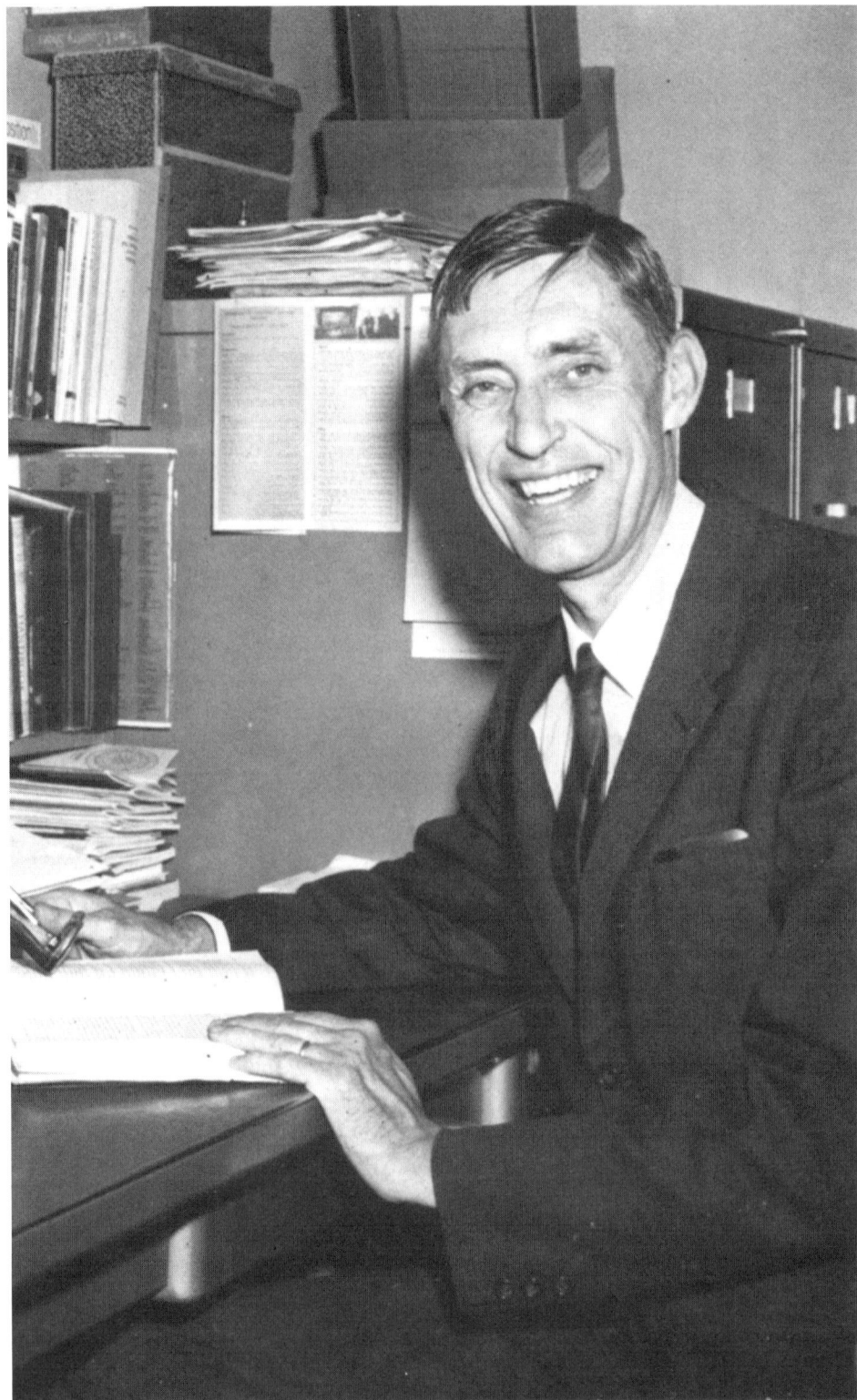

A. JAMES PRINS
A Life in Literature

Edited by Kathleen Verduin
and Christopher James Prins

ℬℬℬ

Hope College, Holland, Michigan

2006

ISBN 10: 0-9655709-1-6
ISBN 13: 978-0-9655709-1-6

This book is printed on recycled paper.

Printed by Thomson-Shore, Inc., Dexter, Michigan

IN MEMORIAM

ALBERT JAMES PRINS

June 11,1916   May 27, 2003

I am a teacher who believes that no piece of literature can ever be taught in an artistic vacuum. Great literature is always morally relevant to human living, any time.

—A. James Prins
Lecture on *Huckleberry Finn*, 1965

DEDICATION

Monica Michelle Bakker

Trevor Jon Bakker

Emma Jeanette Prins

Alexa Joy Bakker

Lillian Rose Prins

Clara Rose Bakker

CONTENTS

ESSAYS AND REVIEWS

Preface

David J. Klooster

HOW TO REMEMBER a teacher, a colleague, a father? How to name the meanings of a career in the classroom, a devotion to novels, a life?

In this collection of writing by and about A. James Prins, Kathleen Verduin and Christopher Prins have given us provocative materials to think about these questions. From 1946 to 1981, Jim Prins was Professor of English at Hope College, introducing several generations of students to the novels of the United States, England, Europe, and Russia. More importantly, he introduced them to the peculiar and powerful ways of knowing human life that the novel offers, knowledge of life's beauty, joy, longing, and loss.

The collection provides many examples—in lecture notes and scholarly writing as well as in the many personal reminiscences of his students—of the power of Prins' thinking and teaching. His believing and doubting, his mirth and his melancholy, his rigor and his compassion, his sharp intelligence and his broad, empathetic humanity—all of these qualities emerge from the collection. Readers who knew and revered Prins will be reminded of all the reasons he mattered so deeply to them. Readers like me who never met the man will be grateful to spend these pages in his company.

One value of this collection is the lens it provides on the significant changes in college teaching from Prins' day to our own. Could anyone today expect to teach a major novel every week, as Prins did, year after year? I assign half the reading Prins did, and still my students, who have grown up without a habit of reading, can barely keep up. Does anyone, in this era of class discussions and small group projects and PowerPoint presentations, prepare lecture notes as eloquent, thorough, and wise as those found in this book? Prins' New Critical readings, beginning with analysis of structure and symbol systems and leading to meditations on universal human truths, speak of an era less ironic and detached than our own, an era when words like "wisdom" and "truth" never had quotation marks around them. His lecture notes remind us of a time when college professors could devote their full attention and their best intellectual energies to classroom teaching; they did not have to ration their time and their intellectual energies for their scholarship. When college faculty today talk about "my own work," they mean their current research and publishing projects, not their teaching. Prins and the professors of his generation gave their all in the classroom, and what a gift of intellect and eloquence and insight it was.

Yet in other ways, the collection also reassures us that not all that much has changed in college classrooms. Young adults, in their first brush with intellectual freedom, still thrill to *The Scarlet Letter* and *Moby-Dick* and *Madame Bovary* and *Anna Karenina*. Professors still return to these novels each year as if revisiting dear friends. When everything is working right, the college classroom still combines the intense thinking and feeling we find described here, as well as the joy and the danger Prins' students describe in his classes. Even in the informality of our time, there can still be the kind of student-professor relationships that mix respect, curious attraction, a bit of fear, and a willingness to talk about what matters most. The college literature classroom is still an oddly intimate space, one of the few spaces in our culture where an adult man or woman can speak about phallic symbols or characters' sexual desires with a room full of teenagers, and where that discussion can lead to honest exchanges about love and power and sex and death. Although much has changed in the twenty-five years since Jim Prins retired, the classroom life and the literature that he so clearly loved remain much the same, and therefore the many writings collected here illuminate the abiding challenges and joys of college teaching.

How to remember a man and his life's work? From reading these pages, I suspect that Jim Prins would be happiest if we remembered him by rereading, alone and together, the novels he loved and taught over the many years of his distinguished career. We remember Prins best when we turn back to *Moby-Dick* or *Huck Finn* or *Wuthering Heights*, with his notes fresh in our mind, and learn to love afresh what he loved: the power of the novel to illuminate the rich, sweet, sad life we share with the characters on the page.

Department of English
Hope College

 ℗℗℗

Foreword

Christopher James Prins

MY FATHER was a passionate and complex man.

Raised in the Dutch Reformed faith, he struggled all his life with questions of religious belief and tolerance. Dad despised dogma for dogma's sake and rebelled against closed ways of thinking. His service in World War II exposed him, like many of his time, to places far away from what he had known and to hardships he perhaps had not imagined. He met my mother in England and returned to the United States changed in many ways. Holland, however, remained his true home, and he chose to live the rest of his life there in an uncomfortable truce with many of the values that had formed him.

In literature my father found an exciting forum in which to satisfy his intellectual hunger, to explore new ideas and discover whole new worlds. As a professor of English at Hope College for over forty years, Dad entertained and inspired generations of students. He changed lives. My dad had charisma. The trademark Prins grin, the infectious energy he brought to his classroom, and his ability to be both clever and provocative were all legendary among those who loved him on the Hope campus. They remember his appetite for truth, his integrity, and his ability to make the literature he taught come alive. His students appreciated the very personal way in which he educated both their hearts and their minds.

My father firmly believed that literature is the artistic fulfillment of important ideas and attitudes and that it allows the reader to experience them in living form. As one former student wrote to my mother in remembrance and gratitude after his death, "He lingered over every line until it disclosed a revelation." In the characters created by the great American, English, European, and Russian novelists, my father found the resilience and ultimate victory of the human spirit, and my father brought these truths to the classroom, giving a great gift to the many thousands of students he taught over the years.

At the same time, my father was a melancholy man, sometimes overwhelmed by a sort of sadness. He was deeply moved by human frailty in its many forms and feared himself his own limitations. Perhaps this is why he could never be certain and rest securely in a knowledge of right and wrong. Perhaps also this nervous edge of uncertainty that accompanied his passion for literature and his lack of arrogance or pretension helped to make him such a great teacher.

The writings in this volume attest to the affection many of my father's students felt for him. They capture his spirit and ideals. This volume also serves as an important history of the period during which my father taught at Hope College. Much of his essence, of course, cannot be captured in print. And he himself did not write a great deal. My father often was told by his students that he should write a novel. He never did, and it is a shame. He did not think of himself as a scholar or critic and did not publish much. Instead, Dad devoted his energies to the classroom. Fortunately, his painstakingly prepared class notes were preserved, and some of these notes are included here as an effort to capture his ideas and approach to teaching.

Nothing was as important to my father as his family. I remember him telling me that he served on the Holland Board of Education, to which he was elected for three terms, so that he could ensure that the voice of an educator was heard in the decisions that influenced my education and because he wanted to be on the podium when I received my high school diploma. Yet it was in my father's professional life, through teaching the novels that he loved, that he could express himself best. Like too many men, he could not express his affections easily to those he loved and tell them what he felt. I think also that depression sometimes interfered with his ability to communicate with those he loved most.

My father is absent now, but he still is with me each day. He is part of my very fiber and being. I hear him in my voice when I speak and see him in the mirror when I shave in the morning. I often find myself wondering what my father would do when I have an important decision to make. Like many sons, I want to be different from my father in some important ways, but I am inspired by the strength of his intense, unspoken love for my sister and me, and I try to give the same to my children and tell them so. Dad taught me how to think—the greatest gift of a liberal arts education—to see that there exist so many ways of viewing the same object or idea, to appreciate uncertainty, and to see that so much is beautiful in this world. To be tolerant and have empathy. I lack Dad's charisma, but I aspire to his passion.

ᔕᔕᔕ

PROFESSING LITERATURE

Novels are stories. But great novels are also the artistic fulfillment of important and significant ideas and attitudes. It's a particularly good way to be exposed to those ideas and attitudes, because you're getting it in a living form. Sometimes I couldn't believe that students would cry about a novel, but they do sometimes. Because it's real.

—A. James Prins
"Reflections of a Literature Prof," 1975

ℒℒℒ

Reflections of a Literature Prof

Eileen Verduin Raphael, Class of 1970

Hope College Magazine, 1975

DR. JAMES PRINS does not particularly like the idea of an interview. He fears a dearth of material. Besides, he says, "Good quotes come only spontaneously when something occurs in a classroom, and then they become mythical. But they don't happen in cases like this, where we say, 'Let's put it down in words'—it doesn't happen."

He likes even less the idea of being photographed. He is concerned that former students may see his image spread on the pages of the alumni magazine and deduce that he is not well. "A person gets old and dowdy, and I'm a lot more stooped than I used to be." He reveals that his wife, Iris, objected to his appearance when he left the house that morning, pointing to his untrimmed hair, the absence of a suit and tie. "My wife said, 'How do you dare!'" He accents each word and then pauses before deciding to finish, "'How do you dare to have an interview the way you look today?'"

But one must protest. The years seem to have been rather benevolent in dealing out their ravages on the person of Prins. His slenderness remains intact; his longer hair seems to shorten his face a bit; the cranberry V-neck sweater relaxes the angularity of his frame.

And, in time, the "good quotes" do come, as Dr. Prins begins to lapse into the manner of speaking which has made his classes immemorable for the thousands of literature students who have enrolled in his courses since he first came to Hope as a faculty member in 1946. Perhaps a former student best described the intrigue when he pinpointed Dr. Prins as the only teacher he had ever studied under who lectured in stream of consciousness.

It is somewhat in this form that we begin to discuss his now nearly sixty-year-long life, and from the stream a pattern emerges, a pattern of what Dr. Prins describes as the "accidents" of his life which have defined his now nearly thirty-year-long career as a member of the Hope faculty in the department of English.

A Holland, Mich., native, he enrolled in Calvin College in 1934. He transferred to Hope the following year as a pre-law student, majoring in English. He graduated in 1938, "poorer than poor." Faced with the financial impossibility of attending law school, Prins opted instead for graduate work in English at the University of Michigan. He received the M.A. degree in 1939. For the following three years, he taught at the Shepherd, Mich., High School.

He entered the Army in 1942 and served in the military police division. While stationed in

Southampton, England, he met his future wife, Iris. They were married in 1949. (Dr. and Mrs. Prins have two children. Christopher is a sophomore at Harvard, possessing what his father unconvincingly describes as "appalling interest" in literature. Robin is a high school junior.)

After his discharge in the early winter of 1946, Prins came back to Holland, where he planned to bide his time until fall when he would enter the University of Michigan to obtain his Ph.D. degree.

Instead, he was approached by then Hope president Irwin J. Lubbers and Professor Clarence De Graaf, who were attempting to prepare for the monumental postwar enrollment jump. Without great enthusiasm, Prins agreed to teach English for a semester. The semester completed, he was anxious to begin his work at the U. of M., where he had been offered a teaching fellowship.

Instead, Dr. Lubbers' noted powers of persuasion were directed toward this young English instructor. Prins eventually received his Ph.D., but he did so while a professor at Hope.

At this point, as well, circumstances redefined Dr. Prins' intentions: "I think that you ought to believe that my original motivation in literature was creative. I always thought that I would like to write. As I look at it now, I don't think I'd be a very good writer. But when I started teaching here, I had the idea that perhaps teaching was the best way into writing that a person could find. But that's very false. It probably hurts a person. I find that before I can dare to teach anything, I have to read everything I can get . . . all the critical material and all the novels by that person, before I would dare go into a class and utter any words that I think are important enough to utter. It takes so much time.

"But I think you should know that I'm not unhappy," he continues. "The accidents that occurred in my life occurred the way that they did. I'm not sorry it happened this way. I mean, what's a more wonderful thing that to be in touch with the things you like—the literature and the people who are young. They're young!" he says emphatically. "You get paid for staying in touch with young people.

"It's been wonderful. It's almost embarrassing sometimes that students remember you, remember you in a kindly way," he says. "People come back and search you out, you get a letter once in a while. It's always been reciprocal. I've always enjoyed the students very much. You get old, things do change, but this contact with the young people remains as something very important to me."

What has changed most for Dr. Prins? Small things mostly—the informality of the times, the addition of a Saul Bellow novel on the reading list for American Novels, slightly smaller classes the past few years. He believes that former students remember him best for the stance he always assumed while teaching—*sans* chair, with one long foot flung over the desk top. "That's changed," he says. "I sit down now almost all the time. I'm still animated, but I'm much more deskbound than I used to be."

And probably Dr. Prins is right—one remembers the small things: his teaching posture, the free-flowing manner of his lectures, the way he pronounces "literature" to come out more like "litrature." Many students, majors in varied fields of study, also remember, however, the uncanny way Dr. Prins had of making the study of literature in the genre of the novel a very meaningful experience. And that has not changed.

"I hope that this general interest holds," says Dr. Prins, "that the preseminary student, or the sociology or the history or the philosophy student does think that coming into contact with ideas as they're dramatized in novels is a significant thing to do. It's a way to approach life. What can you take for credit that's more fun than to read novels that have dramatic and narrative situations in them?

"But they're serious," he continues. "I think literature is a means to make us feel about how we think. It's an approach to life in a vicarious way. It has a dimension that is more than cerebral. Literature shows the individual that he is a feeling as well as thinking mechanism.

"Novels are stories. But great novels are also the artistic fulfillment of important and significant ideas and attitudes. It's a particularly good way to be exposed to these ideas and attitudes, because you're getting it in a living form. Sometimes I couldn't believe that students would cry about a novel, but they do sometimes. Because it's real."

What does Dr. Prins hope students gain from his teaching? "I suppose what every teacher hopes he can do is exactly what happens to Strether [in *The Ambassadors* by Henry James]—the gradual awareness, the growing up, the ability to suddenly be able to say 'Ah!' As Shakespeare said, 'Ripeness is all,' having people see things as they've never seen them before, the way Strether sees things as he never saw them before."

Dr. Prins is now a senior faculty member. The unwritten Prins novel will probably remain un-written, rightly or wrongfully so. He speaks of all the unread novels which continue to beckon. And so this rawboned man continues in much the same way. Ripeness is all.

⚘

Last Chance Talk

In the mid-1960s students at Hope College initiated an annual lecture known as the "Last Chance Talk": a chance for professors to address an audience as if it were their last opportunity to speak. The designated speaker was also the recipient of that year's HOPE (Hope's Outstanding Professor-Educator) Award. A. James Prins received this award in 1966.

> We grow stoneblind and insensible to life's more elementary and general goods and joys.
> —William James

IT IS TRUE that a hypothetical last chance is never far from actuality and always very close in the imagination, especially when one has already embarked on his second half-century of human existence. My barns are filled with goods, my brain is filled with wisdom, my heart and veins are filled with desire—so I am ripe for last chances. I could be struck dead or dumb tomorrow, or I could lose my job. I could even be snatched from amongst you by the long arm of federal law. It has happened here, you know. To be sure, then, the uncertainties of life make it easy to imagine hypothetical possibilities. So it is reasonable that you ask me, "What would you say if or if or if?" I can only answer as truly as my imagination tells me.

Behind the idea of a Last Chance Talk lurk unpleasant assumptions that the Last Chancer has never said before what he will say now, or that, faced with extinction or separation, his vision will be sharpened to an illumination it did not have before, or that, worst of all, he will dare to say something he did not dare to say before, since imminent departure guarantees him immunity to reprisal in the world from which he is shortly departing. It is good that my last chance here tonight is hypothetical and that therefore my immunity is hypothetical and irrelevant—because I like to believe that in twenty years of teaching at Hope College I have said the most important things I know over and over. I like to believe that after fifty years of thinking and feeling my vision doesn't need sharpening by the drastic threat of extinction. I like to believe that I have always dared to say what I thought important to say, without meanness of spirit. None of this is wholly true, perhaps not even most true, but I am aiming at the clarification of a Last Chance Talk in terms of what ought to be, to define it as simply the next opportunity to repeat what is important enough to repeat.

What is it that I have tried many times before to impart and now wish to say over again?

I could make the burden of this talk my intellectual and scholarly opinions on the study of literature. I could give you my philosophy of life or of teaching. These are truly important matters, but likely to be deadly. I could be more exciting with a talk about protest. I have very strong views on Vietnam, on Civil Rights, on the drafting of college students. Some of them might surprise you. I can be passionate, one way or another, about *Anchor* rights and *Opus* rights, about compulsory Chapel and compulsory Culture. The idea of protest appeals to me very much. I believe that without the spirit of protest the teacher and the student and the college will die.

None of all this that I could do would be the simple truth for this moment. It would not be true to what I can imagine myself saying if this were really my last chance. It would not be right on an evening like this one, when the magic of April is creating the magic of May: "when April with its sweet showers/The drought of March has pierced to the root . . ."

> And small birds make a melody
> That sleep all night with open eye—
> So Nature pricks them in their corages—
> Then folk long to go on pilgrimages . . .

Tonight Nature pricks us in our hearts. We desire to move out.

But I *will* in the correct sense of the word protest. For to protest is to affirm and to say positively. I protest once again that life is full of joy and wonder. It is very much worth living, particularly when looked at from the extremity of a last chance. I mean life lived with the open heart, the life responsive to the world of the senses and not isolated in a dungeon of selfish despair. We do not make the most of it, and we miss a lot of it.

In a well-known paragraph, William James states that

our judgments concerning the worth of things, big or little, depend on the *feelings* the things arouse in us. Where we judge a thing to be precious in consequence of the *idea* we frame of it, this is only because the idea is itself already associated with a feeling. If we were radically feelingless, and if ideas were the only things our minds could entertain, we should lose all our likes and dislikes at a stroke, and be unable to point to any one situation or experience in life more valuable or significant than any other.

James' plea is for revitalization of the heart's response to the world that lies around us and is open to our senses, for a renewed joy in the common and ordinary and plain that we have disdained or forgotten in abstract thinking, abstract living. "Life," he says,

is always worth living if one have such responsive sensibilities. But we of the highly educated classes (so called) have most of us got far, far away from Nature. We are trained to seek the choice, the rare, the exquisite exclusively, and to overlook the common. We are stuffed with abstract conceptions, and glib with verbalities and verbosities; and in the culture of these higher functions the peculiar sources of joy often dry up, and we grow stone-blind and insensible to life's more elementary and general goods and joys.

James' prime example of these awakened responses, the sense of life, is Tolstoy's Pierre Besukhov in *War and Peace*, fat and good-natured and indolent Pierre once master of millions, now a cold, hungry, and lousy prisoner of the French:

Here only, and for the first time, he appreciated, because he was deprived of it, the happiness of eating when he was hungry, of drinking when he was thirsty, of sleeping when he was sleepy, and of talking when he felt the desire to exchange some words. . . . Later in life he always recurred with joy to this month of captivity, and never failed to speak with enthusiasm of the powerful and ineffable sensations, and especially the moral calm which he had experienced at this epoch. When at daybreak, on the morrow of his imprisonment, he saw the mountains with their wooded slopes disappearing in the grayish mist; when he felt the cool breeze caress him; when he saw the light drive away the vapors, and the sun rise majestically behind the clouds and cupolas, and the crosses, the dew, the distance, the river, sparkle in the splendid, cheerful rays—his heart overflowed with emotion. This emotion kept continually with him, and increased a hundredfold as the difficulties of his situation grew graver. . . . He learnt that a man is meant for happiness, and that this happiness is in him, in the satisfaction of the daily needs of existence, and that unhappiness is the fatal result, not of our need, but of our abundance. . . . When calm reigned in the camp, and the embers paled, and little by little went out, the full moon had reached the zenith. The woods and the fields roundabout lay clearly visible; and beyond the inundation of light which filled them, the view plunged into the limitless horizon. Then Pierre cast his eye upon the firmament, filled at that hour with myriads of stars. "All that is mine,'" he thought. "All that is in me, is me! And that is what they think they have taken prisoner! That is what they have shut up in a cabin!" So he smiled and turned to sleep among his comrades.

I do not want to philosophize or moralize upon what James says except to note what is needful to say, to emphasize what must not be forgotten, what must always be remembered: that every single thing we do rests on the importance of living, on our sense of life. Every burden of thought, every philosophy and theology and doctrine and dogma and moral system, every "course" we take in college rests on the primary assumption that the experience of living is significant. Every mode of expression serves this assumption. We protest the denial of Civil Rights, because life is very much worth living for *all* people; we protest war in Vietnam because the importance of life is at stake. We *affirm* the importance of life. Evil, I think, is the denial of life and protest a sensitive response to life. When we cease to protest we are dead indeed. Yet protests, like doctrines and dogmas, too soon become abstract, stale and sterile ends in themselves, and the sensitive response itself is too easily darkened and overcome by pain and anger and despair.

That is why I must say over and over again, if only as an idea, that life is very much worth living. Those who say this best are the poets, all those who see imaginatively into the heart of things, those who attack the sense and pierce the heart. It is their function to find where joy resides and to give it a voice in our vital responses, to awaken the sense of life. It is just because the poet is peculiarly sensitive to joy that he is peculiarly vulnerable to pain and anger and despair. By sense of life I do not mean an undifferentiated sensuality or a starry-eyed sensibility that embraces no darkness. In fact, the sense of life I am talking about is a kind of true realism, call it a romantic realism, a *feeling* that cannot be divorced from *thinking* about darkness and the end of life. It cannot be divorced from the ultimates and last chances that we must confront in our imagination. In Camus' *The Stranger*, the hero

Mersault, a prisoner faced with the certainty of death, "hears the tin-trumpet of an ice-cream vendor in the street, a small, shrill sound cutting across the flow of words" in the courtroom. He thinks,

And then a rush of memories went through my mind—memories of a life which was mine no longer and had once provided me with the surest, humblest pleasures: warm smells of summer, my favorite streets, the sky at evening, Marie's dress and her laugh.

Whatever the differences in the final assessment of life by Camus and Tolstoy, Mersault and Pierre Besukhov, in the extremity of their position, have the same sense of the importance of life, the importance of the common and ordinary and plain. They have the same understanding that life is very much worth living.

All the poetry in the world, rightly felt and rightly understood, could be summoned to my aid; all the poets in the world have celebrated the joy of life, have sung the same sense of life, or they were not poets. Here is Dylan Thomas, singing his boyhood Spring in "Fern Hill," when "the Sabbath rang slowly/In the pebbles of the holy streams."

All the sun long it was running, it was lovely, the hay
Fields high as the house, the tunes from the chim-
neys, it was air
    And playing, lovely and watery
        And fire green as grass
    And nightly under the simple stars
As I rode to sleep the owls were bearing the farm
away,

All the moon long I heard, blessed among stables, the
night-jars
    Flying with the ricks, and the horses
    Flashing into the dark.

Here is Stephen Spender, singing his praise of
the "truly great," those "who hoarded from the
Spring branches/The desires falling across their
bodies like blossoms."

What is precious, is never to forget
The essential delight of blood drawn from ageless
springs
Breaking through rocks in worlds before our earth;
Never to deny its pleasure in the simple morning light
Nor its grave evening demand for love.
Never to allow gradually the traffic to smother
With noise and fog, the flowering of the spirit.

And here is Alfred Housman, singing Spring
with cherry blossoms:

Loveliest of trees, the cherry now
Is hung with bloom along the bough,
And stands about the woodland ride
Wearing white for Eastertide.

Now, of my threescore years and ten,
Twenty will not come again,
And take from seventy springs a score,
It only leaves me fifty more.

And since to look at things in bloom
Fifty springs are little room,
About the woodlands I will go
To see the cherry hung with snow.

Perhaps these lines from Housman are not so good as those from Spender and Thomas. They sing too little. They "say" too much. They are too much an idea. But there in them is my whole Last Chance Talk—first chance, last chance, every chance.

And so my Last Chance Talk turns out to be a defense of Poetry, a defense of Spring, a defense of Life. I am taking this last chance to tell you not to forget the first thing of all, the importance of life itself. I am telling you not to be narrow, to open your eyes and to respond with feeling to all that is in life, to all that may now seem common and ordinary and plain. If you respond to life with awakened senses, you will not be careless of life. You will be a lover of life. You will be a lover of others. For you will know what other men can feel of pain and joy, and you will not be careless of them and their feelings. And if you have such responsive sensibilities, life will always be worth living. You will reverently pray this "Prayer in Spring":

> Oh, give us pleasure in the flowers today;
> And give us not to think so far away
> As the uncertain harvest; keep us here
> All simply in the springing of the year.
>
> Oh, give us pleasure in the orchard white,
> Like nothing else by day, like ghosts by night;
> And make us happy in the happy bees,
> That swarm dilating round the perfect trees.
>
> And make us happy in the darting bird
> That suddenly above the bees is heard,
> The meteor that thrusts in with needle bill,
> And off a blossom in mid air stands still.

> For this is love and nothing else is love,
> The which it is reserved for God above
> To sanctify to what far ends He will,
> But which it only needs that we fulfill.

I am inclined to suppose that you consider these lines quite banal, trite, sentimental. Perhaps they are. They happen to belong to Robert Frost. You are likely to respond, "Don't you know that conditions in the world today are pretty grim! Don't you know that literature today is nihilistic! Don't you know that life is absurd!" *I know.* Here is the way a Berkeley professor puts it:

Time and again absurdist plays carp at us that the human condition is absurd, as though the confrontation of absurdity were some sort of agonizing process that paralyzed our ability to act, that corroded our will, destroyed our hope, and sapped our imagination of all vigor. Generally, they present human action in a particularly depressing and dreary light, as though all life suffered from spiritual and emotional leukemia.

It is partly because of this "spiritual and emotional leukemia" that I am taking the line I am tonight—not just because it is Spring, or to defend Poetry. Of course, it's all of a piece. Lately, it seems to me, there has been enough darkness of mood, meanness of spirit, bitter spitefulness, destructive protest—or merely apathy—on this campus, without my contributing more tonight. That is not what one does with a last chance.

I'll conclude by returning to a point I made earlier: that the sense of life I am talking about is a kind of romantic realism, a *feeling* that cannot be divorced from *thinking*—cannot be divorced from the extreme position of a last chance, the end of life. Camus, who popularized the philosophy of the Absurd, always took this extreme position. If you have wanted a tone more somber than the one I have taken tonight, at least listen to the words of this *optimistic* Absurdist:

As for me, it has always been from the word and from the idea of fruitfulness that I have drawn my hope. Like so many men today, I am tired of criticism, denigration, and meanness—in short, of nihilism. We must condemn what needs condemnation; it should be done with vigor and then put aside. But what deserves to be praised should be exalted at length. After all, it is for this I am an artist, because even when what the artist creates is a denial, it still affirms something and pays homage to the magnificent life we live.

So keep your eye open and bright to the wonder of life. Remember Chaucer's birds "that sleep all night with open eye." But don't take those birds too literally. Chaucer is speaking poetry.

𝕊

Huckleberry Finn: Racism and Christianity

Delivered as a class lecture in 1965, the following remarks are better categorized as a public address, an exercised protest against the kind of complacent bigotry
Prins deplored. They exemplify as well his consistent
drive to project literary study beyond the classroom and
to engage the real issues of the day.

I WANT TO BEGIN with a point made by one of
you on the day we began our discussion of *Huckleberry Finn*: the point was that I was being unre-
alistic about people because I did not take into
account (both in Twain's satire on Christians and
in my own caustic remarks) that certain people
do think of Negroes as animals and therefore
cannot regard their inhumanities as inhumanities.

I desire to say that, quite the contrary, I was
being very realistic. I know that what my critic
said is true. And it is right to my point and
Twain's. The real question is: how does it happen
that people from specifically Christian communities have gotten these attitudes (both in *Huckleberry Finn* and in the U.S.A., 1965)?

First, of course, the argument could be called irrelevant. My primary attempt was to show you Twain's use of ironic understatement to bring out his theme.

But, second, I am a teacher who believes that no piece of literature can ever be taught in an artistic vacuum. Great literature is always morally relevant to human living, any time. If Twain's ironic technique is morally irrelevant to the church, then the church is irrelevant, too. Even some church leaders say that: because the church hasn't done what it should have done in the world, it has become morally irrelevant in today's world.

So let me tell you a few things that make me sick, not love-sick, or heart-sick, but anger-sick, the kind of sickness that sometimes causes people to turn their faces from the only hope the world has, Christianity.

- It makes me sick that in Alabama and Mississippi and many other places whites and Negroes can be openly and cold-bloodedly murdered and that just as often as the murders occur white juries acquit the murderers. These murderers and these juries are usually church people and it is well known that the attitudes I am talking about are most prevalent in Bible-belt areas, churchy areas, South and North. In the last instances of the kind of murder I am talking about, the murderer (I call him such and I trust so does the Lord) was acquitted because he performed a service to the community he had to perform.

- It makes me sick that these attitudes are often ("usually" is a better word) held by right-wing, conservative, fundamentalist (call them what you wish, even "sincere" if you want to) religious groups and preachers of the Gospel, they claim. They are the ones who denounce the National Council of Churches and put up signs on national highways for the impeachment of Earl Warren.

- It makes me sick that the mayor of a large city near Detroit pledges to keep Negroes out of the city, and wins big every time. His campaign slogan is "Keep Dearborn clean"—you know what this Christian gentleman means.

- It makes me sick when the wife of a Reformed Church pastor in a small New Jersey town (she being a former student of mine) writes to tell me what the unanimous attitude of her husband's parishioners is to Negroes.

- It makes me sick when another former student of mine writes (just last week) from Ann Arbor to tell of obstructions good church people— especially real-estate dealers—put in the way of improving Negro housing. I get the same reports from Grand Rapids.

- It makes me sick when a minister reveals what problems have to be faced in Holland with Christian leaders in the Chamber of Commerce when it comes to Negro employment in new industries that come to Holland.

- It makes me sick to have to disagree with students (many of them) who write freshman themes that argue that the Negro is inferior, dirty and cursed by God from the time of Noah. I remember particularly one pious bright girl from Chicago who must hate me to this day for giving her some well-meant advice about how to say her prayers.

- It makes me sick when an elder of the church tells me without any irony whatsoever, "You know, Jim, we don't contribute money to missions to bring them [you know who] over here but to keep them over there"; it's the last part of the statement that's significant.

- It made me sick when two Ph.D. chemists from Texas who attended the Science Institute here at Hope last summer told me they liked the idea of the Holland Christian schools. It was a way, they said, of avoiding the school desegregation problem. A bit expensive, they said, but think of the advantage of keeping your children clean and Christian. Incidentally, I speak with no malice; I am an HCH graduate.

- It even makes me sick to see some people (not many, I hope) in Civil Rights marches at Hope—faculty and students—who actively supported national candidates whose only victories came in Southern states for anti-civil rights stands. There were even two (not students) who I had heard derogatively use the word "nigger." A march like that with an issue already settled by a huge majority in Washington, and no possibility of skin being bruised or somebody helped, becomes a Public Relations gambit, a picture in the *Milestone*. We too!

- It makes me sick that at Hope I am asked to listen to people like Senator Tower of Texas—and very often people of his stripe.

- It makes me sick when a seminary student tells me that a suburban Detroit church was formed to get away from Negro infiltration of the church community. My uncle is pastor of that church, and my own church financially supported the building of the new church. This uncle married my wife and me, and no one has been more sympathetic to the problems of me and my wife (unnecessary religious problems) in this Christian community than he has.

The thing that made me most recently sickest of all was a meeting I attended. I am a committeeman for a social organization that is supposed to help very young people on their way to democratic citizenship. Let's call them the Bluebirds, something like that. Over the inevitable coffee and cake afterwards, the committeemen started to discuss the deplorable, they thought, infiltration of the public schools by Negroes and (I suppose) Mexicans who would lower standards. One man said that if things got worse he would have to send his children to the Christian School. All were in agreement (and took it for granted I would be too). To a man (except for my own wicked self), these men were all elders and deacons of churches.

No, I am very realistic. I believe men are very sinful and very much in need of redemption. Does this mean that no soul-searching is necessary, and that no one should be critical of what the churches haven't done that they should have done? And the record of the church in this matter is pretty sad, as every high-churchman (or low) of any decency has admitted. Christ's words on the necessity of Christian love were pretty blunt; he didn't give anyone much chance without it (or the grace of God that allows it).

One last thought that makes me sick. Too often, around here, if one emphasizes human rights over property rights, spiritual advantage over material advantage, he is in trouble. Stick to your subject, they say, teach English! How does one teach *Huckleberry Finn* without making Twain's own point? To some the subtle artistry is highly effective, to others a chance to avoid the truth. Remember the second strand of Father Mapple's sermon. Maybe this will turn out to be my Last Chance Talk. (Incidentally, I don't talk behind people's backs; for four years I have averaged two hundred students/semester, and 75% of the class of 1965 had been in a class of mine one time or another.)

⅋

The Fall: Guilty or Not Guilty?

This essay appeared in the Hope College *Anchor*, 26 March 1964, in preparation for a campus-wide discussion of *The Fall* by Albert Camus.

THE SETTING OF CAMUS' *THE FALL* is a sad and sunless Amsterdam, under a gray Dutch sky. The dark atmosphere of the city, the system of canals, the Zuider Zee ("a dead sea") are meant to suggest a dank hell of the soul, a nether-land, to which the narrator has descended. "Are you familiar with Dante?" he asks a silent listener. The whole narrative is a monologue, or series of monologues, addressed to this mute companion by a man who calls himself "Jean-Baptiste Clamence, play actor," "a double face, a charming Janus." To his shadowy auditor Clamence relates the adventures that have brought him from a loftier role in Paris to the foggy streets, the dingy bars, the bleak little room he haunts in Amsterdam. Camus cleverly plants the idea that Clamence is talking to no one but himself, an idea that turns to our realization that he is talking to no one in particular because he is talking to everybody—condemning the whole world in his profession of "judge-penitent." His name is significant: the Christian name Jean-Baptiste suggests

John the Baptist, preaching "repentance for the remission of sins"; the sound of the surname, Clamence, suggests not only the French for crying and shouting ("clamant") but also the French for clemency and mercy ("clemence").

Confession of Guilt

Clamence's recital is a confession of guilt: the progress of his monologue is a "fall," a descent into a hell of private introspection. Once, he tells his listener, he lived blissfully in a kind of Eden of self-complacency, one of the most respected lawyers in Paris, the protector of widows and orphans, in his own estimation. He had been at the height of his powers, successful, assured of his own righteousness and virtue—until one night he had failed to risk his life to save the life of another. He had failed to plunge into the icy waters of the Seine to save a desperate young woman from suicide. He failed in an encounter with human misery and thereafter he has been plagued by an unidentifiable laugh that follows him everywhere, the ironic laughter of self-judgment. He confesses, "I, I, I is the refrain of my whole life, which could be heard in everything I said." "Modesty helped me to shine, humility to conquer, and virtue to oppress." "In short, for me to live happily it was essential for the creatures I chose [to love] not to live at all. They must receive their life, sporadically, at my bidding."

Clamence's further discoveries about himself are even more shattering to his complacent self-righteousness. He rips off layer after layer of duplicity. "After all I have told you, what do you think developed? An aversion to myself? Come, it was especially with others that I was fed up. The prosecution of others went on constantly, in my heart." The truth is that the whole purpose of Clamence's confession of guilt is selfish—to gain from his listener a recognition of the listener's common involvement in human guilt and thereby lift the burden of guilt from himself. Clamence is a "judge-penitent," he tells his story so that he can accuse and judge through confession and penitence. There takes place in his recitation a gradual shift from "I" am guilty to "we" are guilty.

Covered with ashes, tearing my hair, my face scored by clawing, but with piercing eyes, I stand before all humanity recapitulating my shames without losing sight of the effect I am producing and saying: "I was the lowest of the low." Then imperceptibly I pass from the "I" to the "we." When I get to "This is what we are," the trick has been played and I can tell them off. I am like them, to be sure; we are in the soup together. However, I have a superiority in me that I know it and this gives me the right to speak. You see the advantage, I am sure. The more I accuse myself, the more I have the right to judge you. Even better, I provoke you into judging yourself, and this relieves me of that much of the burden.

With self-satisfaction, Clamence states: "I am for any theory that refuses to grant man innocence and for any practice that treats him as guilty."

Guilty or Not Guilty?

Because *The Fall* is a monologue delivered just from the point of view of Clamence and because it quite possibly is ironic, it is the most puzzling of

Camus' novels, with an ambiguity, probably intended, at the very heart of it. It is possible to look at the novel as affirming the idea of man's guilt; it is also possible to regard it as denying the idea of man's guilt. According to the first view, Clamence's descent is something like what has been in called in Christian tradition, or at least in the criticism of Milton's *Paradise Lost*, a "fortunate fall." That phrase is intended to suggest that the fall of Adam (the fall of man) proved to be fortunate for mankind since it made necessary the extending of divine grace through the entrance into human history of God as man; it made necessary the Incarnation. The phrase "fortunate fall" also suggests that the fall from innocence or virtue can have a fortunate, a providential (determinism is implicit in both adjectives) effect in the fallen individual's new recognitions as to the nature of evil and his own guilt. Thus, by his fall, Jean-Baptiste Clamence becomes true prophet for man: his "clamant," his crying in the wilderness, is a proclamation of man's wickedness and guilt, man's need for penitence and grace ("clemence," "clemency"). Strangely enough, the doves that circle in the dark Dutch sky never descend: "there is nothing but the sea and the canals, roofs covered with shop signs, and never a head on which to alight." The only grace that Clamence offers is the innocence of universal guilt.

Irony

The idea that Camus is stressing the guiltiness of man goes against the grain of the rest of his work. The contrary view is that *The Fall* is pure irony: far from seriously expressing a view of universal wickedness and guilt, Camus is satirizing this belief. Concerning the doctrine of original sin, Camus once said: "People have insisted too much on the innocence of creation. Now they want to crush us with feelings of our guilt." Note that the two extremes attacked here contain the course of Clamence's "fall." Clamence speaks of his original condition of self-assurance as a state of Eden, of innocence. He is a monster of pride in his own perfection. When he is struck with a sense of guilt, when he loses faith in his own virtue, when he can no longer look down on other people, he subdues them by making them feel guilty, drawing them into a quagmire of remorse and self-abasement from which they cannot rise—so that he may judge them, satisfy his contempt for them to recapture his pride. According to this second interpretation of the novel, Camus is attacking a view that stresses the dominance of evil, that robs man of his capacity for moral choice, takes away his freedom and makes him wait till the doves of some external grace alight upon him to rescue him from his hell of depraved humanity for some other world than the one in which he lives. Clamence is thus a false prophet: his "clamant," his crying in the wilderness, is a weeping moan of self-pity and hypocritical pride. His "clemence," his clemency of grace, is justification by guilt, a new kind of innocence that props his pride in an alienation of condemnation: if everyone is equally wicked and guilty, everyone is equally good and innocent—and no one is personally responsible.

Devil?

I think the second interpretation of the novel is
nearer to being correct. When Mlle. Germaine
Brée, close friend, critic, and biographer of Albert
Camus, spoke on this campus two years ago, I
approached her on the question of Clamence. Her
reply was emphatic: "Clamence is the devil!" She
meant that Clamence, from beginning to end, is a
monster of self-pride, his guilt just another form
of perverted ego, hypocritical pride of self that
seeks to enslave men. This is the kind of devil
Clamence is, and this, I think, is the image of
contemporary man that Camus deplores.

But take your choice. Guilty or not guilty?

ℤ

Teaching Melville's *Moby-Dick*

In the summer of 1982 A. James Prins received and filled out a questionnaire from Professor Martin Bickman of the University of Colorado, who was then at work on editing the Modern Language Association's collection on teaching Melville's great novel (1851). Prins' answers reveal not simply his view of *Moby-Dick* but his vision of teaching literature.

Name: A. James Prins, Professor of English, Emeritus
School and address: Lubbers Hall, Hope College, Holland, Michigan 49423

Courses in which you have taught Moby-Dick. *Please give course titles and levels, average class sizes, and kinds of students (e.g., "mainly undergraduate nonmajors"):* THE AMERICAN NOVEL. Twelve novels from Hawthorne to Bellow. Upper undergraduate level. Majors and non-majors. (Hawthorne, Melville, Twain, Howells, James, Dreiser, Fitzgerald, Hemingway, Faulkner, Steinbeck, Wright, Bellow.)

Please answer the following in as much specific detail as you can, using the backs of these pages or other sheets if necessary. If you teach MD *in*

*more than one kind of course, please make clear
the course for which your answers are applicable.*

1. Which edition(s) of MD *do you use, and why?*
NORTON CRITICAL EDITION. Very good text,
notes, and criticism, but very expensive in a
course which requires that the student buy
twelve novels. RIVERSIDE EDITION. Excellent
format, very readable type. NAL SIGNET. Inex-
pensive. I have used the RIVERSIDE EDITION
through most of thirty-five years. Lately, because
of cost, I have moved to NAL Signet.

*2. What would you like to see in an ideal class-
room edition of* MD*?* Large type, clear print, accurate text, non-esoteric (intellectually available to
the student) critical foreword, low cost.

*3. How do you feel about teaching only selections
from the book in a survey course? If you do this,
what selections do you use, and what do you try
to do with them?* Emphatically not. My critical
approach has always been to show the relation of
form and content in a novel—to demonstrate how
point of view, narrative structure, setting, character, atmosphere, images, symbols, diction, etc.,
release human significance. Even for the "baggy
monsters" like *Moby-Dick* and *Bleak House* (in
THE ENGLISH NOVEL) I assert their unity, that
the meaning (human, or, rather, "humane," significance) is fulfilled in the total work of art.

*4. Do you ask your students to consult back-
ground materials (e.g., historical or critical studies,
biographies, other works by Melville)? If so, list ti-*

tles, indicating whether they are required or rec-ommended and the reasons for your choices. No. Twelve novels are more than enough reading in a 3-hour course. In my first lecture ("talk" about the novel) I synthesize what I consider to be the best available critical views of *Moby-Dick* (or any novel), and I relate the novel to the development of American fiction (techniques, etc.), American history, American ideas. I do provide bibliography: Willard Thorp, Henry F. Pommer, Charles Olson, Leslie Fiedler, Richard Chase, R. W. B. Lewis, Charles Feidelson, Jr., Lawrance Thompson, Howard P. Vincent, M. O. Percival, Warner Berthoff, Milton R. Stern, Randall Stewart, Harry Levin, Leon Howard, William Braswell, Murray Krieger, Richard B. Sewall, and others. I do not teach any novel without considering the author's other works and all significant critical and biographical materials.

5. *Which articles and books would you recommend to a beginning teacher? Which ones do you find yourself most often rereading and consulting? Feel free to annotate your lists, with special attention to each item's relevance for teaching.* NORTON CRITICAL EDITION. Richard Chase, *Herman Melville.* Charles Olson, *Call Me Ishmael.* Lawrance Thompson, *Melville's Quarrel with God.* Howard P. Vincent, *The Trying-Out of* Moby-Dick. M. O. Percival, *A Reading of* Moby-Dick. Randall Stewart, *American Literature and Christian Doctrine.* Milton R. Stern, *The Fine Hammered Steel of Herman Melville.* Harry Levin, *The Power of Blackness.* William Braswell, *Melville's Religious*

Thought. Murray Krieger, *The Tragic Vision.* Richard B. Sewall, *The Vision of Tragedy.*

6. *If you have found any aids (e.g., films, illustrations, maps) helpful in teaching* MD, *please give titles and specific dates about availability.* I have never used so-called study aids. The text of *Moby-Dick* is my primary tool. Oh, maybe a woodcut or two by Rockwell Kent.

7. *How much time do you usually allow for teaching the book? How do you coordinate the students' reading with the class sessions (e.g., do you ask them to finish the entire book before the first meeting, or assign specific chapters for specific classes?* 4-5 class sessions of about an hour apiece, 1-2 weeks in an M W F sequence. The student begins reading immediately with each new novel and reads as rapidly as possible. Course readings are posted before the beginning of the course.

8. *How do you discover and evaluate student response to the book (e.g., discussions, exams, papers)? What pedagogical uses do you make of these responses?* My questions almost invariably call for critical responses: "essay," or "thesis," or "thought" questions. I don't call for "facts" for themselves or for recall of my lectures. Often I use a significant scene or quotation (and ask for identification to ensure reading), which the student must relate, with specific references to the content of *Moby-Dick,* to the art and meaning of the whole novel. Sometimes I employ a challenging critical statement (or counter statements) and

require the student to defend/ refute/ choose between. Responses are judged for critical sensitivity and clarity of expression, not right or wrong.
Possibilities of response are discussed in a class
period.

9. *What do you see as the major difficulties in
teaching* MD? *What ways have you found to miti-
gate these difficulties?* Time and evaluation are
my biggest problems. In a course designated THE
AMERICAN NOVEL, twelve novels are almost
minimum coverage, so the student is hard
pressed for reading time. Short cuts like CLIFF
NOTES become a temptation, requiring that I do
some missionary work on the values of humane
letters. Students today want quantitative evaluation, not judgment on the quality of their thinking. Sensitive and perceptive reading is a primary
goal in every course I teach.

10. *What do you see as the central concerns of the
book, and how do these concerns shape your approach in the classroom?* I emphasize the philosophical (cosmic, theological) and psychological implications of *Moby-Dick* over the social and political (all are related). I raise the question of Ahab's
character in pursuing a malignant (or benevolent)
deity (the whale as God-figure)—whether Melville
affirms or condemns Ahab's quest, or is neutral,
in the total form of the novel. I follow Ahab's development in the text, then make a counter case
for Ishmael as central character. (SEE EN-
CLOSED MATERIAL)

11. *Do you see the book as a unified and coherent text? If so, what are the sources of this unity, and what uses do you make of it in the classroom? If not, how does this view affect your teaching of the book?* Yes, see #3 and ENCLOSED MATERIAL. I approach the unity/coherence of *Moby-Dick* through the relation of point of view, narrative structure, settings, the texture of images, symbols, language, etc.—all creating a consistent theme/meaning/message. I probably stress the developing counter perspectives of Ahab and Ishmael, and the imagery/symbolism in the novel.

I don't understand the reference to "it" in this question (2nd sentence). If "it" refers to unity, my purpose in the classroom is to show Melville's artistry in using the techniques of fiction to create a significant comment (unified ambivalence) on human life.

12. *In teaching the book, do you stress more its continuities and connections with other works of literature or its uniqueness and anomalies? What kinds of relations do you find yourself most often making with other works?* Probably the latter, since my approach is a critical concentration on the text of each novel in the course (THE AMERICAN NOVEL). However, from Hawthorne to Bellow, I relate the novels to show the development of fictional techniques (point of view, for example, in Melville in contrast to James) and American ideas (innocence and perfectibility, moral freedom and responsibility, for example, from Hawthorne and Melville to the realism and naturalism of

Howells and Dreiser). I cannot do all things, but I attempt to open minds to everything.

13. *Describe in detail the class structure(s) and format(s) you use in teaching* MD. *Be specific about the amount you talk as compared to the amount the students talk, the kinds of interactions, the nature of the questions you and they ask. How does this relate to your vision of the book?* (SEE ENCLOSED MATERIAL) The first class period (sometimes a bit more) is spent on formulating a theme (meaning, human significance) or possible themes and introducing the important techniques (point of view, narrative structure, images, etc.) that create this view of life. All this is presented very tentatively and meant to be tested through concentration on the text of the novel in remaining class periods, with discussions on propositions made concerning the relation of theme and technique. Students may (should) reject my tentative reading of the novel, but their job is to test questions in the world that the novel creates for internal validity and for relevance to their own lives.

14. *How would you describe your own stance as a critic and scholar, and how do you see this as shaping the specific ways you teach* MD? Eclectic and synthetic. Though I do not presume to teach any novel until I am in control of the author's other works and all significant critical and biographical materials, I think of myself as a teacher rather than as a scholar or critic. The insights of scholarship and criticism regarding *Moby-Dick* are important only in so far as they make the

novel relevant to the student's education in life. Obviously, my stance is zealous in promoting clear critical thinking about and sensitive emotional (aesthetic) response to the world of *Moby-Dick* (or any novel I teach), Melville's vision of life. That vision matters immediately, for much more than literary criticism or scholarship. The humanities humanize, are imperatively needed in any civilized education.

15. *Describe the aspects of your teaching of* MD *that have slipped through the net of this questionnaire. What do you feel is the most important thing you do in the process of teaching the book?* No questionnaire gets close to bringing out what happens between me and my students in the process of teaching. In my every reading and teaching of *Moby-Dick* (or any other significant piece of literature), I have gained new insights to the experience of living, and my students have every time discovered truths I did not see before. Not "know" before, but "see" before—vicariously experience, live, feel. To communicate a vital sense of meaning and purpose and discovery and vision in mutual human enterprise is my most important objective for the teaching of *Moby-Dick*. What Ishmael discovered, saw. Or what Ahab saw. Or ambivalence.

16. *Any comments on this questionnaire or suggestions for the project?* Very exasperating, between the lines. All neatly rationalized and objectified, coldly and dryly, but not at all what happens in the classroom, I certainly hope. See previous question.

17. *As mentioned in the cover letter, I am soliciting responses from a cross-section of students on the experience of reading* MD, *and would be grateful if you could supply names and summer addresses of willing subjects. Perhaps the easiest procedure is to pass around a sign-up sheet in the classes in which you have taught* MD. *Please indicate below if you have enclosed such a sheet or would be willing to send one along later. Also, feel free to make suggestions for this short questionnaire.* I am a Professor, Emeritus, retired, so I have not had a class in THE AMERICAN NOVEL since last summer. But, should you want it, I can provide a list of students, past and somewhat present, with addresses. Hundreds have become teachers: elementary and secondary teachers, college and university teachers in all disciplines. My best gift to them, I hope, has been enthusiasm, fervor, inspiration.

℘℘℘

LECTURES ON THE NOVEL

How do the structures of the various novels in this course develop the relation of self and society? How do they expand your own experience in the world, help you to find yourself? To me, this last is the most important question of all, but one that will (can) never be asked in a test—the question behind all other questions.

—A. James Prins
Introduction to The English Novel, 1965

ঌঌঌ

Prins the Teacher

Christopher James Prins

MY FATHER'S TEACHING NOTES, which we discovered after his death, are a treasure indeed. In addition to serving an important historical purpose, they are as alive today for students of the novel as they were thirty-forty years ago when they were written. Perhaps nothing more in this memorial volume comes as close as these teaching notes to capturing the essence of A. James Prins the teacher, and to recording the energy and ideas he imparted to the thousands of students he taught at Hope College. A. James Prins felt intensely about the material he taught—in his American, English, European, and Russian novels courses particularly. He had the charm, wry sense of humor, and vision to engage his students as they together explored new worlds through great literature. Prins the teacher brought these works alive by placing them in historical perspective, emphasizing their timeless qualities, and integrating his personal views with those of the great literary critics of his era.

To some students in the classroom who witnessed my father's command of the material and "stream of consciousness" style, it may have seemed that A. James Prins needed to prepare little before he taught. These teaching notes, however, tell a very different story. They are the product of extensive research on each and every novel and were carefully crafted—complete with references and selected passages to elaborate on points my father wanted to make. In fact, the typed notes I found carefully filed in the basement of our home amount in some cases to fully-conceived essays. These detailed class notes are the product of a man who was intent upon being fully prepared to justify his ideas and approach to teaching.

The teaching notes, as presented in this memorial volume, have been organized by course in a manner similar to the way they originally were used: the American Novel, the English Novel, the European Novel, the Russian Novel. Although my father's selection of texts for these courses changed slightly over time, the syllabus for one year was chosen to represent each course, and, in a few cases, the teaching notes for a text not in the given syllabus are included. Only in the instance of a few novels were teaching notes not found. Except for Tolstoy's *Anna Karenina*, the notes on Russian novels taught both in the European Novel and Russian Novel courses have been placed for organizational purposes with the Russian Novel.

Although my father used no uniform method in constructing his teaching notes, attention both to theme and style can be found in the notes for almost all novels. Titles to organize the material have been added and formatting changes have been

made to assist the reader. Bibliographical material
in the notes has been retained. Certain references
(e. g., page references to editions of novels being
used) have been deleted.

ℒ

THE AMERICAN NOVEL

ᘒᘒᘒ

THE AMERICAN NOVEL
English 332, Fall 1978

1. Hawthorne: *The Scarlet Letter* (1850), NAL Signet
   August 30, September 1, 6, 8
2. Melville: *Moby-Dick* (1851), NAL Signet
   September 11, 13, 15, 18
3. Twain: *Huckleberry Finn* (1884), NAL Signet
   September 20, 22, 25

September 27: Test on Hawthorne, Melville, Twain

4. Howells: *The Rise of Silas Lapham* (1885), NAL Signet
   September 29, October 2, 4
5. James: *The American* (1887), NAL Signet
   October 6, 9, 11
6. Dreiser: *Sister Carrie* (1900), NAL Signet
   October 16, 18, 20

October 23: Test on Howells, James, Dreiser

7. Fitzgerald: *The Great Gatsby* (1925), Scribners
   October 25, 27, 30
8. Hemingway: *A Farewell to Arms* (1929), Scribners
   November 1, 3, 6, 8
9. Faulkner: *As I Lay Dying* (1930), Vintage
   November 10, 13

November 15: Test on Fitzgerald, Hemingway, Faulkner

10. Steinbeck: *The Grapes of Wrath* (1939), Bantam
    November 17, 20, 22, 27
11. Wright: *Native Son* (1940), Harper Perennial
    November 29, December 1, 4
12. Bellow: *Henderson the Rain King* (1959), Fawcett Crest
    December 6, 8, 11

December 19, 10:30 am: Test on Steinbeck, Wright, Bellow
YOU ARE EXPECTED TO ATTEND ALL CLASSES

Nathaniel Hawthorne, *The Scarlet Letter*
(1966)

THEMES IN HAWTHORNE

First, let me give you some points on what to look for in Hawthorne, not only in *The Scarlet Letter* but in his other stories:

Human Nature. Hawthorne believed in the reality of sin and the immanence of evil in human nature. He did not believe that man is naturally good or that man is innocent of evil or that Americans were naturally predisposed to the attainment of what has been called the American Dream for the New World. Hawthorne believed in the reality of sin in the human condition; he believed in the mixture of good-and-evil in the human heart (good-and-evil should be hyphenated to show their interrelation to Hawthorne). Listen for a moment to what Austin Warren has to say. Warren asks, "Why was Hawthorne so obsessed by sin and guilt?"

Though he did not become an orthodox theologian or churchgoer, he found more intellectual satisfaction in the older Calvinist faith with its dogmas of the Fall (the total depravity of the natural man) and Predestination (theological determinism) than in its nineteenth-century liberal alternatives. Like Melville, his friend and literary peer, he had no confidence in the characteristic achievements of his century and no ready answer to human ills.

You should read the rest of what he has to say. But here is what another Hawthorne critic has to say on the point of Hawthorne's belief in man's sinfulness, man's dark nature:

It has been suggested many times that Hawthorne temperamentally found the seventeenth–century Puritans more congenial than the nineteenth-century Unitarians and Transcendentalists. In no respect is this more true than in his recognition of sin as a vital and incscapablc rcality in life. Though he did not accept Calvin's doctrine of original sin in its full theological sense, he nevertheless felt that the universality of sin could be empirically supported. The Calvinistic doctrine of predestination finds some counterpart in Hawthorne, too. To be sure, he does not suggest that every act can be ultimately traced back to the mind of God, but he demonstrates with the utmost rigor that every sin has its inescapable consequences far beyond the immediate circle and generation of the sinner. Indeed, if Dimmesdale's last words are to be taken as a cue, these consequences extend beyond the grave and color our relation to the hereafter.

At any rate, Hawthorne had no easy or optimistic view of man's natural goodness or freedom to choose an innocent destiny. In *The Scarlet Letter*, Hawthorne's dark view is supported from the beginning by the dark images of human society which are drawn from the cemetery and the prison on the opening page of Chapter One. In the opening, too, appears Hawthorne's other dominant tone: the color red, imaging the dark stain of passion in human nature. But red is an ambivalent symbol for Hawthorne: in the red rose, in the scarlet A, and in the scarlet A's correlative in the child Pearl. Red signifies not only sin but the natural impulse to creation, the flame of life; it signifies the tragic and paradoxical mixture of good-and-evil in nature and human nature.

The Human Heart. Hawthorne sympathized with what he called "the truth of the human heart." By "truth of the human heart" Hawthorne meant an inner felt truth. He leaned toward intuition as a source of truth over against intellect, the head. Ideally, Hawthorne believed in the equilibrium of heart and head—in a balance his characters never achieve. Hawthorne's "unpardonable" sin is the exclusion of the heart by complete reliance on the mind. This is Chillingworth's premeditated and cold-blooded violation of the human heart. Hawthorne did not think of what the heart felt to be always good and pure. The heart of fallen man is, according to Hawthorne's own words, a "foul cavern," capable of great deception, and Hester and Dimmesdale are sinners, led astray by natural passion, an imbalance of feeling. But the heart offers man's only possibilities for happiness and is to be trusted over the head, the mind. Thus, Dimmesdale's and Hester's sin of natural passion, the excess of human feeling, is a lesser sin to Hawthorne than the dehumanizing, cold-hearted, and calculated torture of Dimmesdale's heart by Chillingworth. Reflecting on his own love for Sophia Peabody, Hawthorne wrote, "We are not endowed with real life, all that seems most real about us is but the thinnest substance of a dream—till the heart be touched. That touch creates us—then we begin to be."

Fusion of the Natural and the Supernatural. Hawthorne fused the natural and the supernatural; he intermixed the actual and imaginary worlds. The world of *The Scarlet Letter* is one in which reality and fancy slide in and out, each world imbued with something of its own nature (e.g., in Hawthorne's treatment of the rosebush at the prison door, the mark on Dimmesdale's breast, and Mistress Hibbins). Hawthorne cannot technically be called a novelist, if by definition a novelist is a writer of realistic literature. By his own description he was a "romancer," writing in the symbolic, imaginative mode rather than the realistic mode. One cannot say that Hawthorne's work is realistic, for there are in it too many suggestions of the fanciful, imaginary, supernatural. This does not mean Hawthorne was contemptuous of reality: the point is that he was less concerned with accurately representing external facts than he was with suggesting some truth about man's inner nature.

Images as Symbols. A symbol is a thing or a person or a situation that stands for or suggests a different plane of meaning than the fact, or facts, presented. Thus, in giving us images for Dimmesdale and Hester, for Chillingworth and Pearl and Mistress Hibbins, for the scarlet A and the mark on Dimmesdale's breast, for the three pivotal scaffold scenes,

Hawthorne is less interested in realistic detail than in searching out an inner truth, a psychological truth, a truth of the human heart.

MEANING OF *THE SCARLET LETTER*

In the sense of significant human experience, what then is the meaning of *The Scarlet Letter*? What inner truth? What deep truth of the human heart does Hawthorne mean to express with his story?

Violation of the Human Heart. I think it would be superficial to say that the central meaning of *The Scarlet Letter* is primarily an attack on the sin of adultery, or, going in the opposite direction, to say that the novel is primarily an attack on Puritan intolerance for Hester's sin. There is some truth in both attitudes, but there is something deeper at issue. I think it is getting closer to the central meaning of *The Scarlet Letter* to say that for Hawthorne the adultery of Hester and Dimmesdale, because of its dark and secret nature, represents a breach of personal integrity. Its lawless passion violates the true respect that each individual heart must have for every other human heart, including the unborn; the act of Hester and Dimmesdale violated the deepest truth of the human heart in its original spiritual purity. It is the hidden quality of that sin of Hester and Dimmesdale that compounds the darkness that separates the hearts of mother and father and child and husband and community. Hester and Dimmesdale, unlike Chillingworth, are not heartless, but in excess of passion they, too, have violated the human heart. In their heart of hearts, where there is something left of God's image, Hester and Dimmesdale know this, but in different ways they hide it and deny it. Adultery, the adulteration of love in human relations, is not all right, though sexual love cannot in itself be called bad and the connections between flesh and heart and spirit are subtle and mysterious.

The Effects of Sin on Character. It is only when Hester and Dimmesdale recognize the fault to each other's hearts, when they are inwardly penitent and openly acknowledge the fault, that they are whole again and the black veil of sin which has hidden the hearts of Hester and Dimmesdale and Pearl from each other is lifted. So *The Scarlet Letter* has something to say about the effects of sin on character, on the human heart. It has something to say about the importance of personal integrity and inner truth and conscience. It has something to say about "being true" to the truth in the human heart that should bind together hearts in love and light, something to say about forgiveness of sin and compassion for the frailty and imperfection of the human heart, something to say about the need for inner and open penitence and the futility of external punishment and penance that keeps hearts dark and secrets hid.

Yet all this is only suggestive and still superficial. There are contradictions in *The Scarlet Letter* that cannot be cleared by the intellect: for in the mysteries of the human heart are the paradox of the spirit's relation to the flesh, the paradox of the rela-

tion between good and evil, the paradox of the relation between human freedom and necessity, the
law.

ॐ

Herman Melville, *Moby-Dick*
(1966)

MELVILLE, HAWTHORNE AND THEIR RELATION TO AMERICAN LITERATURE

An Historical Perspective. Melville and Hawthorne were friends. In fact, *Moby-Dick* is dedicated to Hawthorne. Both men were concerned with the problem of evil in this world. Neither was well received in the time he wrote. They had a darker view of human nature and the conditions of human existence than was permitted by the prevalent optimism of their times: the mood of optimism and innocence. Subsequent history seems to have vindicated Hawthorne and Melville; at least, today, we have no easy confidence concerning the conditions and ends of life. Today, the vision of Hawthorne and Melville seems truer to our human experience than that of, say, their contemporaries Emerson and Whitman. At any rate, Hawthorne and Melville now stand at the forefront of American literature. *Moby-Dick* is probably the only American work that is admitted to great world literature along with the works of Homer, Dante, Shakespeare, Dostoevsky, etc.

Similarity and Difference in _The Scarlet Letter_ and
Moby-Dick. There is a difference in the focus of
Hawthorne and Melville. One's focus is more psychological, the other's more philosophical. Hawthorne is more concerned with the impact of sin on
the human heart, with a consideration of character.
Melville's focus is more philosophical: he is concerned with metaphysical questions, the why and
the what of evil. "Sin" is a personal word; "evil" is
more objective. Melville is also more ambiguous
than Hawthorne. That is not to say that Hawthorne
is perfectly clear or that being ambiguous makes a
writer less true or significant. But in Melville's consideration of the cause of evil in the world, in _Moby-
Dick_, one is never quite sure whether Melville is on
the side of those who affirm or those who rebel
against the powers that be. One is never sure
whether he is God's advocate or the devil's. He often
seems to be on the side of the rebel apostate in
man.

SUGGESTIONS OF MEANING IN _MOBY-DICK_

Deep Meaning. _Moby-Dick_ is a novel with a deep
meaning, I insist. That was Melville's intention for
sure. In a letter to Hawthorne, he wrote, "A sense of
unspeakable security is in me this moment, on account of your having understood the book." Obviously, Melville is not rejoicing because Hawthorne
was able to follow a simple sea story about a whale;
there is something in the book to be understood, to
have challenged Hawthorne's intelligence in a way
that made Melville happy. In the same letter, Mel-

ville continues to Hawthorne: "I have written a wicked book, and I feel spotless as a lamb." *Moby-Dick* must have something to do with man's relation to the powers that be.

Human Pride Ends in Destruction. Let us say, tentatively, the theme of *Moby-Dick* can possibly be stated this way: human pride that defies God and his providence for this world (or, human pride that rebels against the conditions of human existence in nature), even if that providence or the conditions of human existence is unintelligible, and seems evil, ends in destruction. I want to make a strong caution about accepting this statement of theme. If it is correct, the lesson in it (the lesson of Father Mapple's sermon) does not come easily and piously for Melville in the novel; it comes out of a heart full of angry rebellion at personal injuries and deep sympathy for what seems to be man's unjustified suffering (the novel has similarities in theme to the Book of Job). It may be that the theme of *Moby-Dick* is exactly the opposite of what I have stated; it may be that *Moby-Dick* is an ironic and bitter protest against God's ways with men, or against the conditions of human existence. Whether the ambiguity in the novel is resolved affirmatively for the powers that be, or negatively, or remains unresolved—ambiguous or ambivalent—is for you to decide.

Ahab. The key figure in the novel is, of course, Ahab (but don't neglect Ishmael)—Ahab who is described by Captain Peleg as a "grand, ungodly, godlike man." Ahab is, in attitude, a close parallel to Milton's rebellious Satan in *Paradise Lost*. Ahab has been scarred by Providence, or Fate, or Nature—however you wish to see it, in the form of Moby-Dick, the white whale. Ahab's wound is psychological as well as physical; it is a personal injury, he thinks, dealt by an intentionally malignant force, whatever purposefully evil force rules the world. And Ahab is hot for revenge; he is determined to strike through and beyond the reality of appearances, through what he calls the "pasteboard mask" of Moby-Dick, the external appearance of nature. Moby-Dick is for him a symbol, in fact a form of the malicious evil power that has caused his suffering. Concerning the white whale, Ahab says to his first mate Starbuck in Chapter 36: "He tasks me; he heaps me; I see in him outrageous strength, with an inscrutable malice sinewing it. That inscrutable thing is chiefly what I hate. Talk not of blasphemy, man; I'd strike the sun if it insulted me." Mad, monomaniac Ahab is obsessed with one idea and hell-bent for damnation if need be, and near the end invokes the powers of darkness, the very Devil, to aid his cause.

But Ahab is, nevertheless, truly a "grand, ungodly, godlike man," as Melville makes him. And what human being cannot sympathize with him and identify with him as he defies in his egocentric madness the cosmic injustice that batters him, he thinks. In this he is like Lear, and you may have noted by now that two of Melville's grandest sources are Shakespeare and Milton. Ahab stands against, even pursues, his fate, his destiny, his necessity he calls it, magnificently to destruction, even as Milton's Lucifer, particularly in the early books of *Paradise Lost*. There are critics (chiefly Lawrance Thompson in *Melville's Quarrel with God*) who believe that *Moby-Dick* is really a blasphemous blast at God, the source—or, at least, the permitter—of evil in the world. In taking up the problem of evil in the world, Melville, by his ambiguity, is thus courting blasphemy. Evidently, when Melville wrote to Hawthorne that he had written a "wicked book," he meant that he had grandly presented a man in prideful rebellion against the conditions of human existence—perhaps against the God whose providence those conditions are.

BRIEF COMMENTS ON MELVILLE'S ART IN *MOBY-DICK*

Point of View. The point of view, that is, the mind through which we get the story, the content, of *Moby-Dick*, is a first-person point of view. The author, Melville, takes the *persona* of Ishmael as character-commentator on the story of Ahab's pursuit of the whale. I consider this highly significant. The story is told by the moody, philosophic, speculative Ishmael, a wanderer on the face of the earth (or sea). "Call me Ishmael," he says, and his experience runs counter to that of Ahab.

Literary Mode. The literary mode of the novel, like that of *The Scarlet Letter*, is not completely realistic (though the novel contains more factual detail on whaling than you will find almost anywhere). The mode is fundamentally symbolic; the story becomes symbolic, suggestive of a universal human myth—the myth of good-and-evil (hyphenated). There is the sea, which is a mirror of life, of human existence; there is the voyage, a journey into the unknown meaning of life and the self that starts on Christmas day, significantly a kind of anti-quest of hate; there is the ship, the *Pequod*, savagely named, loaded with humanity of all colors and creeds, all attitudes toward life; there is the quester, the challenger, the pursuer, Ahab-man, searching for meaning in the wide world of oceans and the perilous seas of his own soul; there is the pursued, the question, the problem of good-and-evil, the enigma of human suffering and cruel power all symbolized in the ambiguous form of the white whale—the color white which suggests both good and evil and the mysterious interrelatedness which they have. Every detail of whaling, every incident and encounter in the novel, has more than one level of meaning—every bit is relevant to the big question. Remember, Ahab's quest, he says, is for love, as well as meaning. Is the universe framed in terror, not love? Or worse, is there no purpose, meaning—no purposer—behind it all? Maybe one thrusts through the pasteboard mask to discover nothing, meaninglessness.

The Structure. The structure of *Moby-Dick* is epic, heroic, not dramatic, like that of *The Scarlet Letter*. The swell of the sea runs through it, and it is as big and broad and deep as the sea, symbolically as deep as the depths of life and the soul. It is not confined to time; it contains an archetypal myth of human existence, and the structure of the novel is the breadth and depth of the sea that mirrors human experience eternally and internally, in nature and the self. For Ishmael, the end of *Moby-Dick* is just the beginning of knowledge and wisdom.

NOTE: The theme I have stated reflects the critical tendency at present. See such men as Newton Arvin, Richard Chase, Willard Thorp, Howard P. Vincent (in our library), with, of course, psychological, psychoanalytical, anthropological, theological variations. I have simplified, perhaps, quite naturally, according to my own religious inclinations.

REVISED STATEMENT OF THEME

Alternate Thesis. The man who takes the conditions of painful human existence as a personal injury and spends his life (being) in a mad, monomaniac, obsessed pursuit of a private intellectual and spiritual vengeance (vindication) to the point of losing his human bonds (his humanities) destroys his self and affirms evil (Ahab). Thus Mapple's sermon on submission of self to a higher authority points the prow of the ship in search of self on the sea of life in the right direction. Father Mapple says the hardest thing to do is to disobey oneself. Life is a predestined paradox of good and evil; but a man can rescue a measure of freedom and meaning from it by loving his brother (Ishmael). To Melville this is the point of a voyage that starts on Christmas.

You will notice that Father Mapple's injunction to obey God and disobey self is opposite to the direction of Ahab's individual will. Ahab asserts his own divinity and immortality, the possibility of overcoming God, Nature, Necessity—the conditions of human existence in life. Ahab knows at the end that he is doomed by (or to) Necessity, but struggles on to his annihilation by the white whale. He represents, of course, in one way of looking at the novel, the heritage of American individualism, a rational and social optimism, romantically heightened, that is in conflict with another American heritage, that of American theology: the idea that mortal man is fallen and doomed in the natural world, can only hope for redemption beyond natural life.

MOBY-DICK: INTRODUCTION TO ISHMAEL THEME

I want to begin today's thoughts by reading a quotation from Josiah Royce (American philosopher) concerning the problem of evil in the Book of Job:

Job's world, as Job sees it, is organized in a fashion familiar to us all. The main ideas of this cosmology are easy to be reviewed. The very simplicity of the scheme of the universe here involved serves to bring into clearer view the mystery and the horror of the problem that besets Job himself. The world, for Job, is the work of a being who, in the very nature of the case, ought to be intelligible (since he is wise) and friendly to the righteous, since according to tradition, and by virtue of his divine wisdom itself, this God must know a righteous man. But—here is the mystery—this God, as his works get known through our human experience of evil, appears to us not friendly, but hopelessly foreign and hostile in his plans and doings. The more, too, we study his ways with man, the less intelligible seems his nature.

I have read this statement of Job's problem, be-cause it is Ahab's problem also—and Ishmael's, and ours. This is the way God seems to Ahab, as the powers that be are symbolized in the form of the white whale. The powers that be, masked by *Moby-Dick*, are to Ahab evil, malignant, formed in fright—and Ahab pursues the whale to his own destruc-tion. And in the egocentric agony of his obsession (monomania), Ahab completely loses his humane sympathies.

But there is a counter-movement in *Moby-Dick*. Ishmael, like Ahab, is a speculative alien, peering into the mystery of the universe. Though Ishmael does not overlook the reality of pain and suffering in the world, his progress through the novel is differ-ent from Ahab's. It could be said that the white whale comes to symbolize for him good-and-evil (hyphenated), or even good in evil. In contrast to Ahab's narcissism, self-absorption, and solipsism, compare Ishmael's relations with Queequeg:

- The whole relationship begins rather humor-ously in Chapter 4 ("The Counterpane") as a mar-riage ritual: "Upon waking next morning about day-light, I found Queequeg's arm thrown over me in the most loving and affectionate manner."
- "You had almost thought I had been his wife" (Chapter 4). See the rest of this paragraph, for, sig-nificantly, Queequeg is hugging Ishmael through a patchwork quilt of many colors—like a bridal lover (hugged in a "bridegroom clasp . . . as though naught but death should part us twain").
- In Chapter 10 ("A Bosom Friend"): "I began to be

sensible of strange feelings. I felt a melting in me. No more my splintered heart and maddened hand were turned against the whole wolfish world. This soothing savage had redeemed it."

- "I'll try a pagan friend, thought I, since Christian kindness has proved but hollow courtesy."
- "He . . . clasped me round the waist, and said that henceforth we were married; meaning, in his country's phrase, that we were bosom friends; he would gladly die for me, if need should be."
- In Chapter 72 ("The Monkey Rope"): "[T]he monkey-rope was fast at both ends; fast to Queequeg's broad canvas belt, and fast to my narrow leather one. So that for better or for worse, we two, for the time, were wedded; and should poor Queequeg sink to rise no more, then both usage and honor demanded, that instead of cutting the cord, it should drag me down in his wake. So, then, an elongated Siamese ligature united us. Queequeg was my inseparable twin brother; nor could I any way get rid of the dangerous liabilities which the hempen bond entailed." "So strongly and metaphysically did I conceive of my situation then, that while earnestly watching his motions [Queequeg is on the slippery back of the whale], I seemed distinctly to perceive that my own individuality was now merged in a joint stock company of two: that my free will had received a mortal wound; and that another's mistake or misfortune might plunge innocent me into unmerited disaster and death."
- In Chapter 94 ("A Squeeze of the Hand"), the washing of hands in sperm and the marriage rituals both symbolize affirmations of love, fertility in the

human relationship—physical, creative life and love: "[A]s I snuffed up that uncontaminated aroma,— literally and truly, like the smell of spring violets; I declare to you, that for the time I lived as in a musky meadow; I forgot all about our horrible oath; in that inexpressible sperm, I washed my hands and my heart of it; I almost began to credit the old Paracelsan superstition that sperm is of rare virtue in allaying the heat of anger: while bathing in that bath, I felt divinely free of all ill-will, or petulance, or malice, of any sort whatsoever." And: "Oh! My dear fellow beings, why should we longer cherish any social acerbities, or know the slightest ill-humor or envy! Come; let us squeeze hands all round; nay, let us all squeeze ourselves into each other; let us squeeze ourselves universally into the very milk and sperm of kindness."

Thus, through Ishmael, Melville asserts the interdependence of things, of men, in their natural condition, and the need to accept the realities of human existence. There is even a paradoxical polarity in the natural condition of human existence, a close connection between good-and-evil in which good comes from evil, life from death. In the affirming bond of man to man, Ishmael is saved in the coffin of Queequeg by the *Rachel* searching for its dead children, and is cast back into life. Contrariwise, Ahab in monomaniac self-absorption rejects all bonds with man and nature, and tragically plunges into self-immolation. Noble?

LOOKING BACK AT *THE SCARLET LETTER*

Looking back, you should see that Hawthorne in *The Scarlet Letter* represents the same conflict— between the natural impulse to life and creation, and the conditions of mortal existence that restrict that impulse. Unfortunately, in *The Scarlet Letter* the Puritan community dogmatically enforced the laws of life, too rigidly, without compassion, often hypocritically—unsympathetic to the joy of life. But don't forget that Hawthorne and Melville saw clearly the law that hedges us in our mortal condition—call it the law of God, Nature, or Necessity. It is futile to blame systems, societies, establishments, father and mother, for denying us divinity, immortality, absolute freedom. We are not any of these: divine, immortal, or free, even standing on the moon with a transplanted heart. By any new adjustment to natural law we only accept it further and enforce its immutability and ultimate control over us. What we can rescue from our conscious knowledge of material reality—and *Moby-Dick* says so—is love and compassion for each other born from our mutual dependence upon and interdependence in our mortal condition. That is a kind of heaven we can have now—and perhaps one we can have later, if we don't put the later before the now.

LOOKING AHEAD TO *HUCKLEBERRY FINN*

Looking ahead to *Huckleberry Finn*, you will be able to see that it carries the same conflict as *The Scarlet Letter* and *Moby-Dick*: the dream of a natural state of innocence and freedom held up against the knowledge that deterioration and corruption accompany coming of age. By the time of *Huckleberry Finn*, the United States has grown up through a fratricidal war, though still carrying the illusions that are rebutted in the fratricide of today. Huck's is a dream that belongs only to innocence and youth—to a child of a young country. Huck, in the novel, cannot, is not permitted to, grow up, become a man. He must keep running. His alternatives in adulthood are poor. They are the vicious and hypocritical codes of the civilized society he instinctively abhors. But if you think Twain is plugging for the other alternative, anarchic freedom from society in adulthood, you are wrong. Look at Huck's father, who is even more rebellious, resistant to society, intent upon his individual freedom than Huck is. He utterly rejects law and society. He is an instinctive animal, inhuman and inhumane, violent and murderous, degenerate in his death. He is harder to accept, as an example of freedom to be, personal integrity, than Captain Ahab. No, between civilized society and uncivilized Pap, Huck can't grow up, because the dream of freedom and innocence belongs only to youth. The American Dream is the young dream of a young country—the latest form of an old hope, to be reborn and to remain perfect, without knowledge of evil or mortal decay. You can measure the dream by defining what is meant by "success" in American society today. Hawthorne and Melville and Twain reflect doubts about a perfect democracy in America's growing up. They do not solve the problems inherent in conscious life, except to define and clarify them with images of life. A growing knowledge of our mortal state, without the hope for transcendence once held, is why we "grow up absurd" (Paul Goodman) today—despite a pretense of "progress."

Mark Twain, *Huckleberry Finn*
(1966)

ROUND AND ABOUT THEME

The Natural Man *Versus* the Civilized, Conventional Man. Let's start with a statement of theme for *Huckleberry Finn*—a theme which to you may sound farfetched in that it concerns a flight from the slavery of human institutions. It concerns the natural man *versus* the civilized, conventional man. It concerns the quest of the natural human being for freedom from the restraints of society. And, in relation to the development of American society, *Huckleberry Finn* dramatizes the fact that the American Dream of innocence and freedom and success, the dream of a Perfect Society in the natural world, has gone sour on the Mississippi frontier. (Hawthorne, first, and Melville, second, were skeptical of this dream, as you must have noted.) Anyway, so sophisticated a way of stating the theme of *Huckleberry Finn* is not far-fetched when one stops to note that the instinctive goodness of Huck and Jim is put in contrast with the more civilized society along the banks of the river. This contrast is structurally enforced by the development of the plot, which follows the course of the river. The novel emphasizes the goodness of the natural man (in the persons of Huck and Jim), living sometimes outside civilization on a raft in the middle part of the novel, *versus* the evils of organized, institutionalized society; the novel is an attack on conventional society and institutions in favor of the natural goodness of the simple man and boy. On a social-political level, the Mississippi frontier puts the naive faith in the democracy of the common man in contrast with the actual conditions of slavery, murder, material greed, and other institutionalized inhumanities.

Mythic Quest for Innocence and Freedom. Huck and Jim's retreat from society, their journey down the river, becomes a kind of mythic quest for innocence and freedom, a release from the encroachments and restraints of evil, a quest for a harmony they cannot find in the society they leave. Nigger Jim's flight from slavery is a part of the same theme as Huck's resistance to attempts to civilize him. Jim is fleeing from a brutal institution that is entirely insensitive to the human suffering involved in his situation. May I caustically note here that Jim's suffering (his being sold away from his wife and children) is caused by good Americans, good moralizing church people, the same people who want to civilize Huck and make a Christian out of him, the people who dominate both ends of the Mississippi, St. Petersburg and Phelps Farm, the Americans who talk the same today, North and South, and act the same way. In contrast, the natural, uncivilized Huck instinctively pities Jim as a person who can suffer humanly, though he wonders at the marvel of Jim's humanness. Although Huck comes to humanly pity and love Jim, he never questions the rightness of slavery, the social institution that has molded his mind, enslaved and corrupted a part of his conscience. He even believes he will go to hell if he helps Jim.

Twain then seems to affirm the brotherly love and freedom that the natural Huck and Jim (white and black) find together in idyllic moments on the river—when they are stripped (literally naked) of social institutions that might deaden the natural impulses of their hearts. Their life on the river, in the middle section of the novel, is a romantic idyll, indeed! But the tension between the romantic idyll, which Twain seeks to affirm, and the reality of evil in society, is never released in the novel. In their most idyllic moments on the river, Huck and Jim are literally living outside the world of society, and the idyll of the river, the romantic dream of youth and freedom and innocence in every heart, is constantly overshadowed by the inhumanities of the society, the people living along the banks of the river.

The American Dream Gone Bankrupt. Actually, though the novel seems to afford a romantic answer in the innocence and freedom of the river, apart from society, Twain was just as aware of the prevalence of evil as Hawthorne and Melville were. Escape from society into a primitive existence is really no answer; nor is Huck's heading for the territory at the end. What lies beyond the frontier always looks like fertile territory for the American Dream, but the frontier society will follow Huck. Twain knew this: he died a cynic and spoke of "the damned human race." In Twain the American Dream is going bankrupt, but it lives on in the myth of the movie and TV Western where there are only white hats and black hats, good people and bad people, innocent and guilty people—nothing in between—and always, with lots of death and violence, the white hats (that is, we good and innocent Americans) prevail over the evil. The idyll of Huck and Jim is a romantic dream, but it doesn't prevail (although Hemingway thought *Huckleberry Finn* the greatest thing in American fiction, he called the end of the novel "cheating" because Twain did not face reality in the freeing of Jim). Twain's vision is most honest in people like Aunt Sally, kindly people but inhumane in their unseeing righteousness, kindly people in whom the conventional evil is rooted (in fact, evil has become institutionalized, as in Vietnam): their kindliness accommodates inhumanities that serve their prosperity (like selling slaves) (like segregation to protect property and white education and superiority).

TECHNIQUE IN *HUCKLEBERRY FINN*

<u>Point of View</u> (the mental, or emotional, perspective from which we get the story). The point of view is sustained and restrained in Huck, a 12-year-old boy. We always see through Huck's eyes; he is a perfect instrument—a naive mirror for the creation of irony. Through him we get two views of things:

Huck's boy's view, which is unsophisticated in evil but realistic, and, in contrast, our own adult, sophisticated view, added to Huck's. All is seen through the eyes of Huck, who knows in his heart he must love, even though, ironically, society has taught him he will go to hell if he responds to his love. Huck reports what he sees in society and accepts what he sees with his head (rationally), but rejects it with his heart (emotionally).

What I am trying to emphasize is Twain's great art in containing the novel within the point of view of a 12-year-old boy, and not intruding a point of view not characteristic of Huck, thus giving us the effect of seeing what a boy sees from our perspective of maturity. The implicit force of the novel is in the difference between what Huck sees and knows and what the adult reader sees and knows. This difference is the same as the difference between what a young reader finds in the book and what the older reader finds, though it is a tribute to the art of Twain that the heart of the older reader still yearns for what the boy found. I remember my first reading. And I still yearn for the innocence of childhood.

Narrative Structure (the way in which the author has arranged the parts of his story for a peculiar effect). The novel has been said to have three units which contribute to theme:

CHAPTERS 1-16. Connections with St. Petersburg— Huck, Tom, Nigger Jim, Pap. Ends when Huck and Jim get beyond their St. Petersburg relations.

CHAPTERS 17-32. This is the largest unit and has to do with the larger world of the Mississippi South that Huck and Jim encounter along the river. It begins when the raft is wrecked by the steamboat, the beginning of the shore episodes. Always, in this unit, the idyllic life on the river is touched by, intruded upon by, the corruption of society on the shore (e.g., the Grangerford-Shepherdson feud; chicanery of King and Duke; Sherburn's killing of Boggs [quelling of the mob]; the village funeral [Wilks]).

CHAPTERS 32-END. This unit has to do with the re-entry of Tom Sawyer at Phelps Farm, a place exactly like St. Petersburg in values, but at the other end of the Mississippi. It has been called a weak unit. Here we are back to conventional, righteous insensitivity through Tom's romantic-heroic fictions (the conventions of sentimental romance according to *Monte Cristo*). Tom's indignities to Jim are really brutal. Tom's is a piety of rules, which is insensitive to human feeling. This is the same insensitivity and brutality as that of St. Petersburg.

∅

Willliam Dean Howells, *The Rise of Silas Lapham*
(1967)

APPROACH TO *SILAS LAPHAM*

<u>Howells as a Realist</u>. Howells is very important to the history of the American novel because he is regarded as the first significant champion of the doctrine of realism in American fiction, not only in his novels but also in his criticism of fiction. In Hawthorne and Melville, and even Twain (who is often described as a local-color realist), the imaginative, figurative mode is very strong. And that is the emphasis I chose to put on *The Scarlet Letter, Moby-Dick,* and *Huckleberry Finn.* I could have put my remarks about these novels under such titles as "The Symbolism of Sex and Sin in *The Scarlet Letter*," "The Allegory of Good and Evil in *Moby-Dick*," and "The Myth of American Innocence in *Huckleberry Finn.*"

Whereas the novels of Hawthorne and Melville and Twain can be classed as "romances" because they often depart from the literal level of experience into imaginative treatment of deep psychological and philosophical problems, Howells' aim was to accurately represent the factual details of ordinary life. Though one can see that the direction from Hawthorne to Melville to Twain has been gradually from felt truth, Howells is bluntly on the side of mind, realistic common sense. He defined realism as "nothing more and nothing less than the truthful treatment of material," involving "fidelity to experience and probability of motive." The novelist, he said, should "report the phrase and carriage of everyday life." Quite obviously, Howells meant something else by "truth" than did Hawthorne and Melville, or even Twain.

The Ordinary Self. Hester and Ahab and Huck represent ideas and attitudes beyond themselves; Silas Lapham is important only for his ordinary self, and the ordinary is primary in every Howells novel. Howells not only illustrates his critical theories of realism through the plots of his novels but also has characters voice those theories. Watch for such statements in *Silas Lapham*. Howells' own term for his kind of realism was "commonplace." Commonplace realism, Victorian realism, Puritan realism, Reticent realism—these are the tags applied to Howells' writing, usually in a derogatory sense. It has been said that Howells never really faced the observable facts of life (not to mention the inner truths) he said it was his job to record. He was always optimistic about ordinary life, in contrast to his successors in realism, the naturalists.

Howells as Pioneer. Whether or not life is actually as he drew it, we must keep in mind that around

1880 Howells was opening up subjects for the novel that had never been realistically explored before in American fiction. He was a pioneer. One of his best novels, *A Modern Instance*, is the first American novel of major structure to deal with the realistic details of an unhappy marriage, and hint at the great gap between ideal hopes and realistic fact. Howells may have been very reticent in his reporting of what he thought to be the ordinary truth of life, but he paved the way for a frankness in American fiction. Yet it must be said finally that Howells explored the outside of reality, not the inside. He feared to look within.

TECHNIQUE: DOUBLE NARRATIVE PATTERN

The Financial-Fall and Ethical-Rise. Silas has a financial rise and fall that closely correspond to a moral fall and rise. Is there any significance in the balance of the relationship? Is there a connection between the financial rise and the moral fall, between the financial fall and the moral rise?

The Tom-Penelope-Irene Love Plot. Many critics have insisted that it is irrelevant to the main plot, which concerns Silas' financial, social, and moral problems. Is it? Does it, perhaps, link Silas' social aspirations to the financial-fall and ethical-rise plot? Do the two plots fulfill a common theme? Does the novel have organic unity? What is the central meaning of the novel?

Stephen Crane, *The Red Badge of Courage*
(1966)

INTRODUCTION TO CRANE

We have now progressed from the psychological "romance" (*The Scarlet Letter*) of Hawthorne to the commonplace "realism" of Howells (*The Rise of Silas Lapham*). The next steps are to naturalistic realism through Stephen Crane and Theodore Dreiser, and psychological realism through Henry James. I would like to approach Crane's *The Red Badge of Courage* from two perspectives: (a) the content aspect (relating to meaning or theme) I will call naturalism; and (b) the formal aspect (relating to means or technique) I will call impressionism.

<u>Naturalism</u>. With respect to content, I must say at the outset that rather than calling *The Red Badge of Courage* and *Sister Carrie* naturalistic novels, it is better to say that they are novels with naturalistic characteristics. But *The Red Badge of Courage* is a forerunner of naturalism in American fiction. Naturalism, defined, is a mode of literary realism which objectively studies man and events as the deter-

mined (in the sense that no free choice is exercised) products of natural causation. Literary naturalism treats man as bound by the natural laws of heredity and environment. Thematically, I think, Henry Fleming in *The Red Badge of Courage* is treated as a victim of nature, both biologically and psychologically. He reacts naturally to a fear of death and a fear of being thought to be afraid. Perhaps the most persistent characteristic of literary naturalism in American fiction is its objective, systematized observation of natural phenomena in the economic, social, biological, and psychological spheres of man's existence. Theoretically, naturalistic fiction objectively and frankly reports rather than interprets life ("slice of life"). Theoretically, it is amoral (since characters do not have free choice, as in the moral commonplace realism of Howells), as well as deterministic, and pessimistic (because there is no freedom to choose one's destiny).

Impressionism. In technique, *The Red Badge of Courage* is a forerunner of impressionistic stream of consciousness. It is an imaginative, poetic recording of the stream of sense impressions that flow through Henry Fleming's mind. The novel is largely a succession of fragmentary and momentary sense images that flash through Fleming's hypersensitive consciousness while he is driven by the fear of death and the fear of fear. The dramatic focus of the novel, unlike that of *Silas Lapham* you just read and *Sister Carrie* you will read next, is not on the external world which is perceived but on the consciousness of the perceiver of the external world—on the mind and feelings of Henry Fleming. We do not get the external world, but rather Fleming's impression of the external world—the external world as it appears to the private consciousness of the hero.

MEANING

Natural Conditioning Rather Than Moral Growth. Now a bit more on the meaning of *The Red Badge of Courage*. I have already hinted that, despite the poetic images, the poetic impressions in the novel, I choose to interpret it naturalistically; that is to say, I regard the process of Fleming's development in war as that of natural conditioning rather than moral growth. Some critics disagree with this interpretation. The question is: Is this a symbolic story of spiritual death and rebirth, a moral regeneration? Or is it a story of instinctive animal adjustment to an environment of terror and violence, an amoral development? I think the latter.

The Use of Religious Symbols in Relation to Meaning. Now let us reinforce some of the points I made by referring to the introduction in your text. I do not agree totally with either Chase or Stallman, though Chase is more right. However, religious symbols are more related to a structure of meaning in *The Red Badge of Courage* than he thinks. But they are used negatively, rather than positively, ironically to reinforce the naturalistic theme in Henry Fleming's development—for example, the suggestions of Christ's passion in relation to Jim Conklin's horribly grotesque death are intended by Crane to be ironic comment on the natural reality and horrible finality in the death struggle, an animal struggle and suffering of Jim Conklin (see the irony in the "resemblance in him to a devotee of a mad religion"). All through the novel there is a structure of Christian symbolism that stands in ironic contrast to the naturalistic development of Henry Fleming's moral character. Crane is mocking the idea of spiritual growth in Henry, rather than accenting it.

<u>Like an Animal</u>. The test of Stallman's thesis is in the lack of spiritual growth after the death of Conklin. What are the consequences of this incident? Fleming compounds his shame by guiltily deserting the barely living Tattered Soldier, who is himself badly in need of help, and sneaks away aimlessly, not desirous of honorable battle. By Chapter XIII, he has received a bloody blow on the head from the rifle-butt of one of his own men, has been returned to his regiment by a friendly soldier, and is being sympathetically nursed with bed and food by Wilson before turning in for the night. While hiding in a lie, he taunts Wilson for a cowardice that has been less than his own. To be sure, on the next day he fights heroically, but the point to be made here is that not only has he not returned to his regiment by deliberate moral choice, but he has also persisted in the convenient deception that he was wounded by the enemy in action. Nor does he ever (except in the movie version) reveal that he had run away from battle and that his wound is spurious. In his heroism he reacts like an animal (as his comrades note) almost automatically, in a survival instinct that is

another step in his natural conditioning, after the flight. He stands and fights like an animal, after having run away like an animal. To say that Conklin's death has sown in Fleming the seeds of heroic resolve, or has initiated him into moral manhood, is to exceed the evidence. Certainly there is no spiritual growth, regeneration, as Stallman asserts.

ℒ

From Howells to Dreiser

"REALISM" AND "NATURALISM" IN THE NOVEL

Before beginning Dreiser I would like to make some remarks relative to such terms as "realism" and "naturalism" in the novel.

<u>Definitions</u>. "Realism" can be defined as observation of the ordinary actuality of experience. Literary naturalism is a kind of realism, theoretical and systematized. Naturalism is a further step in realism in literature.

<u>Origin of Naturalism</u>. Naturalism in literature is the result of the impact of a realistic/rationalistic, materialistic, scientific age in literature—an age which increasingly believed that the essence of reality is to be found in the laws of natural material causation (Darwin in biology, Comte in philosophy, Marx in economics, Taine in literature, etc.). Émile Zola is called the father of the naturalistic novel, his definition of naturalism being "realism held in the current of the progress of science; it is an attempt to assimilate the processes of realistic literature to the processes of science." In writing his novels Zola tried to

follow the same scientific principle that Claude Bernard laid down in his *Experimental Medicine.* Compare Zola's *The Experimental Novel.*

Connections between Realism and Naturalism. *Webster's New Collegiate Dictionary* shows the close connection between the naturalism of philosophical positivism and scientific materialism, and literary naturalism—the dominating emphasis in the modern world of material reality explicable in terms of natural law:

REALISM
1. In *Philosophy:* a. The doctrine that universals exist outside the mind. b. The conception that objects of sense perception are real in their own right, existing independently of their being known or related to mind. OR
2. Preoccupation with material reality, or the objects of sense perception, as opposed to idealism.
3. The theory that art or literature should conform to nature or to real life, that is, the objects of sense perception; the practice of this theory; representation without idealization.

NATURALISM
1. Action, inclination, or thought based on natural desires and instincts alone.
2. In *Literature and Art,* a type of realism emphasizing scientific methods of observation and experiment in the treatment of character.
3. In *Philosophy,* the doctrine denying that anything in reality has a supernatural significance, the doctrine that scientific laws account for all phenomena, and that teleological conceptions of nature (for instance, that divine purpose in nature has precedence over natural law in nature, including natural man) are invalid; loosely defined, materialism and positivism.

4. In *Theology*, the denial of the miraculous and super-natural in religion, and the denial of revelation (including inspiration) as a means of attaining truth.

Characteristics of Naturalism

OBJECTIVITY. The naturalistic writer seeks truth in the spirit of the scientific observer by recording sense impressions objectively. He seeks to answer the problems of human behavior by quantitative re-cording. Compare the procedures in our social stud-ies today, in sociology, psychology, history, or even philosophy. Cf. the qualitative recording of James, interior *versus* exterior.

FRANKNESS. Naturalism records the basic animal facts of natural material causation, of the basic animal drives (sex, hunger, etc.), without regard for convention.

AMORALITY. Naturalism is not concerned with eth-ics or morals, the questions of right and wrong in human conduct; the naturalist merely records what he observes. Theoretically men do things by natural causation, not by free choice.

DETERMINISM. The vital principle which sets natu-ralism off from moralistic realism (compare Howells) is the philosophy that man is caught in the laws of material causation which determine the course of his existence. Man has no choice, no free will. Ordi-nary realism preserves the drama of man as free agent, moral agent.

PESSIMISM. Naturalists tend toward the gloomy outlook on man as caught in a trap of natural causation which he cannot avoid. Man is a victim of natural circumstances beyond his control. The naturalistic writer tends to observe the more sordid "realistic" truths (facts) of life.

CHARACTER TYPES. The naturalist observes abnormal or subnormal mental and physical types because they respond more readily to the study of man as a product of natural causation, man as victim of his natural fate. Sister Carrie is not strong mentally. Compare Tess Durbeyfield in Hardy's *Tess of the D'Urbervilles*, who is a victim of her sexuality and her environment, not strong mentally either.

Effects of Naturalism on American Literature. Naturalism is a particular phenomenon of modern literature, beginning in Europe, especially in France, and spreading to all literatures in some degree. It was never fully accepted by the English realists (compare George Eliot), who continued to respect human freedom of moral choice. Its impact on American literature was greater, maybe because of a reaction against the Puritanic moralism that sought to retard unconventional realism, even of the Howells variety. Naturalism as a literary philosophy is on the wane today, but its effect has been great. Its most persisting characteristic in American literature is its detailed, objective, systematized reporting of natural phenomena in the social, biological, and psychological (yes) spheres of man's conduct, even though the novelist in question might not accept its philosophy of natural determination. Compare such writers today as Anderson, Farrell, Hemingway, Faulkner, Mailer, Jones.

Naturalism and Dreiser. Dreiser is regarded as a good example of naturalism in the American novel. But he is not thoroughly naturalistic, and *Carrie* is regarded as less naturalistic than other of his novels, e.g., *The American Tragedy*. My problem for you is that you test *Carrie* for the characteristics of a naturalist novel. Dreiser has an amoral attitude toward Carrie and Hurstwood. He doesn't condemn them, morally judge them. But he pities them (man) for their (his) inadequacy. They are only what their heredity and environment made them. They have morals which match the mores of their community; they grasp for the glittering material standards which their society sets. Here is social criticism. But how can Dreiser condemn society, how can he hope to change it, if he gives man no moral choice to resist or change his environment, when he considers morals as merely reflective of environment? A vicious circle.

✐

Henry James, *The Ambassadors*
(1966)

LOOKING BACK

To begin Henry James and *The Ambassadors*, let us look rapidly to where we have been in this course:

- Hawthorne, *Scarlet Letter*, psychological romance
- Melville, *Moby-Dick*, philosophical romance
- Twain, *Huckleberry Finn*, local-color realism
- Howells, *Rise of Silas Lapham*, commonplace realism
- Crane, *Red Badge of Courage*, impressionistic-naturalistic realism
- Dreiser, *Sister Carrie*, naturalism

HENRY JAMES: PSYCHOLOGICAL REALISM

These tags over-generalize and are not very accurate in distinguishing between the realistic novel and the romance, but I would like to make one more tag:

- James, *The Ambassadors*, psychological realism

The realistic focus, up to now, broadly speaking, and particularly in Howells and Dreiser, has been on the external-social scene. Of the so-called realist-naturalists Crane could be said to be the most like James in that both focus on the *inner* life of their characters. Both, and each in his own way, could be called forerunners of the stream of consciousness technique. But whereas Crane in Henry Fleming gives us the reactions of Henry in highly emotional states—fear, terror, animal reactions—James in *The Ambassadors* penetrates the highly refined and sensitive intellectual-moral consciousness of Lambert Strether.

TECHNIQUE IN JAMES' NOVELS

So far as technique in the development of the novel, and not only the American novel, is concerned, Henry James is the most important novelist the United States has produced. So next I wish to outline briefly the significant points in James' psychological realism:

- Subjectivism
- Limitation of point of view
- Scenical (dramatic) handling of story

SUBJECTS-THEMES OF *THE AMBASSADORS*

- The developing-expanding moral consciousness of Lambert Strether.
- The awakening of a middle-aged man to the vitality of life.

- The gradual and subtle transformation of a middle-aged man to a more liberal moral sensitivity (from a rigid Puritan outlook—duty—but be careful).
- The cosmopolitan, sophisticated, worldly European outlook *versus* the innocent, moral, provincial American outlook.

Here are James' own words on the subject of the novel. They are contained in his preface to the New York Edition of *The Ambassadors*:

The subject proper . . . is the matter of free intellectual exploration in general, of the open mind in contrast to the mind closed and swaddled in prejudice and narrow views. . . . the contrast between the cosmopolitan and the provincial, between the European and American outlook.

THEME IN RELATION TO TECHNIQUE

Now let me as shortly as possibly relate James' subject-theme to the significant techniques of the novel.

Point of View. James uses the most effective—the inner—point of view for probing the moral consciousness of a character. The dramatic center of *The Ambassadors* is not the outside (social) circumstances, but rather Strether's inner change. Therefore the point of view is the inner; the subject-theme of the novel is Strether's mind, it is Strether's *center of consciousness*. We see and hear and feel and think. We follow his gradual and subtle inner change, *from within him*. This is not yet stream of consciousness, so-called. Strether's center of consciousness is disciplined, controlled, formalized in the intellectual style of Henry James—it is an abstraction of Strether's mind really—but as in stream of consciousness the focus is inner, intellectual rather than affective, mind as abstraction rather than impression.

Narrative Structure. A small note on the novel's narrative structure: that is, on the way in which James presents the material of his story for thematic effect. E. M. Forster in *Aspects of the Novel* (cf. Lubbock, *The Craft of Fiction*) says that *The Ambassadors* "is the shape of an hour-glass": Chad and Strether change places, moral positions. The hour-glass image also emphasizes the relevance of the passage of time to the theme of the novel: youth and middle-age.

The *Ficelle*. Use of the *ficelle* or confidante in relation to characterization, to "sound out" the point of view—which is Strether. In this novel the chief confidante is Maria Gostrey. Relate to scenical-dramatic handling of story.

SIGNIFICANT POINTS IN JAMES' MEANS AND MEANING

James' Psychological Realism or Subjectivism. In revealing his characters James weighted what he called the "scales" on the side of self, rather than society. He wanted the reader to view the character from the character's own view of himself (or herself) rather than from society's view. James is interested in human beings as fine rational-spiritual entities;

he is not interested in superficial facts. His novels' subject is always the fine working of a sensitive mind, like that of Lambert Strether.

Limitation of Point of View, or Angle of Vision. This point is closely connected with the first. James focuses not on external action but on the effects of happenings on his characters' minds, and his tendency is to limit what the reader knows to the consciousness of a single character. For *Portrait of a Lady* he said he would "place the centre of the subject in this young woman's [Isabel's] own consciousness." James did not follow his own rule absolutely in *Portrait*; he allows us to see Isabel on important occasions from the view of other characters. In *The Ambassadors*, one of the novels of his last period, the reader sees only what Strether sees.

Dramatic Handling of the Story. James develops the interior action of his plots through crucial scenes ("occasions") of psychological tension where the main character talks intimately with another character. These characters are more important for their use in dramatic dialogue than for their relation to the plot.

✠

Edith Wharton, *Ethan Frome*

TWO MAJOR THESES IN WHARTON'S NOVELS

Wharton's novels contain two major theses. One is that New York's old *haut monde* of culture and dignity has been for years giving way before a new cheap aristocracy of money and fashion. The other is that whoever breaks a social commandment, no matter how unfair it may seem, must pay for his transgression in the end.

Social rules, even when they are cruel and superficial, are essential to social order, and cannot be violated with impunity. The moral code of Wharton's world has become debased, but the wicked pay for their insurgency; in some way they do penance for their perversity. It is a Christianity of the Old Testament. Wharton leaves no doubt of her ethical convictions. Taken by and large, man is surrounded by forces quite beyond his own powers to control or deny. If he is a little man in the world, little forces can intimidate him; if he is a more primitive creature in a more natural world, forces as relentless as the elements can crush him. The most triumphant of human powers therefore is not the defiance of fate, but the control of self. A frame of convention is at once a restraint and a stimulus to the joy of living.

Whispering the Last Enchantments of the Victorian Age. Wharton remains for us among the voices whispering the last enchantments of the Victorian age. From the first Mrs. Wharton's power has lain in the ability to reproduce in fiction the circumstances of a compact community in a way that illustrates the various oppressions which such communities put upon the individual vagaries, whether viewed as sin, or ignorance, or folly, or merely as social impossibility. Characterized by a sense of human beings living in such intimate solidarity that no one of them may vary from the customary path without in some fashion breaking the pattern and inviting some sort of disaster.

Tragic Passion. In *Ethan Frome,* losing from her clear voice for a moment the note of satire, Wharton reaches her highest point of tragic passion. In the bleak life of Ethan Frome on his bleak hillside there blooms an exquisite love which during a few hours of rapture promises to transform his fate; but poverty clutches him, drives him to attempt suicide with the woman he loves, and then condemns him to one of the most appalling expiations in fiction—to a slavery in comparison with which his former life was almost freedom. Not since Hawthorne has a novelist built on the New England soil a tragedy of such elevation of mood as this.

The Illusion of Reality. Poverty and decorum. Lucidity, detachment, irony. If Wharton had a little less of this pride of dignity she might perhaps avoid her tendency to assign to decorum a larger power than it actually exercises, even in the societies about which she writes. Decorum, after all, is binding chiefly upon those who accept it without question but not upon passionate or logical rebels, who are always shattering it with some touch of violence or neglect; neither does it bind those who stand too securely to be shaken. For this reason the coils of circumstance and the pitfalls of inevitability with which Mrs. Wharton besets the careers of her characters are in part an illusion deftly employed for the sake of artistic effect. She multiplies them as romancers multiply adventures. But the illusion of reality never fails her—no shoddy romantic elements. Nothing is admitted that does not bear on the total tragedy. Event follows event with such a look of iron logic that the reader has no chance to think of possible acts by the characters which might have saved or relieved them. To Wharton, Frome is a simple, easily understood character—not a sophisticate.

Ethan's Struggle to Attain One Moment of Happiness. Zeena's utter selfishness fastens itself upon Ethan's generous nature. One of the chief claims of the novel to importance lies in the skill with which petty circumstances of life bind Ethan to his helplessness. His poverty and his incapacity for a mean action, which prevent him from leaving Zeena and going off with Mattie to begin a new life, the long slow decay of the New England farm, the bitter winters that have sapped the strength from body and will, finally have their way with Ethan. Zeena rises from invalidism to take care not only of Ethan, but also of Mattie, whose broken back takes her out of the reach of Zeena's physical jealousy. It is not misery that makes *Frome* a fine and tragic novel; it is the struggle of Ethan to attain one moment of happiness, and the iron logic of the situation in which a nature like his could not abandon a duty, even if it wrecked his life. There is potential greatness in his soul.

Wharton's irony does not spring from an imagination that contemplates man in his relation to cosmic forces, but as an observer whose irony springs from noting the clash between men and social convention. *Je suis venue trop tard dans un monde trop vulgaire.*

STYLE AND DESIGN

In style and design Edith Wharton is a traditionalist. No technical experiments—no departure from classical rules of unity, coherence, and emphasis. Her stories are delicately balanced, with faultless tone and movement; and her tonic style, rich in biting imagery, lends itself well to the tonic pitch of her mind. There is also a nice articulation of sound and sense in her work, and she has a deft (if sometimes too remarkable) gift for revealing character in sharp lightning flashes of language. She has a rare talent for the *mot juste*. In fact, the only objections that might be argued against her technique are that in her last novels the melodrama on which her work is based shows through too clearly, that her winking jewels of style and epigram draw more attention to themselves than they should, that her satire now and then edges over into "cattiness"—and that her plots are made to hinge on too many coincidences (such as the sled in *Frome*). Both Wharton and James (and Howells?) deal, above all, in situations artificially constructed to evoke certain reactions from their characters, as a chemist might adjust the background of a test for the purpose of producing the desired result, or the writer of a "problem play" stacks the cards to bring out his thesis. In order to secure their purpose, they have to warp the irregular outlines of reality into invented symmetries, and make use of more than the number of coincidences warranted by chance. The hand of Wharton peeps through.

NOTE: Edith Wharton belongs to no movement or group. Wharton does not think of *Ethan Frome* (1911) as her greatest novel. Begun as an exercise in French.

ℒ

Sinclair Lewis, *Babbitt*
(1963)

SOME BACKGROUND ON LEWIS

I am giving you this background because Lewis became the most important commentator that American fiction has produced on American society and mores in the first thirty years or so of the twentieth century. His importance as a novelist has steadily declined, but his significance as a social critic remains. We are now between two wars.

He was born February 7, 1885, in Sauk Center, Minnesota, which became famous as the Gopher Prairie of his fiction. His father was a village doctor. He graduated from Yale in 1907. He did a lot of bumming around in the United States, and twice worked his passage to Europe on cattle boats. He was a newspaper editor, reporter, and doer of less important journalistic jobs. He did all kinds of menial work in his travels about the country, including that of janitor and soda jerk. I tell you of these occupations in declining order of importance because Lewis was an acute observer of the American scene, top to bottom.

Lewis wrote a lot of rather trashy stories, ghost-wrote for more important writers, and did five pretty poor novels before he became something of a sensation with *Main Street* in 1920. It took the country by storm because of its attack on the center of American life—on the dullness of the American small town—what Lewis called the "village virus," placid, hypocritical conformity. *Main Street* established the reputation of Lewis. In 1926 he was awarded the Pulitzer prize for *Arrowsmith*, but declined it. This rejection was either courageous or a good publicity stunt. In 1930 he was the first American to receive the Nobel Prize for Literature. Although the prize is never awarded for a specific novel, it is generally agreed that the prize came as the result of a powerful character portrayal and the somewhat exaggerated idealism of the hero in *Arrowsmith*, belatedly (cf. Sholokov, 1965). *Arrowsmith* is somewhat different, better if less spectacular, than his other novels because of the influence on it of Paul de Kruif.

LEWIS' CRITICAL APPROACH

What Lewis attacks are the values of American middle-class material progress, values that are closely related to those of the small town, the so-called grass roots. But it would be wrong to think of Lewis as an anti-materialist. In fact, Lewis' ideal is a material one. What he attacks are what he considers the side effects of the American conquest of the material: conformity, standardization and sterility of mind, the hypocrisy and inferiority of values. Lewis decries the shoddiness of daily American life as an unnecessary concomitant of technological achievement; he berates the dullness, intellectual dishonesty, sham, irrationality, and the mechanized, standardized, advertised conduct. His liberal philosophy is based on an individualism that caters to discoveries in the physical and social sciences. He hates any kind of institutionalization that limits individual persons. He dislikes the deterioration of the individual American soul that has accompanied American material progress and technological advances. But he doesn't dislike that material progress itself: his ideal is scientific truth, pure science. Lewis is typical in his idealization of the material, typically American, that is. As a disillusioned romanticist (abstract idealist, if you wish), he probably fails to see to the heart of the matter: that conquest of the material world and technological advances are inevitably tied to a standardization of mind and values that limits personal freedom. "Where your treasure is . . . ." We are looking ahead to that interesting American, Gatsby, and his Daisy Fay.

NOTE: Lewis taught me the mind of America more than any other novelist. He is still more relevant than is ordinarily thought. Then why do I not find him so today?

REALISM IN THE AMERICAN NOVEL

Since Howells, we have been watching the progress of "realism" in the American Novel, from the "commonplace" realism of Howells, through the naturalistic realism of Crane and Dreiser, to the psychological realism of James. These men were deeply interested in the theory of realism, as a philosophy that explained the natural and social and psychological forces behind the actions of their characters, and as an artistic creed for their writing, even though their moral philosophies might be as different as those of Howells and Dreiser, their artistic philosophies as different as those of Howells and James.

Lewis' Realism

Well, how about the "realism" of Sinclair Lewis, the first post-World War I writer we are studying, the first American novelist to win the Nobel Prize for Literature? (Note that all our remaining novelists are Nobel Prize winners.) Of Lewis' realism this much can be said, I believe:

- His realism lacked the intensely serious commitment to the ideas of his predecessors in the line of realism, lacked the commitment to art or social criticism or moral philosophy.
- Yet Lewis gave the most accurate and comprehensive picture (caricatured and exaggerated, perhaps) of American society and the American character and values that any writer has ever given for any period. I myself believe that the picture holds true even today. (Follow through, for example, on the manner in which Virgil Gunch dictated conformity.)
- Lewis fell short of greatness because he failed to see or apply the serious implications of his realism for the American character. In the end George F.

Babbitt is really a nice guy and we love him. We recognize him and Gunch and the other Lewis characters as true to American society and small-town values, but neither Lewis nor we want deeply to see what is the matter with Babbitt and the others, and with us today—though some may be beginning to see.

Fitting the Times Perfectly

Lewis is pretty clever at drawing Babbitt's picture, and my points may be exaggerated, but Alfred Kazin (*On Native Grounds*) makes them better.

Lewis fitted the times so perfectly that he became almost invisible *in* that scene; he had worked over the surface world so thoroughly that he became a part of it. A more profound writer would not have so assured a success; a less skillful one would not have been so influential in his success. But Lewis hit a certain average in art perfectly, as he hit off the national average—or what Americans like to think is the national average—so well in his characters, and that was at once his advantage and his misfortune. As his characters become public symbols, he came to seem more an influence than a novelist; as his jokes against the old American ways became new American ways themselves, the barriers between his books and life in America came down altogether. George F. Babbitt had entered as completely into the national imagination as Daniel Boone, but with his emergence, as with every archetype of American character Lewis brought in, some part of his usefulness seemed to be over.

There is a certain irony in Lewis's career that is now impossible to miss, and one that illustrates it as a whole. Here was the bright modern satirist who wrote each of his early books as an assault on American smugness, provincialism, ignorance, and bigotry; and ended up by finding

himself not an enemy, but the folksiest and most com-
radely of American novelists. Here was the American rebel
who had begun *Main Street* as his spiritual autobiography,
who even wrote dashingly in its foreword that it preached
"alien" doctrines and who painted the whole world of endless Main Streets where "dullness is made God"—and
found that people were delighted over how well he had hit
off the village butcher, the somnolent afternoons on Main
Street, the hysterical Sunday-night suppers, and the genteel money-lender's wife, with her "bleached cheeks,
bleached hair, bleached voice, and a bleached manner."
Here was the crusading satirist who spared none of the hy-
pocrisies by which Babbitt and his group lived, least of all
their big and little cruelties, and gave Babbitt back to his
people as a browbeaten, noisy *goodfellow.*

Babbitt, George F., became, and still is, a sentimental
folk hero.

F. Scott Fitzgerald, *The Great Gatsby*

For *Gatsby*, I wish to reverse my usual procedure by first looking at the novel itself, then making some summations on its method and meaning. But first, let us start with this idea:

THE SUBJECT OF THE NOVEL

Jay Gatsby's Dream. Jay Gatsby is a pathetic, perhaps tragic, figure because the dream he pursues is unworthy of him. Jay Gatsby has a romantic imagination, but the real materials from which he must shape his dream in the society around him are not worthy of his idealizing potential.

In general, Gatsby's dream is the American Dream—the way it was at the beginning of American history and in boyhood, unspoiled and virginal, at least in his Platonic conception. More particularly, in historical process, it is the American Dream of Success (with a capital S). Most specifically that dream is symbolized by the superficial (even vulgar) beauty of Daisy Fay which Gatsby pursues. The pathos of Gatsby's pursuit lies in the difference between Gatsby's idealized-romanticized conception of Daisy Fay, symbolized by the green light burning at the end of her dock (which links with the green breast of land, the green breast of the New World/Long Island when first sighted by the Dutch sailors also across an expanse of water), and the actuality of Daisy in the American society of the 1920s. And thus Gatsby's dream is not worthy of his dreaming.

As Nick Carraway and the novel put it: "Gatsby turned out all right at the end; it is what preyed on Gatsby, what foul dust floated in the wake of his dreams that temporarily closed out my interest in the abortive sorrows and short-winded elations of men." And, Gatsby "sprang from his Platonic conception of himself. He was a son of God—a phrase which, if it means anything, means just that—and he must be about his Father's business, the service of a vast, vulgar, and meretricious beauty." This is a religious ideal of American Success, the romanticizing of material reality, which in the end proves not amenable to idealization.

Fitzgerald's Critique of the American Dream. *The Great Gatsby*, then, is a kind of critique of the American Dream, focused on the American 1920s, a critique of the romantic capacity for the wonder of life in a new land, that has become corrupted by a kind of meretricious material splendor (seen in the moral emptiness of Daisy Fay, Tom Buchanan, Jordan Baker), a corruption that has been potentially intrinsic to the dream from the American beginning (from de Crèvecoeur, through Franklin, to the 1920s, to now). The pity of Gatsby is that he cannot even tell the difference between his dream concept and its unworthy object—he cannot even see himself for what he is. Gatsby's dream, the American Dream, the American Dream of Success, has become so confused (in the 1920s) that Gatsby believes the dream can be purchased, recaptured from the virginal past, with money: money, in fact, criminally gained from his vaguely hinted gangster operations ("gat").

But Gatsby's dreaming, at least, is pure, the capacity for wonder is there, and that is why the narrator Nick Carraway (Carraway me back to old Virginny) thinks Gatsby is better than all the rest: "You are worth the whole damn bunch put together." He is better than the phony treachery of Daisy Fay Buchanan, the narrow-minded moneyed snobbery of Tom Buchanan, the cheating of Jordan Baker. The novel has an extra dimension of irony in that Fitzgerald's life was like that of Jay Gatsby: like Jay Gatsby's, Fitzgerald's dream, his capacity for wonder, was fouled (in his writing) by pursuit of a meretricious dream of success. But in *The Great Gatsby* Fitzgerald is true: in this novel he knows his dilemma of being Gatsby (as he said in a letter). The mysterious "Owl Eyes" or "Four Eyes" (who is a writer) is really Fitzgerald commenting on Fitzgerald, particularly when he says at Gatsby's funeral: "The poor son-of-a-bitch."

In Owl Eyes, and particularly in the sentimental honesty of Nick Carraway, Fitzgerald recognizes the paradox of the American Dream of Success, the conflict between the ideal and the material in the American Dream. In this recognition, Fitzgerald, I think, is superior to Lewis' simplistic idealization of the material in *Arrowsmith,* and inferior to James' analysis of the American dilemma in *Portrait of a Lady,* which goes deeper than *Gatsby* even. In this same connection we must not forget the problem of Carrie and Hester.

One more thought: Gatsby's dream is not merely American: it is universal. Like Lord Jim's conflict between illusion and reality in Conrad's novel (from which Fitzgerald said he learned much for *Gatsby*), it is a yearning for a lost innocent past which cannot be recaptured in the pursued future. It is the dream of the lost Eden, the dream of the sought-after Paradise on Earth, both impossible in the fallen world of reality. Van Wyck Brooks puts it this way:

You put the old wine [Europeans] into new bottles [the American continent] . . . when the explosion results, one may say, the aroma passes into the air and the wine spills on the floor. The aroma or the ideal turns into transcendentalism and the wine or the real becomes commercialism.

TECHNIQUE IN *THE GREAT GATSBY*

Point of View. How are we to interpret the narrator, Nick Carraway, for he himself is a romantic sentimentalist? Some have said that he is the central figure of the novel, at least the moral center. If so, how much value has his dream, his respect for Gatsby's dream over the others? Can a person or a nation retreat from reality, mature recognition of the world as it is—head for the territory or the Middle West?

Can we go back to Eden or the womb of innocence?
Did Nick (Carraway) think so at the end?

Narrative Structure. Nick is also central to the narrative structure of the novel: through Nick, Fitzgerald tells Gatsby's story, not chronologically, but as
it can be most effectively presented: present to past,
to present, to past, to—using Nick's guesses, what
Jordan Baker and Gatsby tell him. Narrative structure is closely bound up with the characters, good
and bad: Nick, Gatsby, Tom and Daisy Buchanan,
and Jordan Baker. For Nick's story really complements Gatsby's: he is bound up with the good and
bad; Gatsby's dream, which transcends (ironically)
the material and sexual, is a comment on Nick's
complicity with corruption and evil: his careless acceptance of a casual sexual affair with Jordan, the
congenital liar, whom he rejects in the disgust engendered by Gatsby's worth. Was that a realistic decision?

Symbol and Image. Above all think of the way the
novel achieves by symbol and image the status of
myth on both individual and national levels, with its
imaginative, poetic presentation of innocence and
corruption: the green light at the end of Daisy's
dock; Gatsby's stairway to the stars in Louisville;
the Dutch sailors' sight of the green breast of the
new world; the sightless, faceless eyes of Dr. T. J.
Eckleburg that brood over the wasteland valley of
ashes; the gaudy car and clothing and house and
parties of Gatsby; the tawdry love affair of Tom Buchanan; the quick, sudden violence with which

Myrtle's nose is broken and in the flapping breast and ripped mouth at her death; the incurable dishonesty of Jordan Baker; Gatsby's vaguely-hinted criminal activities and his unheroic death (like Sweeney's death in T. S. Eliot's "Sweeney among the Nightingales"); Nick's El Greco dream of the East at the novel's end.

SUMMARY REMARKS: IS THE DREAM VIABLE?

I meant to sum up the formal aspects of the novel at the end, but I have said enough about them along the way—so I'll sum up a bit differently from what I intended. And probably lose you.

The large question which *The Great Gatsby* asks is this: Is the dream viable? That is, is it workable, or, in the central meaning of "viable," can the dream, the Ideal, live in the world, be incarnate, born into the world?

In any existential sense, a simple "yes" or "no" to the question would destroy the experience the novel contains. But a kind of tentative judgment is possible. Certainly, Fitzgerald and his spokesman Nick Carraway are pessimistic about the viability of the dream—I think, just as are Hemingway and his spokesman Frederic Henry in our next novel, *A Farewell to Arms*. The reason (or, rather, what I believe to be the reason) for this pessimism I want you to see.

I believe the reason for the failure of the dream in Fitzgerald and Hemingway (and maybe in America) is that it springs from what can be called romantic individualism. The ideal and material aspirations of Nick Carraway and Frederic Henry—of Fitzgerald and Hemingway—are basically selfish. And their frustrations and disillusionments are private pains: most of all, they feel sorry for themselves.

Of course, both Nick and Frederic Henry show considerable unhappiness about the suffering of others, and even some insight about their romantic dilemma. Nick's last conversation with Jordan Baker is ironically revealing, especially in view of what Nick had previously said about his honesty: "I am one of the few honest people I have ever known." Jordan Baker calls him on this point. Nick is very angry about the Buchanans' carelessness for other people. But there is nothing morally honest about carelessly taking a girl, even though she carelessly offers herself—and then being morally scrupulous afterwards. Nick, I think, does get Jordan's point about careless drivers and careless people: he took her on the careless basis and then backed out. That is why Nick says Gatsby is better than the whole damned bunch. He means to include himself: Gatsby did better by Daisy than he by Jordan.

But even with this insight, there is nothing very mature about Nick's nostalgic retreat to Minnesota, or Frederic Henry's retreat into expatriation, alienation, disaffiliation—or, ultimately, Fitzgerald's crack-up and Hemingway's suicide.

Is the dream viable? Can it live in the world? Not, I think, for the romantic individualist, the romantic idealist. What is wrong with romantic individualism is that it makes the world bear the burden of one's romantic ego. The job is to create out of whatever there is in the world an ideal one can serve. I think Jesus indicates this alternative when he says that he who professes to love God but hates his neighbor lies. The fallacy is in the private assumption of intimacy with godhead, personal or national. I am not being pious. Melville pointed out the same alternative to the dangers of imposing a romantic ego on the natural world and others in the story of Ishmael and Ahab.

TRANSITION TO HEMINGWAY

In this course, from Hawthorne and Melville to James and Fitzgerald, I have been trying to get at some deep things in the human consciousness, Western or American. We do grow up, we do grow older, in fuller knowledge through a consciousness of time passing. We all hold, or once held, I suppose, the dream of immortality, the hope that we can live forever in this world, the hope that time, as the human consciousness measures time, can be forgotten, or be endless. This is an illusion of innocence, which shatters when we grow into the maturity of knowledge and find what the world of reality and our own human flesh hold in store for us. The American Dream is no different from this universal dream—just another form of it in another time and place, "the last and greatest of all human dreams" (Nick Carraway).

At this deepest level of meaning, Hester and Dimmesdale, Ahab and Ishmael, Newman [in *The American* by Henry James] and Nick and Gatsby, all dream the same dream of innocence, a dream of timelessness and perfection and immortality in this world. And Hawthorne and Melville and James and Fitzgerald knew that the dream, for any person and any people, must fade with the knowledge that comes from maturity. The dream incarnate must perish; the rose withereth on the stem.

But still the dream persists, the idea of a rose remains, and what makes one writer greater than another, perhaps, is what, in the form of literature, his art, what of the human spirit he rescues from our mutability, from the knowledge of our perishability, from the knowledge that man, after all, is but mortal. How does he celebrate the human spirit, in the face of human mortality? You remember, at the beginning of great literature, Odysseus chose mortality over immortality, Penelope over Calypso. Odysseus had the mortal scar, the mortal flaw, like Achilles, a quite different man. Despite their human limitations—or because of them—they struggled magnificently.

In this frame of reference, we look ahead to Hemingway, a pessimistic writer; and Steinbeck, an optimistic one; and Faulkner, one of questionable optimism.

✠

Ernest Hemingway, *The Sun Also Rises*
(1973)

INTRODUCTION

At the beginning of *The Sun Also Rises* I want to say some general things. Consider that from *The Scarlet Letter* to *The Great Gatsby* the question has been, in every novel, "What happens when the idea, the ideal, the dream is born into the world, the word becomes flesh, reality, incarnate?" Is it possible to make the dream immortal, perpetuate it in the reality of temporal existence? This is a peculiarly American question, because of American emphasis on the wealth of the material world.

In *Gatsby* we watched the dream bloom (the incarnate blossom) as James Gatz joined his "unutterable visions" to Daisy's "perishable breath." Nick Carraway, and possibly Fitzgerald, clung to the dream by dissociating it from material reality (Gatsby's criminal operations). I think that Hawthorne, and maybe Melville, reconciled reality, one in the saving child Pearl, the other in the saved child Ishmael. Gatsby had no child (the child was Tom's). He kept his dream pure of reality, his conception immaculate, "faithful to the end," says Carraway. "Immaculate conception" is an ironic combination of words in what they suggest. The immaculate conception of love into the real (the mortal) world is exactly what is being attempted in *The Great Gatsby* (and in the American Dream). And the attempt fails—at least there is an impasse.

Note that *The Great Gatsby* and *The Sun Also Rises* are both post-World War I novels. There is, I think, a greater darkness in *The Sun Also Rises* than in *Gatsby*. In *The Sun Also Rises*, the loss of love—in fact, the death of love—is accompanied by a loss of faith. The romantic hero, Jake Barnes, and his Lady Brett, too (in her own way), have lost the ability though not the power to generate love. It is necessary for me at this point to risk grossness by asking you to think about the particular symbols used by Hemingway in *The Sun Also Rises*. It is worth remembering, too, that the culminating images in Hemingway's *A Farewell to Arms* are a stone-cold mother and a child that is stillborn. In *The Sun Also Rises* the central image is the war wound of Jake Barnes. Hemingway has made it clear that Jake has not lost his *power* to generate physical love. Put crudely, we can say that Jake is not precisely a steer—he has simply lost the instrument for communicating physical love. It's an important point, and I am not punning. It's not funny, but darkly symbolic, like Myrtle's flapping severed breast—grotesque.

In the mysterious relation of mind and flesh, words like "conception" and "generation" are ambiguous. For all of his Platonic conception, Gatsby does not really conceive, nor does Jake generate, for all his power and desire to generate. Jake has lost the ability to communicate love, the ability to make love incarnate in the world.

There is an even greater darkness in *The Sun Also Rises*. (Note the significance of "also rises," which puts an implicit stress on the sun's going down.) There is not just frustration in this novel: there is a loss of faith. At the very end, Brett says, "Oh, Jake, we could have had such a damned good time together." "Yes," replies Jake, "Isn't it pretty to think so." The emphasis here is on "think." Jake has no faith that there would have been any more fulfillment even had he been more capable in a sexual way. He has no faith in the idea of love. Or, Jake could simply mean thinking about having Lady Brett is not quite up to having her in the flesh. Anyway, he'll never know. And it must be noted that Brett, after her short fling with Romero, has come to her own death of love—recognition of impotence. In this death of the love ideal (love is eternal, and all that rubbish), it is important to realize that Jake has actually played the pimp for his lady—prostituted his love. Brett can say that their love would have been different, but she and Jake know it isn't so. They are both over thirty and cannot lie to themselves (though Nick Carraway and Jay Gatsby can. Nick says he can't lie to himself, but Jordan Baker knows he can).

The ultimate sickness of Hemingway's romantic hero, Jake Barnes, is his ironic pity for himself (the same irony and pity he and Bill Gorton spoof on their fishing trip). Jake feels sorry for himself and hides it with irony (the "tough" Hemingway exterior). What he seems to rescue from his lost faith in the idea of love is a smart satisfaction in his knowledge of reality. He is, of course, a much more compassionate person than Daisy Buchanan, but it doesn't take too much imagination to hear him smirk, "God, I'm sophisticated." Even Gatsby does better than that and that's why Nick Carraway thinks Gatsby is better than the whole damned bunch, including Nick himself.

APPROACH TO *THE SUN ALSO RISES*

<u>Voice</u>. *The Sun Also Rises* is a hard book to interpret. Its theme, tentatively, is the death of romantic love, but it is not necessarily a novel of despair. Think back to what I said about the artistry of *Huckleberry Finn*. *Huckleberry Finn* is seen totally (and naively) through the sensibilities of Huck, in his voice (first person point of view). As with *Huckleberry Finn*, the meaning of *The Sun Also Rises* depends a lot on the point of view. Hemingway was a great admirer of *Huckleberry Finn*, of what it said and the way it was said:

All modern American literature comes from one book by Mark Twain called *Huckleberry Finn*. If you read it you must stop where the slave Jim is stolen from the boys. . . . The rest is just cheating. But it's the best book we've had. All American writing comes from that. There was nothing before. There has been nothing since.

Hemingway liked Twain's way in *Huckleberry Finn* of presenting his material matter-of-factly through the mind of a rather simple hero, in the hero's own voice, with the effect of understatement and possibly irony. Hemingway also liked the greater part of *Huckleberry Finn* because it didn't cheat: in Hemingway's words, "telling it the way it was."

Hemingway presents *The Sun Also Rises* through the voice of Jake Barnes in the first person. We get the whole experience of the novel through him, and we pretty much get his reactions on the physical level in basic, elementary speech. There are few deeply mental observations; we get sensuous experience apparently objectively reported, with suggestions of understatement and irony. We have to interpret for ourselves what the experiences of Jake and his friends mean. A point to remember is Hemingway's warning not to take it for granted that any of his heroes speaks for Hemingway.

The Usual Interpretation. The usual interpretation of *The Sun Also Rises* is that it is a study of sexual and spiritual frustration, the one symbolizing the other: Jake's war wound (his emasculation) suggests a deeper wound, the spiritual wounding of the post-World War I generation to which Hemingway belonged. Jake's sexual impotence symbolizes the spiritual emptiness and lostness of a generation disillusioned by the war. Jake has desire but no capacity for sexual love; he has desire to believe in spiritual values but no belief (in *The Wasteland* T. S. Eliot similarly uses sexual impotence to symbolize spiritual emptiness). According to the usual interpretation, the theme of *The Sun Also Rises* is the death of illusion about the way things are, particularly, the death of romantic love. Without belief, one must learn to live with toughness and honor and dignity—with grace and *sang froid*. Robert Cohn is a fool, a butt of jokes in the novel, because he refuses to give up the idea of romantic love, does not see Lady Brett for what she is, a bitch. But one has to be careful in looking at Cohn this way—because the toughness and irony of those who mock Cohn verge on self-pity: "'Oh, Jake,' Brett said, 'We could have had such a damned good time together.' 'Yes,' I said. 'Isn't it pretty to think so.'"

Here is clinging to the illusion of romantic love in self-pity, and even the recognition of all that. Maybe Jake's and Brett's is the greatest sentimentality, after all—the romantic illusion of self-pity; they don't believe, yet they pity themselves for their loss, with smart sophistication. It could be that Hemingway intended us to see Jake and Brett that way, as pitying themselves too much, with make-believe toughness. All Hemingway heroes, like Hemingway himself, cry beneath their tough understatement. Cry, like Carraway, for what is lost.

Certainly *The Sun Also Rises* does report the adventures of a group of people who have lost a spiritual excuse for existence, the lost and wounded and damaged souls of a generation of Americans Hemingway knew after World War I. *The Sun Also Rises* does concern spiritually empty people, but to say "lostness" and "despair" is the ultimate tone of the novel might be going too far. As I said, the difficulty lies in interpreting the rather flat reporting of Jake Barnes, discovering what lies beneath the understatement or suggestion of irony.

A More Optimistic Reading. Facing the title page in the original edition Hemingway placed two quotations, one from Gertrude Stein in conversation, the other from Ecclesiastes:

You are all a lost generation.

One generation passeth away, and another generation cometh; but the earth abideth forever . . . . The sun also ariseth, and the sun goeth down, and hasteth to the place where he arose . . . . The wind goeth toward the south, and turneth about unto the north; it whirleth about continually, and the wind returneth again according to his circuits . . . . All the rivers run into the sea; yet the sea is not full; unto the place from whence the rivers come, thither they return again.

Put together, these quotations can be read in more than one way. They can be taken as supporting each other, or as contrasting each other. The piece from Ecclesiastes can by itself be read two ways: as thorough pessimism about the meaningless and repetitious order of nature, or as a qualified optimism about the stability and endurance of nature. The writer of Ecclesiastes was pointing up the vanity of material things. But Hemingway, in a letter to Maxwell Perkins, his editor, said that he did not mean *The Sun Also Rises* "to be a hollow or bitter satire, but a tragedy with the earth abiding forever as hero." And he disagreed with Gertrude Stein that his generation was a lost generation. So I shall take Hemingway's word for it and look in *The Sun Also Rises* for what is optimistic.

Romantic love is dead, but from this recognition springs a tough realism that takes full sensuous stock of all human existence, and reckons neverthe-less that one's short span on the "abiding earth" is good. Something can be salvaged. For Hemingway (and Jake) the bullfight is a symbol, an image taken from life, with tragedy and death at the center of its meaning. But there is a significance and a satisfaction in physical existence: life, the reality of physical existence, can be faced honestly, fairly, cleanly, bravely, even beautifully, with respect, maybe even with compassion for one's adversary. The bullfighting of Pedro Romero is exemplary of the way to live one's life where only the earth abides forever, exemplary of how to live bravely and gracefully, without cheating, with only the facts of life, with the *only* fact of the abiding earth.

The only characters who know how to make a realistic art of life are probably, to Hemingway, Jake Barnes and Bill Gorton and Pedro Romero, especially the last, who makes a graceful art out of dangerous living, faces the tragic meaning of life in the bull ring, with honesty and dignity and honor, cleanly. And that's the way Hemingway wants to make his art of the novel. Jake and Hemingway know what the score is: they are essentially religious men who would like to believe what they can't. They are physically and spiritually wounded men, hurt men who have lost faith in the romantic ideal but have come to terms (at least they put on a tough exterior) with the conditions that nature, the adversary, imposes. They can't sleep nights but they wring a certain satisfaction from strenuous physical activity: basketball, boxing, trout fishing in cool mountain streams—a satisfaction in "the abid-

ing earth." This attitude, lifestyle, if you like, sometimes seems a superficial front, a studied athletic
toughness underneath which is the whimpering of
self-pity.

TECHNIQUE, SHORTLY

Point of View. The whole novel is told through the
objective, almost cold reporting of the sensations of
Jake Barnes, Jake's reactions to life as told by
Jake. Underneath the tough, cynical exterior of
Jake is the man who can't sleep nights, the man
physically and spiritually hurt but not beaten, the
man who can live with his disillusion, according to
the rules of the game. This man tells the story.

Symbolism. The whole story symbolizes the condition of human existence (see epigraph) as seen by a
disillusioned post World War I generation (disillusioned but maybe not lost). Particularly, Jake's
wound symbolizes spiritual emptiness, sterility and
frustration. The bullfight and Pedro Romero symbolize the tragic conditions of human existence and
how to face them. Hemingway gives a similar image
in the old man fighting the marlin in *The Old Man
and the Sea* (Hemingway nearing the end).

Structure. The structure of the novel goes like the
passage from Ecclesiastes: the sun goes up and the
sun goes down, but the earth abides forever. The
story runs its course without meaningful consequence, but the mountains and the cool streams
and landscapes of France and Spain remain.

<u>Style</u>. Hemingway's style is simple, clear, concrete—
a prose fitted to basic elementary physical-
sensuous experience. Hemingway believes that
whatever meaning there is in life must be found in
the physical contact with life, not on a conceptual
abstract level of two-bit words and idealistic cheating. If there is LOVE it must be found where we
touch it, where it makes us feel good, or hurts.

⌖

William Faulkner, *As I Lay Dying*

THEME OF THE NOVEL

The whole novel deals with an almost endless agony, a prolonged suspension between life and death. The novel is concerned not so much with death as the process of dying, not so much as a brute fact as its mute presence in the very heart of life. *As I Lay Dying* works from the start with the double paradox of a dying life and an active death.

All the book's action revolves around the unburied remains of Addie Bundren. *As I Lay Dying* is first and foremost the story of a family struggling with a corpse, the story of an unburiable cadaver, and most of the ordeals encountered on the journey stem directly from the material difficulties of carting the body to the graveyard at Jefferson. Death therefore comes to impinge on the banal practical problems of everyday life. For the Bundrens, the corpse is not so much an object of horror and revulsion as a nuisance. By their continual manipulation of the coffin, they almost reach the point where it is considered a mere load to be carried. They are too absorbed by their immediate task to realize how shocking the unduly prolonged presence of a rotting

corpse may be to others; they even forget its nause-
ating smell, which attracts buzzards and repels
people. To this guileless scorn of decorum and convention, this obstinate failure of realization, this
seemingly unruffled innocence in the face of death
the story owes much of its baffling extravagance.
Apart from Darl and perhaps Cash, none of the
Bundrens appears to be conscious of the outrageous nature of the journey. Behind their blindness, however, we discover another form of blindness: the feigned blindness of the author, pretending not to see the scandal. For, all the way, Faulkner's humor keeps death at a distance. As in the
grotesque wake scene in *Sanctuary*, he desacralizes
the corpse by treating it as a mere object and de-
fuses the Gothic potential by farce.

For these primitives there is no dividing line between life and death. In the magic universe which is
theirs, "every death is analogous to a change of
birth, every birth analogous to a change of death,
every change analogous to a death-rebirth—and the
cycle of human life is analogous to the natural cy-
cles of death and rebirth." The whole of Faulkner's
work revolves in the ever-renewed cycle of gesta-
tions and agonies, but in few of his novels are death
and birth as closely interwoven as in *As I Lay Dying*.
And none perhaps is as firmly rooted in the primal
earth of the archaic mind, for it is, as we shall see,
to archetypal image patterns that the death-birth
theme owes its most eloquent symbols.

SYMBOLISM IN THE NOVEL

Ambiguous symbolism not only pervades the imagery of the novel; it also underlies its narrative pattern. *As I Lay Dying* is the tale of journey—a symbol of death for the primitive mind as well as for child or dreamer. From this archetypal metaphor derives, parallel to the real action, the symbolic and ritual action which gives the novel its mythical dimension. "The structural dimension in *As I Lay Dying* is," as Hyatt H. Waggoner puts it, "a journey through life to death and through death to life."

Madness. As with death, madness is always just around the corner throughout the novel. If *The Sound and the Fury* is "a tale told by an idiot, full of sound and fury," *As I Lay Dying* is a tale of madness told by a madman. Madness is everywhere present. It is in the apocalyptic disorder of the world and the unbridled violence of its elements. It is also in the unreason of man: could there be a more senseless undertaking than that of the Bundrens? As in *King Lear*, human madness thus parallels the madness of the world. Echoing and questioning each other, the multiple forms of madness draw us into another vortex of ambiguities and ironies. The Bundrens' expedition is a fool's errand in the eyes of the community; in the eyes of Vardaman, the child, it is the folly of adults. Yet it is also, paradoxically, madness in the eyes of Darl—who is himself thought to be mad. There must be reason, then, in his madness, a reason that challenges the reason of reasonable people. Hence the difficulty, fully recognized by

Cash, of discriminating between reason and unreason:

Sometimes I ain't so sho who's got ere a right to say when a man is crazy and when he ain't. Sometimes I think it ain't none of us pure crazy and ain't none of pure sane until the balance of us talks him that-a-way. It's like it ain't so much what a fellow does but it's the way the majority of folks is looking at him when he does it.

In the Western sensibility, the shift from the theme of death to the theme of madness was not, as Foucault [in *Madness and Civilization*] points out, a clean break:

What is in question is still the nothingness of existence, but this nothingness is no longer considered an external, final term, both threat and conclusion; it is experienced from within as the continuous and constant form of existence.

In *As I Lay Dying* the two themes are intimately linked; they crystallize around the two most significant figures in the novel: Addie and Darl. Addie embodies the obsession with death: "I could just remember how my father used to say that the reason for living was to ready to stay dead for a long time." And throughout the book the concrete presence of her rotting corpse acts as a reminder of nothingness as "an external, final term," as "threat and conclusion." In Darl's madness, on the other hand, nothingness is experienced "from within as the continuous and constant form of existence":

How do our lives ravel out into the no-wind, no-sound, the weary gestures weary recapitulant: echoes of old compulsions with no-hand on no-strings: in sunset we fall into furious attitudes, dead gestures of dolls.

The Scandal of Existence. The real outrage, the genuine scandal is in everything that humiliates and crushes man, in all the violence which fate makes him suffer. Its most visible manifestation in the novel is in the series of catastrophes which shower down on the Bundrens in the course of their journey, and first of all the rain so often referred to in the opening sections. This rain is expected by everybody and known to be imminent. Yet when it finally starts to fall, Anse looks thoroughly dumb-founded: "from behind his slack-faced astonishment he muses as though from beyond time, upon the ultimate outrage." The astonishment provoked by the outrage is not the shock of the unexpected but the stupefaction at the occurrence of the inescap-able: "again he looks up at the sky with that ex-pression of dumb and brooding outrage and yet of vindication, as though he had expected no less." As-tonishment in Faulkner, then, does not preclude foreknowledge. Anse expected "no less"; he knows what happens was due to happen. The event con-firms his expectation, and his outraged air suggests an uncanny wisdom beyond thought: "his humped silhouette partaking of that owl-like quality of awry-feathered, disgruntled outrage within which lurks a wisdom too profound or too inert for even thought."

Astonishment at outrage is the encounter of in-nocence and evil. Whether paralyzed by stupor or driven to fruitless rebellion, Faulkner's characters are above all victims. An obscure curse seems to weigh on them, but they are not guilty. To explain their misfortunes, one could no doubt look for those responsible and incriminate Addie's destructive pride or Anse's massive egoism. But in fact, as Faulkner himself pointed out, there is no villain in the story other than the absurd convention which makes the Bundrens drag the corpse as far as Jefferson and all the evil forces let loose against them during their agonizing journey. Evil here is on the world's side. It also lies within man, but it does not spring from man. In *As I Lay Dying*, Faulkner's pessimism—insofar as such a label can be used to define his tragicomic vision—is less moral than metaphysical.

The themes of sin and guilt appear only marginally, and the historical, social, and racial context of the South in which these themes are treated in most of the novelist's other works is hardly perceptible here. *As I Lay Dying* is an almost timeless fable. The human beings it presents seem to date from before history; yet they have already been exiled from Paradise, and are already doomed and damned. The effects of the primal curse are indeed strongly felt, but Faulkner does not here, as in his other novels, raise questions about the origin of the malediction. What we are shown instead is the naked scandal of existence revealed through the extremes of madness and death. The decomposing corpse dragged along the road is the *memento mori*, a grim reminder of the radically contingent and irremediably finite nature of man; death is, as Addie soon learned, what invalidates all life. As for madness, the other aspect of the scandal, it designates here—like Benjy's idiocy in *The Sound and the*

Fury—the intolerable paradox of utter degradation linked to absolute innocence.

LANGUAGE AND STYLE

<u>Voice</u>. In *As I Lay Dying* every character speaks in his own voice, and the reader is soon able to distinguish between Darl's taut, tense metaphorical style, Anse's placid sententiousness, Cora's cant and cackle and Vardaman's helpless stutterings. Faulkner has orchestrated all these voices with admirable skill and effectiveness, sometimes counter-pointing them, playing them off against one another to emphasize contrasts (putting Addie's monologue, for instance, between Cora's and Whitfield's), sometimes using their resemblances to point out affinities which bind one character to another (as Cora to Whitfield in the above example). This chameleonic, plural style gives the measure of Faulkner's prodigious gifts for verbal mimicry. Yet, sharply individualized as they are, the characters' voices seldom possess the objective author's voice throughout the novel.

<u>Vocabulary</u>. The rustic vocabulary serves essentially to designate the concrete and familiar world of everyday life. But whenever these country people experience the need to express ideas or feelings, we see them turn naturally to the Bible. In *As I Lay Dying*, the biblical tradition, with all that Southern fundamentalist religion in such a rural community adds in the way of violent emotionalism, shows through time and time again.

The characteristics we have noted so far—nearness to the spoken word, reliance on the plain diction of common speech, occasional use of biblical phrases—can all be related to the tradition of the vernacular narrative initiated in American literature by the humorists of the old Southwest and by Mark Twain. That Faulkner's prose is indebted to this tradition, no one will dispute. Yet the lexical resources it draws upon are by no means limited to the fund of colloquial speech. At the risk of forfeiting credibility, the novelist does not hesitate to endow at least some of his uncouth farmers with a richer and more refined vocabulary whenever it suits his purpose. The curious combination of rough-edged spoken language and an ostensibly literary language that may be detected in the diction of *As I Lay Dying* is present as well in its syntax.

Metaphor is the figure of figures in this novel, consubstantial with the vision and art of the novelist. Of all the demons which presided over Faulkner's work, analogy was without doubt one of the most intrusive, and in this novel his presence is as strongly felt as in any other. Through the multiplicity of unexpected connections and reverberations they introduce into the book, metaphors reinforce the interrelatedness of its parts; by carrying its meanings beyond literal significance, they expand the fictional world beyond the narrow boundaries of realistic convention and make room for the imagination. Their function within the novel's texture is very similar to that of the symbols within its structure: both transmute the factual into the poetic.

NARRATIVE

Organizing Principles. As the account of a series of events, *As I Lay Dying* is one of Faulkner's simpler works. Unlike most of his other novels, it does not disrupt the basic chronology of events nor does its narrative indulge in digressions. With a few hardly perceptible exceptions, the unity of action is respected from start to finish and the whole tale is perfectly circumscribed in space and time.

These are the space and time of a journey: the space is measured by the distance separating the country from the town, the Bundrens' house in the hills from Jefferson, the end of their trek; the time is the ten days they need to prepare and undertake their journey. *As I Lay Dying* is first and foremost the account of an expedition. The journey determines both the theme and the form of the book. As well as constituting one of the focal points of the novel's meanings, it provides the narrative with one of its main organizing principles. As is the case with most travel accounts, the novel consists of a series of episodes. The preparation and departure, the river crossing, the barn fire, the arrival at Jefferson—these are the major sections of the tale. They are presented in their time sequence. Manipulation of them occurs primarily in the distribution and orchestration of narrative voices; it hardly affects the narrative itself, whose arrangement remains broadly chronological. It will also be noted that, like any episodic novel, *As I Lay Dying* shows little plotting.

The Journey. In a sense, the action certainly results from the development of the initial situation, namely the Bundrens' obligation to go and bury Addie in Jefferson cemetery, but neither the mishaps of the journey nor their succession are predetermined by that situation. Among the obstacles they meet on the way, some are purely fortuitous (e.g., the swollen river, the broken bridges, losing the mules, Cash's accident) and others are brought about voluntarily by human agency (e.g., the barn fire started by Darl), but the episodes arising from the confrontation with these obstacles are not likely by any requirement inherent in the logic of the tale itself. Their order could be reversed, their number increased or decreased, without the structure's being seriously altered.

The journey of the Bundrens is no random wandering along chance paths, however. It is an expedition taken for precise reasons: for Addie it is the realization of a wish—to be buried at Jefferson—and perhaps, too, a posthumous act of revenge; for the family as a group, it is the fulfillment of a promise. To these, private motives are added—a new set of teeth and a new wife for Anse, an abortion for Dewey Dell, a "gramophone" for Cash, bananas and an electric train for Vardaman—motives which, in spite of their disparity, strengthen the Bundrens' determination to go to Jefferson, but whose self-interested nature throws suspicion on the act of family piety they are supposed to be accomplishing. Yet two of Addie's children, Jewel and Darl, are notable exceptions in this respect. Jewel's personal motivation coincides exactly with the official reason for the journey; Darl, on the other hand, stands out from the rest of the family by his indifference, then by his hostility, to the project, and he is the only one who tries at one point to prevent its being carried out. Both of them perform an essential function in the narrative strategy of the author: the first appears as the main hero of the story, the one whose fierce energy pushes the action forward and whose exploits and sacrifices allow the enterprise to succeed; the second, because of his critical detachment, assumes in essence the peripheral role of narrator or, as one critic has aptly put it, of antiheroic intelligence.

Reciprocal Illumination. The central object in the story is Addie's corpse both as a material thing, as the constant mainspring of and object at stake in the physical action, and in its symbolic function, as a reminder of the event which has just upset the existence of the Bundrens, as a visible sign of the great void left by Addie's death, which each member of the family after his fashion tries to fill. The circle around the object is made up of all those still alive who gather around the body, suddenly brought face to face with the enigma of death. Each consciousness caught in the novel's sweep is one of those little lamps of which James speaks; each one, in its flickering light, illuminates one particular aspect of the central figure and situation. But instead of lamps one might also suggest a comparison with reflecting mirrors: most of the sections, in addition to throwing an oblique and intermittent light on Addie's personality, testify to the persistent effects of her dark radiance. It is precisely in terms of reciprocal illumination that one could define the relationship between Addie's single monologue and the rest of the novel. Were it not for this monologue, the book would lack focus, and much of the meaning would be lost on the reader, since the family drama can be understood only by reference to the personal tragedy suggested by the dead woman's confession. But conversely, Addie's monologue needs the echoing space of the whole work for its significance to be fully grasped.

Centrifugal and Centripetal Movements. A double movement is thus set up. On the one hand, within the circle there is a simultaneous centrifugal and centripetal movement, a nonstop to-ing and fro-ing between circle and center; on the other hand, there is a circular movement governing the whole novel and making it turn around its fixed axis. That this circular pattern possesses thematic significance hardly needs to be stressed. In this connection it is interesting to note that the circle also appears in the imagery of the novel. The whole story of the journey is punctuated by the repeated evocation of the circles traced in the sky by the buzzards which follow the funeral cortege, and the circling vultures ceaselessly intersecting the straight line of the Bundrens' progression could almost be seen as an emblem of the book's structure.

In addition, it is significant that Darl associates his dead mother with a wheel: "the red road lies like the spoke of which Addie Bundren is the rim." In her soliloquy, Addie herself refers to the circle of her solitude; by Cash's birth, she remarks, her "alone-ness had been violated and then made whole again by the violation: time, Anse, love, what you will, outside the circle." The metaphor of the circle would apply almost equally well to most of the other Bun-drens. If the pattern of *As I Lay Dying* suggests first a moving circle whose center is Addie, it could also be described as a series of waves and eddies: it is as if a handful of pebbles were thrown into still water, rippling its surface, making concentric circles which overlap and interact in unexpected ways as they expand. Everything starts again and nothing is the same. The end of the novel is a false restoration (just as Anse's new teeth are false), a ludicrous de-nouncement echoing with Darl's mad laughter: am-biguity is given a final twist and irony is raised to its highest pitch.

<u>Time and Tense</u>. The discourse of the novel is as-sumed to be contemporaneous with reality—or, if you prefer, the fiction of reality—it presents to the reader; it purports to be its immediate, moment-by-moment transcription. It is quite evident though that the dramatization of certain events is not com-patible with exclusive use of the present tense. The present is perfectly appropriate for reporting the scenes of action, where events are shown as they happen. But as soon as it become necessary to make time elapse, to link scenes to one another, to span whole days in a few pages or even a line, the novelist has to fall back on retrospective narration. *As I Lay Dying* is no exception to this rule. The pre-sent is far from being the only tense used by Faulk-

ner. The manuscript shows, indeed, that he was aware of the difficulties involved in his narrative mode and sometimes hesitated between present and past. In fact, out of the fifty-nine sections, only twenty-four are written in the present, and there are many in which past and present are interspersed (the shifts being marked at times, as in *The Sound and the Fury,* by the use of italics), and some twenty may be counted where the past clearly predominates.

Points of View. The distribution of sections is as follows: Darl 19; Vardaman 10; Vernon Tull 6; Cash 5; Dewey Dell 4; Cora Tull 3; Anse 3; Peabody 2; Addie 1; Jewel 1; Whitfield 1; Samson 1; Armstid 1; Moseley 1; and MacGowan 1. Seven of the narrators belong to the Bundren family (actor-narrators); the eight others are outsiders, either episodic participants in the action or mere witnesses (spectator-narrators). Yet if the two categories of narrators are numerically almost equal, the share of sections given to the Bundrens (43) is far in excess of that of the outsiders (16). It is noteworthy, too, that Darl, with nineteen sections, takes on single-handed one-third of the narrative and thus occupies a highly privileged position as narrator. Like the dramatized narrators in Conrad and James, Darl is the one who sees and knows the most, and it is through him that we are most completely, if not most reliably, informed, not only of the external development of the action but also of the secret links which bind the Bundrens together and of the hidden motivations which guide their behavior.

Of all points of view, Darl's is by far the most flexible and complex. Darl, as we have seen, is the principal narrator, but his monologues are far from being a mere record of events. Nothing is less objective than his narrative. Its transparency is almost constantly blurred by the welter of descriptive touches, epithets, comparisons, and metaphors; images, thoughts, and memories well up at every turn of the narration, sometimes bursting out with short-lived brilliance, sometimes lingering for meditation and reverie. Darl's mind is so supple and fluid that it slips effortlessly from one thing to another and changes place and time in a trice.

Consider, for example, section 3: the very short opening paragraph is both descriptive (of Tull and Anse sitting on the back porch) and narrative (with Darl dipping his gourd in the water bucket to drink); a conversation is started by Anse's question to Darl ("Where's Jewel?"), but the answer is delayed for a page by the past suddenly breaking in on the present ("When I was a boy"). Darl, drinking, reflects on the taste of the water and remembers scenes from his childhood. The return to the present is marked by a close-up on "Pa's feet": the narrative is then resumed ("I fling the dipper dregs "), and the question about Jewel is finally answered ("'Down to the barn,' I say. 'Harnessing the team'"). Darl's answer induces the superb description of Jewel and his horse on which the section ends. Darl's mind is seen working in four registers—perceptions, reflection, memory, and second sight—and passing from one to another with no other logic than the unpredictable one of free association.

Not all his monologues, to be sure, contain so many breaks and bifurcations. Yet all he says and describes bears the hallmark of an intensely personal vision. Almost every time Darl starts speaking, reality is transmuted: space begins to waver, the scenery takes on a disturbing life of its own, and everything stands out against an indistinct and shifting background with the strange clear-cut quality and fierce colors of a bad dream. Hyperconscious and hypersensitive, Darl is always perfectly at ease with language. There is even in him a kind of intoxication with words. The same is not true of the younger Bundrens: Jewel, Dewey Dell, and, particularly, Vardaman.

It is true that by probing innermost thoughts in Faulkner's way, there is a risk of reviving the absolute viewpoint of the traditional novel, but the author's self-effacement in *As I Lay Dying* is in any case only a clever pretense. Giving up, apparently, the privilege of the novelist-god, Faulkner most often hides behind his characters, and pretends to listen to them and let them tell the tale in his stead. Yet how could anyone without uncommon powers of divination transport himself into the minds of fifteen different narrators? Is the extreme multiplicity of points of view not, in the end, omniscience in disguise? The technique used in *As I Lay Dying* is by no means a guarantee of realism; it is simply a creative method suited to the writer's purpose. Far from encroaching on the novelist's prerogatives, it makes him all-powerful by making him invisible.

CHARACTERIZATION: THE BUNDREN FAMILY

In order to see better how characterization is effected in this novel, it is necessary to return to the interior monologue and to reconsider its significance as an instrument of psychological revelation. In *As I Lay Dying*, at the same time as being face, body, attitude, or action, the character comes to life through his inner speech. He exists in the silent discourse addressed to no one but himself, and which at first one would not be able to ascribe to a subject were it not for the name preceding it. In the monologue the character thus grows gradually from the inside. Not *seen* from without but *heard* from within, he cannot be identified at once. Transported without warning into secret inner recesses, where most intimate thoughts and most carefully hidden desires and obsessions are avowed, the reader at first gains little knowledge from his closeness to the character; in fact he is too close to discern his contours and too unfamiliar with the workings of his mind to interpret them correctly.

Yet, though we cannot see the monologuing character, we see the world through his eyes and temporarily share the way he responds to it. And after several immersions in his stream of consciousness, we manage at last to link this vision to an eye, this speech to a voice. Then we can stand back and identify the character as a person.

Half *voyeur*, half *voyant*, Darl is nothing but his look, and this look probes people's hearts as easily as it covers distances: "It's like he had got into the inside of you, someway. Like somehow you was looking at yourself and your doings outen his eyes." No secret escapes him. Before his eyes, Dewey Dell feels stark naked: "The land runs out of Darl's eyes; they swim to pin-points. They begin at my feet and rise along my body to my face, and then my dress is gone: I sit naked on the seat above the unhurrying mules, above the travail."

Like Lena Grove in *Light in August*, Eula Varner in *The Hamlet*, or the anonymous woman in "Old Man" (*The Wild Palms*), Dewey Dell belongs to Faulkner's mammalian fertility symbols; she is *natura naturans*, and the life forces quickening in her belly are no different from those that speed the harvest. So Darl, in a "metaphysical" conceit worthy of Donne, compares his sister's leg to Archimedes' lever that moves the world: "her leg coming long beneath the tightening dress: that lever which moves the world; one of that caliper which measures the length and breadth of life."

While it may be tempting to compare Addie and Dewey Dell to Demeter and Persephone, or to other fertility goddesses, it must also be recognized that this symbolism tends to be reversed and that once more irony prevails. Unlike Lena Grove, Dewey Dell stubbornly refuses maternity and thinks only of having an abortion. As for Addie, she is indeed a mother figure, but she embodies motherhood associated with death rather than life, hatred rather than love. In *As I Lay Dying* it is the "wicked mother" who eventually predominates. The children she bore were not only unloved or ill loved in her lifetime; she seems to be hounding them even after her death by the ordeals she inflicts upon them, and it almost looks as if she were reaching out from beyond time to drag them after her into the nether world. In her unrelenting vindictiveness, she is a cruel stepmother rather than a mother, Hecate or Medea rather than the all-loving Demeter. The novelist endows Addie with attributes of head of the clan and the virtues of the totem traditionally reserved for the male. She is at once a mother in flesh and a father in spirit—the matriarchal sovereign.

In the words of Cleanth Brooks, <u>Anse</u>

is one of Faulkner's most accomplished villains. He lacks the lethal power of a Popeye and the passionate intensity of a Percy Grimm, but the kind of force he embodies has to be reckoned with. It is deceptively slight, as delicately flexible as a root tendril but, like the tendril, powerful enough to break a boulder. Anse resembles most nearly Flem Snopes—in his coolness, his sheer persistence, his merciless knowledge of other human beings and how much they will put up with.

Whether <u>Darl</u> is mad or not at the outset is a debatable question. If Faulkner is to be believed, "Darl was mad from the start." Indeed, it does not take us long to discover how precarious his mental balance is, and though there is little to suggest plain insanity in the first monologues, they provide enough clues for the reader not to be surprised by his ultimate breakdown. All the classic symptoms of schizophrenia are soon discernible: withdrawal from reality, loss of vital contacts with others, disembodiment and splitting of self, obsession with identity, sense of isolation and deadness, armageddonism (the sense that "the end of the world is nigh" apparent in Darl's account of the river scene). It is scarcely surprising therefore that, with the ordeals of the journey to help, he ends by succumbing to madness.

Yet Darl's madness is actually something other than a case for psychiatrists. It is distress and disorder certainly, but it is also knowledge and poetry; it is as much a breakthrough as it is a breakdown. Of all the characters in *As I Lay Dying*, it is surely this rustic Hamlet who has the closest affinities with his creator. Faulkner makes him his principal narrator and to some extent one of his alter egos: if Cash is an image of the craftsman-novelist, Darl represents the novelist-poet. Of the gifts it takes to be a creative novelist Darl possesses the most precious: the faculty of vision, the "negative capability," the power of speech. In a way Darl is Faulkner's portrait of the artist as a young madman.

Jewel is attached to his wild horse in a way surprisingly similar to the way his mother is attached to him. He cherishes it as a prized possession; he never leaves it, often sleeps with it, and permits no one except himself to take care of it. The horse becomes the object of his love and hate. Jewel brutalizes and caresses it in turn, and curses it, in Darl's words, with "obscene ferocity." With his usual shrewdness, Darl does not fail to identify the treasured animal as a mother surrogate: "Jewel's mother is a horse." This strange transference (parallel in some ways to Vardaman's equation of Addie with a fish) is obviously a defense mechanism indicative of the incestuous nature of Jewel's love for his mother. Like Quentin Compson's, his is in some measure a forbidden love, an impossible love the reverse of which is hatred for the other members of the family. The fantasy which closes his single monologue leaves no doubt about the fierce intolerance of his feelings for Addie. Just as Quentin wanted to isolate Caddy "out of the loud world," Jewel would kill father and brother to be alone with his mother and so be assured forever of exclusive rights: "It would just be me and her on a high hill and me rolling the rocks down the hill at their faces, picking them up and throwing them down the hill faces and teeth and all . . . ."

Dewey Dell's consciousness, unlike Darl's, is not dissociated from her body, but becomes ensnared and lost in it. The image Dewey Dell paints of herself is that of a "little tub of guts," and her whole universe is one mass of viscera. Hers is a world trapped in flesh, an almost mindless world of sensory contacts and blind tropisms; her monologues drag us into a muddy limbo where life and death are inextricably tangled. Naked flesh, warm breath, dampness, darkness, all the images associated with Dewey Dell are organic, sensual, cosmic. In *Ulysses*, Joyce had made Molly Bloom's sex talk. Here it is seemingly Dewey Dell's body which speaks. Yet a voice is heard at times above this confused murmur, one which is not simply the body, an anxious and faltering voice expressing at one and the same time the wish to be something other than flesh and the vanity of that wish, a voice which tells both of the terror and the fascination of surrender:

The dead air shapes the dead earth in the dead darkness, further away than seeing shapes the dead earth. It lies dead and warm upon me, touching me naked through my clothes. I said You don't know what worry is. I don't know what it is. I don't know whether I am worrying or not. Whether I care or not. I don't know whether I can cry or not. I don't know whether I have tried or not. I feel like a wet seed wild in the hot blind earth.

The fish is in the first instance a metaphor of the mother; it is perhaps not going too far to consider it also a regressive image of the child. Is a fetus not physiologically a fish in its mother's womb? And would it be so surprising that the loss of his mother reactivated in Vardaman the desire to be at one with her, the wish to revert to the sheltered life of the embryo? If we retain this hypothesis, it follows that the fish represents both mother and child, and the image should then be read as an expression of prenatal nostalgia, an emblem of the primal union of child and mother, what Vardaman is unconsciously yearning for. Such an interpretation seems all the more plausible as it fits perfectly into the overall symbolic pattern of the book.

It is obviously no mere chance that the family is the privileged object of Vardaman's fumbling attempts at analysis. Vardaman is trying to unravel the web of family relationships and determine his own position with the family and with respect to each of its members. In him the apprenticeship of reason goes hand in hand with the search for identity. Is his search as futile as Darl's or Dewey Dell's? Vardaman doubtless ends by discovering his identity, but in the grief of a further loss: "Darl is my brother. Darl. Darl." These are his last words, this last cry. And all the endeavors of this child's intelligence have in no way lessened his perplexity and powerlessness, for they can do nothing against the incurable madness of adults: "He was a child trying to cope with this adult's world which to him was, and to any sane person, completely mad. . . . He didn't know what to do about it" (Faulkner, quoted in Gwynn and Blotner, *Faulkner in the University*).

THE SETTING

Few of Faulkner's novels give so intensely the sensation of a seething world, and rarely does the novelist keep his paradoxical wager better: "to arrest motion, which is life, by artificial means and hold it fixed so that a hundred years later, when a stranger looks at it, it moves again, since it is life."

The riddle of motion and immobility is the spatial and physical translation of the metaphysical enigma of time and timelessness. This is probably the reason that Faulkner finds it so exciting. Again and again he reverts to it and attempts to capture it in words. And there are moments indeed when revelation seems near. In *As I Lay Dying*, as in the opening pages of *Light in August* depicting Lena Grove's progress on the road to Jefferson, it happens that the paradoxical conjunction of motion and stasis reaches a kind of perfection, that motion becomes so slow as to become the mere tremor of immobility. Then space and time exchange their attributes; time becomes space, space time—not the time of events but a time accumulated like that of memory, bewitched like that of dreams, fluid and static, a time marking time: "We go on with motion so soporific, so dreamlike as to be uninferant, as though time

and not space were decreasing between us and it."
Similarly, at the time of the crossing, when Darl is
looking at his family on the other bank, the separating interval seems temporal rather than spatial:

It is as though the space between us were time: an irrevo-
cable quality. It is as though time, no longer running
straight before us in a diminishing line, now runs parallel
between us like a looping string, the distance between the
doubling accretion of the thread and not the interval between.

METAMORPHOSIS

Through this baffling dialectic of space and time,
through this giddy interplay of stasis and motion, in
which reality is no sooner mentioned than it is con-
jured away, Faulkner's universe offers us one of its
central paradoxes: dynamic immobility, petrified
turbulence, "fury in itself quiet with stagnation."

The climactic river scene is the most revealing in
this respect. Water, the element of metamorphosis
par excellence, springs to life. Tull, for instance, describes it in the following way:

The water was cold. It was thick like slush ice. Only it kind
of lived. One part of you knowed it was just water, the
same thing that had been running under this same bridge
for a long time, yet when them logs would come spewing up
outen it, you were not surprised, like they was part of the
water, of the waiting and the threat.

The most disturbing feature is not that inert objects enjoy a strange life of their own, but that this
strangeness has something human about it in

which man recognizes obscurely the image of his own destiny. Even the random shapes of nature sometimes resemble human ones, as in this sentence where the configuration of the place suddenly appears like the sketch of some anatomy: "The path looks like a crooked limb blown against the bluff." The human figure in return sometimes seems to reproduce the shapes and forces of the universe. Dewey Dell, as we have seen, is described by Darl as a miniature cosmos: her "mammalian ludicrosities" are "the horizons and the valleys of the earth" and her leg "measures the length and breadth of life." The human and the cosmic are in the relationship of reciprocal metaphor. In this fluctuating world everything thus ends by being absorbed into the unity of single vision.

PRIMEVAL CHAOS

The hallucinating scene, where Cash saws the last planks for the coffin by the feeble light of a lantern, is Shakespearean; the atmosphere is electric noises; lights, shadow, and the whole landscape assume a supernatural aspect, and there is the reek of sulphur. Hell is not far away.

Water rather than fire seems to be the dominant element in *As I Lay Dying*. For it is water that translates most appropriately into the register of the perceptible obsession with chaos and death which wells up from the whole novel. Water is not simply the prime agent for metamorphosis; while allowing changes of form, it also contains the threat of regression to the formless.

All the turmoil in *As I Lay Dying* might presage the birth of a new cosmos. Yet it does not take us long to discover that there is no question here of genesis. The world depicted in the novel is not one emerging from primeval chaos but one preparing to return to it.

BIBLIOGRAPHY: André Bleikasten, *Faulkner's* As I Lay Dying.

ℒ

John Steinbeck, *The Grapes of Wrath*
(1968)

STEINBECK'S BASIC BIOLOGICAL NATURALISM

Steinbeck takes what seem to be two opposing, but common, trends in American thought, transcendental idealism and naturalistic realism, and unites them in an optimistic faith. Steinbeck has been called "naturalism's priest": he builds what is a mystical faith upon a biological base. This biological base is very important to Steinbeck's thinking and art. Edmund Wilson states: "What is constant in Mr. Steinbeck is his preoccupation with biology."

Sex, the Life Impulse. Sex to Steinbeck is a natural, biological function, to be treated objectively. Roughly defined, it is the life impulse to creation and continuance in nature. It becomes a human moral problem only when the rights of others are violated.

Underlying Unity in All Life, All Existence, from Man Down to the Rock. The microcosm contains the macrocosm, as in Whitman's leaf of grass: the smallest unit of life, the smallest organism reflects the largest. On the human level, all men are brothers.

Life as Primarily and Necessarily Collective. Life breeds and dies in groups. Steinbeck's favorite is the tide pool metaphor. Along the ocean, there are locked together in pools many kinds of marine life which must help each other to survive. On the human and animal levels, Steinbeck emphasizes cooperative love among species rather than competition. Compare to Darwin.

STEINBECK'S IDEALISM: HIS OPTIMISTIC FAITH

The Persistent Aspiration and Final Triumph of Life, of the Common Man, of Humanity. In spite of his basic biologic naturalism, Steinbeck invests his characters, at almost the lowest level of economic subsistence, with individual spiritual identities and capacity for love. There is much in Steinbeck of the romantic nature poet and mystic.

Proletarian Interest. A proletarian novel is one that deals primarily with the life of the working classes or with any industrial or social problem from the point of view of the working man. Steinbeck's interest in the working man is not a rational-theoretical concern (that is, Marxist); it is a fundamental human concern for people and a feeling for their miseries and hopes.

Optimism Regarding the Collective Destiny of Mankind. Steinbeck's optimism regarding struggling humanity is not typical of naturalism, although sympathy is. Steinbeck's optimistic faith in the natural life force, in the collective cooperation of natural forces to preserve life, is best illustrated by the symbolic incident which concludes *Grapes of Wrath*: Rose of Sharon's giving her breast, the milk nature intended for her stillborn babe, to the old man dying of hunger. The turtle even more obviously symbolizes Steinbeck's optimism about the natural force of life. Ma Joad, the earth-mother, sums it up for common humanity: "Why, Tom, we're the people that live. Why, we're the people—we go on." Compare to Sandburg's democratic faith in "The People, Yes."

LITERARY METHODS

Epic Structure. Steinbeck uses literary methods that are well suited to his meaning. His narrative structure is an epic structure of people in movement, similar to the structure of Homer's *Odyssey*. The structure moves along a sweep in space, carrying the Joads from Oklahoma to California. Their odyssey, like a turtle's at the beginning, is typical of all life, all humanity: it moves with jerks and starts in short perspective, a steady flow in larger perspective, sometimes faster, sometimes slower, sometimes forward, then a wee bit backward, yet always progressively for life. For humans, there are laughter and tears—joy and pain. There are no pointed climaxes, no highly dramatic incidents that stand above all others. There is more plateau than peak, and the movement is the movement of life. Although the primary story concerns the Joads' involvement in the Oklahoma dustbowl catastrophe and the California migrant labor problem, Steinbeck's epic subject is really life and humanity, the movement of life and humanity.

The Inter-Chapter. Steinbeck's device for bringing out the relationship of the Joads to life and humanity is the inter-chapter. The inter-chapters are thematic generalizations which are sometimes as particular almost as the story of the Joads (migrants in flight), and sometimes as broad as life itself (the turtle parable). They break up the Joad story, relating it to the larger story of humanity, the progress of life. The inter-chapters carry lessons on various themes: the theme of buying cheap and selling dear; the theme of social reform coming into being as necessity requires; the theme of large-scale production for profit that ignores human needs; the theme of spring in California, the fertile earth, fruit trees loaded with life, but people starving; the theme of the blindness of property interests; the theme of common human interests, opposed to private selfish interests, etc.

In the inter-chapters and in the story of the Joads, Steinbeck displays a variety of styles: racy narrative, clipped dialogue, emotive description that is on the verge of diatribe, thoughtful discussion, biblical rhythm. Steinbeck is a very versatile stylist, but right now I will show you an example of how he uses the poetic rhythms of the King James Bible for a contemporary subject. See your text, Chapter 11. Read this text as biblical verse, as four lines of biblical verse:

> The tractors had lights shining,
> For there is no day or night for a tractor
> And the disks turn the earth in the darkness
> And they glitter in the daylight. And continue . . .

Note the King James parallel grammatical structure of parallel meanings, the balance, the concrete details, the summary sentences, the reiterations—all the biblical style is here.

What some have called Christian symbolism in *The Grapes of Wrath* I prefer to call Christian imagery and use of Christian allusions to reinforce Steinbeck's plea for the need for human love. I can save time by simply reading pieces from a paper written on the subject: Martin Shockley's "Christian Symbolism in *The Grapes of Wrath*" (*College English*).

ℒ

Richard Wright, *Native Son*

COMMENTS ON RICHARD WRIGHT

- Richard Wright is probably the most significant black writer this country has had, certainly seminal, influential in themes and techniques. He should be regarded not merely as a black writer but as an important AMERICAN writer. Read the introduction, "How Bigger Was Born"; it's crucial to understanding the novel. Wright regarded himself as an American, an American writer, a "native son."

- Nevertheless, Wright left this country at the height of his career. Whether he rejected the country or the country rejected him is an open question. Both, perhaps. Wright was best at the American scene; it was his heritage. But in alienation he became more and more interested in the international scene, black internationalism, the third world. At one time he was a card-carrying member of the Communist Party, but the Party expelled him. *Native Son* shows why.

- *Native Son* has a lot of autobiography in it: born in Mississippi; father deserted family when Wright was five; mother had strokes when he was very young. The little formal education he got was in a Seventh Day Adventist elementary school. His family moved to Chicago when he was 19. He wrote his first book (*Uncle Tom's Children*) in the WPA Federal Writers Project. His Chicago experience went into *Native Son*, the novel that made him famous. It was written in New York City and was a Book of the Month Club selection.

- In Paris Wright was attracted to communism and existentialism. He knew Sartre, probably Camus. There are many similarities between *Native Son* and Camus' *The Stranger*. *Native Son* was written first. Wright wrote *The Outsider* in 1953 (same as the British title of Camus' *The Stranger*), exploring alienation-existentialist aspects of his blackness. Wright's alienation-existentialist theme was certainly an influence on Ralph Ellison's *Invisible Man*. In fact, Wright's "The Man Who Lived Underground" anticipated Ellison's *Invisible Man* as the account of a man alienated from himself and society. Ellison and Wright both were influenced by Dostoevsky's "The Underground Man."

- Wright played Bigger Thomas in the movie version of *Native Son*, made in Argentina (1940), not Chicago. I saw it in Ann Arbor with my wife about 1951. An artistic disaster.

- In 1950 Wright contributed, with André Gide, Arthur Koestler, and other intellectuals, to *The God That Failed*, the intellectuals' repudiation of communism. Despite not having even a formal high school education Wright was considered an intellectual and included in this prestigious collection of intellectual essays.

- Most critics regard the first and second (existentialist "Fear" and "Flight") parts of *Native Son* excellent but the third part's ("Fate") Marxist ideology of Max a failure, because it is not lived-realized in Bigger's existentialist dilemma.

- Wright died in France (1960) of a heart attack, when he was 52 years old. *Black Boy* is the title of his autobiography.

- Begin with critical statements that make plain the Marxist (naturalist)-existentialist contradiction in the novel.

BIBLIOGRAPHY: T. F. Vandenberg, *Orphan in the Sun*; Michel Fabré, *The Unfinished Quest of Richard Wright.*

☙

J. D. Salinger, *The Catcher in the Rye*

ESME IS ME, ALLIE IS ALL OF US: INTRODUC-
TION TO *THE CATCHER IN THE RYE*

My approach to *The Catcher in the Rye* has to be different from that for any other novel in this course. I
can assume that at least 50% of you read the book
before you signed up for English 63, and I can assume that most of you do already or soon will
greatly admire the views of old Holden and old
Salinger. I can; I really can.

So partly because I am ornery, partly because I
am right, partly because it is a good teaching technique, and partly because it fits the line of thinking
I have laid down for this course, I am going to take
the tack of challenging the rightness of Holden
Caulfield's view of the world and of the men in it.

Few contemporary writers, over the same period
of time, have written so little as Salinger. Most of
what he adds to his writing, after long intervals, is
that which is either collected or rewritten from his
earlier writing. Yet no contemporary American
writer has received anything like the universal critical and popular praise that Salinger has. Pound for
pound, what has been written about Salinger out-

weighs a thousand times what he has written. And only right now has his reputation begun to show signs of decline.

Salinger's Ultimate Intent Is Unclear. That beginning of decline is not because Salinger is a romantic sentimentalist, oblivious to the evils of reality, in contrast to another popular favorite of college or high school students, William Golding (*Lord of the Flies*). The decline more probably comes because Salinger's ultimate intent is a bit unclear, muddled. For if one looks closely at his best stuff (acknowledged to be *Catcher* and stories like "To Esme—with Love and Squalor"), he finds a deep streak of pessimism in Salinger, an impasse to love that contradicts an apparent exterior or clever sentimentalism and a loose religion of Love. If you look closely enough in Salinger you will see that there is no escape from human selfishness and the hate (in "Esme" hate is identified with squalor) (I can assume that most of you are acquainted with much more of Salinger than *Catcher*) in the world. We are left, finally, with a retreat from the whole phony world of society—a retreat by an adolescent boy who winds up in a psychiatric ward, a boy who may or may not make it into the adult world. And there is a further retreat, to the original innocence of the virgin-girl-child, always, whatever her name, Salinger's favorite character. In *Catcher* she is Phoebe, old Phoebe. There she is, near the end, in the rain in Central Park, going round and round, on the carousel, on the golden horse (really, it's brown), reaching for the golden ring (it's really brass) she never gets.

Phoniness in Salinger's Rejection of Phoniness. Further, there is something phony in Salinger's very rejection of phoniness. His characters and audience belong to a class of people who can feel good about their assumed honesty and wiseness about the whole phony world to which they feel superior, and yet not give up this phony world. Salinger manages to make this kind of market big: Holden's attitude toward the working girls and the nuns and many others is also typical of Salinger's admiring readers; he has a condescending sympathy for them that pretends to be Love. Put in terms of another of Salinger's stories, the snotty wise-child intellectual (the Glass family is full of them) is supposed to love the Fat Lady and all the other inferior slobs, and at the same time to laugh at her and them in superior wisdom and clever wit. Salinger's sophisticated audience nods supercilious approval to all of Holden's exposures of phoniness, including themselves; yet, in the end, Phoebe is right when she tells Holden, "You don't like anything." It is certainly hard to be a Lover, a catcher in the rye, if you don't like anything.

The Depth of Salinger's Pessimism. Salinger, of course, knows all this. The depth of his pessimism is not difficult to find. In fact, Salinger killed off his most important spokesman, Seymour Glass, by suicide—quite early in his writing. Sergeant X in "To Esme—with Love and Squalor" and Seymour Glass in "A Perfect Day for Bananafish" are the same person, and continue through the Glass family (particularly Buddy) to be a spokesman for Salinger. In the suicide of Seymour and in Sergeant X we can see that Salinger's cynicism about the existence of hate in the world (squalor) and the near impossibility of love is profound. Having killed off Seymour Glass, and his own optimism, in a cynical fit, it is difficult for Salinger to revive him through Buddy and the Glass family as an apostle of Love. Certainly, the snotty cleverness of the Glass children, who are supposed to be superior to everybody, does not qualify as Love, except for those people who qualify themselves as the only people who love, as the only clever people. All the rest are phonies.

The Theme of *The Catcher in the Rye*. It is also certainly true that Salinger grabs us, with much truth, where our frustrations are today. But the answer is not a clever, snobbish retreat to the Edenic innocence of the virgin-girl-child, grasping for the gold ring in Central Park. It is not finally graspable, and behind the snobbish, misty version of love in the Glass family is easily discernible the all-too-dark alternatives of Seymour's suicide and Holden's psychiatric ward. The evident center of the problem, the theme of *The Catcher in the Rye*, is really the death of Allie (surrounded by all those dead guys, rained on in the cemetery), the recognition of Death and the difficulty of finding love in the adult world—especially in our time. Holden has a hard time growing up (yes, what about old Spencer and the ducks in Central Park?). It is essentially the same problem as the one faced by Shakespeare's Hamlet. But, finally, Hamlet does not lose his rapier in the subway—in the underground world. Hamlet is allowed to grow up to face the adult world; though *Hamlet* is also about Death and the disintegration of Love, the play is affirmative about asserting positive moral values. To me the puny weakness (to be extremely harsh) in Holden's stricken (the clever and biting) gestures of love are just as phony as the phoniness of Hemingway's Frederic Henry's tough, stoic athleticism—which Holden and Salinger both despise.

Comparisons to *Huckleberry Finn*. In Holden's long sustained monologue (soliloquy), there are obvious and numerous similarities to *Huckleberry Finn*. But there are also great differences, both in theme and technique. Although both stories are told by their heroes in the first person and although Huck's physical and mental journeys are analogous to Holden's progress, there is an extreme difference in the point of view. *Catcher* does not have the double perspective (vision) of Twain's novel. Holden Caulfield is almost too aware in reporting the phoniness of everybody. Huck is naive in his response to the corruption of society. The punch of Twain's novel comes from the difference between the naive assumptions of Huck about the morality of society and the sophisticated vision of the adult reader who knows the truth that Huck doesn't see precisely enough to attack. This irony in *Huckleberry Finn* makes all the difference. Holden is anything but naive—even though Salinger's bitterness is closely masked by Holden's pseudo-simplicity.

Therefore, speaking thematically now, Huck is at once more pragmatic (realistic) than Holden and more loving. Through the double vision of Twain's novel (that is, Huck's simplicity joined to the adult reader's insight), we get a sharper, more valid, and less compromised view of adult society. And in Huck's spontaneous love, springing from a very practical view of things, there is never any under-cutting of that love, as there is in the wise-child so-phistication of Holden Caulfield. Huck is never sorry for himself, and it is impossible to always be in sympathy with Holden, unless one is the kind of person who weeps because his sensitive (and clever, too; there is the artistic difficulty in *Catcher*) soul is subjected to the brutality of a phony world. Perhaps the lesson of *Catcher* is that it is not good to grow wise too early. Even old Gatsby, whom Holden ad-mires, never knew the corruption of the dream that Holden knows. It kills me; he really didn't.

In regard to this dream, I leave you to judge be-tween the superiority, romantically speaking, in terms of escape, of winding up in a psychiatric ward out West in California or heading for the territory. Both novels are good, very good; I take a negative line on Salinger, partly because I know what a great guy you think old Holden is. It is possible that Salinger engages you with Holden because, to use Holden's vocabulary, he wants you to examine your own assumptions about all the phony bastards in the four-letter world you are so unhappy to live with and in.

One More Point. All of Hemingway's fictional chil-dren, like Catherine Barkley's child, may prove to be stillborn, in their pessimism. But, anyway, Hemingway did write a lot of dead children. Maybe the difficulty that Salinger has in writing and rewriting the very little he has written proves that his clever love philosophy (so apparently optimistically rewritten in *Franny and Zooey*) was impotent to begin with. It is dead and buried with the subdued knowledge of Seymour Glass, who is Salinger himself.

Try to find light and love in *Catcher* if you can. But remember old Allie with all that poetry in his baseball glove, rained on with all the dead guys in the cemetery. And think of why Holden can't stand old Spencer (who is really old) and his old wife, who will soon join Allie. And give a thought to the ducks on the pond in Central Park; where do we go when winter comes? Growing up in the world of reality is tough. We do not know whether or not Holden will ever get out of the loony bin; he has gone West, one way or another, and it all started with Allie. The fault is more intrinsic than to be explained by identifying oneself as a nice guy surrounded by a bunch of bastards in a phony world. Holden admits this, and, on Salinger's own terms, even though he wants to be a "catcher in the rye," he will find it much harder to bust out of his loneliness than Steinbeck thought it would be for Tom Joad and Casey. The fact is (remember old Sunny in the hotel room) Holden is impotent, afraid of the reality of the world, afraid of life, which is cruel.

NOTE: As I hinted earlier, it is Salinger's habit to rewrite the biographies of his characters backwards: *Franny and Zooey* is actually merely a reprinting of two Salinger stories which first appeared many years before; Seymour Glass is dead before his war exploits, as Sergeant X, are given in "A Perfect Day for Bananafish," and his wedding day is narrated in "Raise High the Roofbeams, Carpenters" by Buddy Glass. More details about Seymour are given in *Franny and Zooey*. And 19-year-old Holden Caulfield is reported missing in action in the South Pacific in a 1945 story, "This Sandwich Has No Mayonnaise." Two other stories about Holden precede *Catcher*. Both of them are incorporated in *Catcher*.

ℒ

Saul Bellow, *Henderson the Rain King*

Henderson the Rain King is Bellow's favorite novel; Henderson, he has said, is most like himself. Henderson is everyman, coming to terms with the realities of human existence.

APPROACH TO *HENDERSON THE RAIN KING*

Henderson the Rain King is a particularly difficult novel to end with. It is hard to assess Henderson the person, speaking in his own voice, and it is hard to assess the tone that Bellow brings to the story, through its very complicated devices: the interrelated animal images, the psychological symbols, the mythological motifs, and the pattern of ironies. Especially the ironies cause a problem in determining if Bellow is making an affirmative statement about Henderson or laughing at him.

General Statement about the Novel. I am going to make a general statement about what *Henderson the Rain King* means, but you should consider what I say very critically, perhaps skeptically. Henderson is a rich, frustrated, violent American. It can be said (and Bellow may be mocking Henderson) that Henderson goes to a symbolic Africa, the source of his instinctive self, the source of life and death, the source of love and hate (the Arnewi and Wariri) to come to terms with himself, with what he is, with what any human is. (Remember how Christopher Newman returns to Europe in peace and how Frederic Henry returns there in war, how Nick Carraway and Jay Gatsby fight in that war and return to the East. Well, Henderson has fought in World War II, but he does not seek his civilized past.) In Africa he is returning to his instinctive past, the collective archetypal unconsciousness of mankind, the springs of life way back—for answers to society.

Henderson is frustrated with the meaninglessness of life, by a horror of the stupidity and sordidness of life, by a fear of non-being and death. In a kind of nose-thumbing, he returns from one war to start another one with his neighbors and to turn his ancestral estate, his heritage, into a pigsty. Death is certainly the central issue of the novel. Henderson must come to terms with the dying animal that he is. Is Bellow saying with his novel that Henderson's experience is a rebirth, that Henderson is renewed and reborn after his descent into darkness? Or is the whole novel a comic, ironic put-on, satirizing the African experience as heroic quest, satirizing, for example, Hemingway's African stories (note the initials of Eugene Henderson, who returns from Africa with a baby lion), satirizing such novels as Conrad's *Heart of Darkness* and Graham Greene's *A Burnt-Out Case*? Is Bellow mocking contemporary literature and criticism that has emphasized anthropology, myth, Freudian and Jungian interpretations of human life? Or is he writing an affirmative antidote to the moods of pessimism, absurdity, and despair in twentieth-century criticism and literature? Perhaps some of all of this is true. Whatever conclusion you come to, do not neglect to observe the humor and comedy, the irony and satire in the novel.

I am going to proceed on the assumption that the overall impression of *Henderson the Rain King* is affirmative—that if rain is a fertility symbol and Henderson is a rain king, Bellow is affirming Henderson's renewal rather than laughing at him in the title. So we'll start with the idea, in one critic's words, that *Henderson the Rain King* "focuses consistently and from many angles upon the single concept of rebirth, and that concept in turn provides the vehicle for the redemption theme."

TECHNIQUE

Before going into the text of the novel, let me make some general observations about the devices (Bellow's techniques) by which the novel is developed. In another way, they are almost as complicated as the structure of Faulkner's *As I Lay Dying*, and what I say is by no means complete or original.

Animal Images. The animal imagery reflects Henderson's spiritual redemption, the transformation of Henderson's essential being. The main steps of rebirth have to do with four animals: the pigs, the abandoned cat which Henderson tries to kill, the frogs in the Arnewi well, and Dahfu's lions (lioness and lion). Henderson identifies with his hogs, assumes their voracious, violent, and crude nature. The cat and the frog incidents are incidents of self-revelation whereby Henderson learns something about the misuse of violence and technical ingenuity (perhaps combined, America) to achieve this rebirth, the Being, he desires. Ultimately, Henderson has to come to an understanding with Dahfu's lions, with violence and death, with the lion in himself, in human nature—assume something of the spiritual strength and nobility the king of beasts represents. I don't know whether I accept this last statement or not, but Henderson does have to move from understanding the "I want" of pig to the "I want" of lion. In psychosomatic psychology, think pig and you are pig, think lion and you are lion. In the lion cub, perhaps the lion strength is domesticated to the social service of medicine (Henderson is going to be a doctor at the end).

Psychological Symbols. The Freudian and Jungian symbols in the novel follow the steps of Henderson's emotional care, the change in his personality. Part of Henderson's frustration is the lingering influence of his deceased father, in relation to his dead brother; part of his striving is his effort to please his father, to communicate with him and receive the assurance that he is living as he should. This longing is represented in Henderson's learning to play the violin, his father's favorite instrument and the medium whereby Henderson feels he can reach his father. It is not surprising that later in Africa, when

Dahfu becomes Henderson's surrogate father figure and Henderson becomes free of the old longing altogether, he gives up the violin, since he no longer needs it. Henderson also has female complexes, problems with his wife and daughter. The obvious mother figure (life and love figure) for Henderson is Willatale (Addie), the obese old queen of the peaceful Arnewi tribe, from whom Henderson learns, significantly, "gru-tu-molani," the will to live, and with her the womb symbolism begins (extended in the cistern). At one point Henderson kisses Willatale's fat stomach and the words "the hour that burst the spirit's sleep" occur to him. Mother and father complexes are combined in Dahfu's dilemma, in his pet lioness Atti and correlative wife-life problems, and the tribe's superstition that Gmilo the wild lion holds incarnate the spirit of Dahfu's father. The most encompassing aspect of the psychological symbolism appears in the scene in which Henderson lifts the idol Mummah and thereby becomes rain king. Henderson initiates his own rebirth; through lifting Mummah he becomes the Sungo, the rain king, the pupil and heir of Dahfu.

Mythological Motifs. The mythic pattern of the novel traces Henderson's release from the weight of the past and his adaptation to a better view of present and future. Henderson's adventures are clearly drawn to conform to the hero myth and the archetypal pattern of the dying king. In the hero myth the hero is involved in adventures and achievements of various kinds, such as the slaying of monsters, overcoming death, and controlling the weather; the hero often has an extraordinary birth; help from animals is a frequent motif; a separation from one or both parents at an early age is usual; antagonism toward near kin is expressed through violent acts; the hero returns with honor and with achievements that are realized by the family and that benefit the family and society at large—all in all, the hero undergoes a moral and spiritual rebirth. Most of this (comically or otherwise) can be applied to Henderson. The myth of the dying king is one of the oldest fertility myths and grew out of annual fertility rites during which the ruler was sacrificed to assure good crops for the ensuing year. The sacrificial aspect is present in the destinies of Dahfu and Henderson the Sungo rain king. Dahfu can remain ruler of the Wariri only so long as he can satisfy his many wives, and Henderson, as the rain king who produces the life-giving water, is next in line for Dahfu's position and Dahfu's sacrificial fate. In his experience with the Wariri, the children of darkness, Henderson experiences a kind of death (the sun go) and rebirth.

Patterns of Irony. By now you are saying what an awful lot of claptrap I am putting you through. I am inclined to agree. Yet there is no doubt that the images and symbols and myths I have mentioned are in *Henderson the Rain King*, and intentionally, almost too intellectually, structured. The question is how Bellow intends us to take them. Does he intend us to laugh at Henderson, at the pretense of rebirth? Ironies abound: I have mentioned the parody of Ernest Hemingway, a man in short pants with a big gun, Bellow called him. "Eugene" means well-born, yet he rejects his good breeding for pig farming. Looking for order, he divorces his first wife to marry Lily, the epitome of sloppiness and chaos. Henderson appears a comic fool throughout the novel: upon meeting the Arnewi tribe in Africa, he puts on a white man's show for them but is approached afterward by a tribesman who addresses him in cultured English. Near the end, balanced on a flimsy platform in the African bush, wearing sun helmet, jockey shorts, and transparent green pants, he watches Dahfu risk his life and lose it, emasculated, in an attempt to net the lion who is supposed to be his father. Really, it's all hilariously funny.

Is the whole novel a put-on for the symbol seekers whom Bellow has more than once attacked? Or is the ridiculous Henderson a kind of holy fool, like Don Quixote, who carries an affirmative lesson? When at the end, Henderson, nursing a lion cub (reversing his early cat shooting), gallops around the ice of Newfoundland airport, carrying the small Persian boy (reversing his attitude to his daughter's orphan black) and wearing rotting socks, Henderson's exuberance is comic—but is it comic in a profound sense: in the realization that life (which ends in death) need not be tragic if one is fool enough to participate in its comic ironies, to live out those ironies and be reborn in the affirmation of human reality? Henderson (now Leo the Lion), paradoxically, has returned to the primitive order to live in the modern present. He has traveled to the "dark continent" to become enlightened. He has practiced the physical order to find the spiritual. He has approached death to find life. And all the time the model of peace for which he has been seeking has been ever-present at his side in his faithful squire and guide Romalayu. Bellow, the alien Jew, who has made America his home, has found in the loud American blue-blooded millionaire a positive parody of America. Henderson is the Sungo. When the sun go the sky darken. When the sky darken, the rain come. When the rains come the plants grow. Fertility, rebirth. Henderson is the rain king. The irony organizes the totality of the redemptive experience as it affects the protagonist and the two cultures that involve him: Arnewi (children of light, love) and Wariri (children of darkness, death).

When I picked *Henderson the Rain King* to conclude this course with a current novelist, I chose it as an end-of-the-American-Dream novel over Norman Mailer's *The American Dream*. Consider that *Henderson* should be regarded as representing the once-romantic America of idealistic individualism, now grown up from childhood, having come through the trauma of disillusion to the recognition that it must not only face but embrace reality with unselfish love, not with anger, frustration, and violence. Critics don't regard *Henderson* as Bellow's most significant novel, but Bellow has said it is his favorite and that Henderson, of all the characters he has created, is most like himself. Bellow's favorite novelist is Conrad, as a seeker of truth and reality, and, like himself, an immigrant. (Bellow began and ended his Nobel speech with Conrad.)

NOTE: Met Ellison, Vonnegut, Mailer, Bellow. Met Bellow at airport, talked over a Michelob, introduced him in Dimnent Chapel, took him to dinner at Point West.

❦❦❦

THE ENGLISH NOVEL

THE ENGLISH NOVEL
English 330, Spring 1980

1. Defoe: *Moll Flanders* (1722), New American Library. January 16, 18, 21, 23
2. Fielding: *Tom Jones* (1749), New American Library. January 25, 28, 30, February 1
3. Austen: *Emma* (1816), New American Library. February 4, 6, 8
Test: February 11

4. Brontë: *Wuthering Heights* (1848), New American Library. February 13, 15, 18
5. Dickens: *Great Expectations* (1860), New American Library. February 20, 25, 27, 29
6. Eliot: *Adam Bede* (1859), New American Library. March 3, 5, 7, 10
Test: March 12

7. Hardy: *Tess of the D'Urbervilles* (1891), New American Library. March 14, 17, 19
8. Conrad: *Lord Jim* (1900), New American Library. March 21, 24, 26
9. Lawrence: *Women in Love* (1920), Viking. April 9, 11, 14
10. Joyce: *Portrait of the Artist* (1916), Viking. April 16, 18, 21
11. Woolf: *To the Lighthouse* (1927), HBW Harvest. April 23, 25
12. Golding: *The Spire* (1964), HBW Harvest. April 28, 30, May 2
Test: May 9, 10:30 AM

Two excellent study aids for historical and critical background are Walter Allen's *The English Novel: A Short Critical History* (Dutton Paperback) and Dorothy Van Ghent's *The English Novel: Form and Function* (Harper Torchbook). Van Zoeren Library has plenty of biographical and critical resources for all authors and titles.

YOU ARE EXPECTED TO ATTEND ALL CLASSES

Introductory Lecture
(Fall 1965)

THERE IS A THEME that I shall stress for all the novels in this course: it is the relation of the novel to the two worlds that people, you and I, live in—the world of SELF and the world of SOCIETY. The world of self is the inner psychological, or spiritual (I prefer "spiritual" to "psychological" because psychology, today, suggests the objective study of mental processes, just as philosophy suggests abstract systems of idealization) world of idealistic, romantic, even fantastic, private imagination; the world of society is the objective, material, so-called realistic world of rational public experience. It is possible, of course, to separate these two worlds in self-consciousness, but the world of self tends to be a *felt* world; the world of society tends to be a *thought* world, a rationalized world: an apprehended-perceived world *versus* a comprehended-conceived world.

Well, what is the relation of the novel to these private and public worlds? It can be said that the novel as a distinct literary genre emerged during transition from a time of emphasis on idealistic truth (spiritual truth) to a time of emphasis on so-called realistic truth, fact. In fact, it is possible to define the novel as a product of tension between real (outer) and ideal (inner) reality, tension between the public and the private worlds. The obvious prototype of the novel, thus defined, is *Don Quixote*. In the words of one critic (Ángel del Río),

the new literary genre in *Don Quixote* (later to be called the "modern novel") arose out of a changed situation of man in history, one in which incongruities between individual intentions and individual capacity for realizing them in the world became apparent, and in which truth became a problem—not in the abstract nor in relation to the transcendental forces but relative to man's own existence.

Another critic (Georg Lukács) has defined the novel as "the search for the expression of the irrational, the soul, in and through an alien and hostile reality"; "the principle of its form," he said, "is derived from the consciousness that 'inwardness' has its own independent value." Lukács was thinking of the fusion of means and meaning in the *form* of the novel. Mark Schorer was even more so when he wrote that the "problem of the novel has always been to distinguish between these two, the self and society, and at the same time to find suitable structures that will bring them together."

In general, the direction of the English novel, from Fielding to Joyce (or Golding), let us say, has been from emphasis on the outer world to emphasis on the inner, from the social to the psychological, from emphasis on society to emphasis on the self. What I want you to watch for in all the novels of this course is the extent to which each novel stresses the self and/or society, and the structures it employs to define and harmonize (perhaps separate) these two worlds. How do the structures of the various novels in this course develop the relation of self and society? How do they expand your own experience in the world, help you to find yourself? To me, this last is the most important question of all, but one that will (can) never be asked in a test—the question behind all other questions.

℘

Daniel Defoe, *Moll Flanders*
(1968)

DEFOE'S POSITION AS FATHER OF THE ENGLISH NOVEL

<u>Moore</u>. John Robert Moore's critical biography of Defoe, *Daniel Defoe: Citizen of the Modern World,* calls Defoe "the father of the English novel." Critically speaking, I don't have a high opinion of Moore's book, but the title is significant. I repeat it.

<u>Schorer</u>. Mark Schorer, author of the introduction to your text edition of *Moll Flanders,* would probably not grant Defoe the honor of being the first English novelist; he thinks that *Moll Flanders* lacks moral integrity and artistic unity. He would say that a novel must be a sustained narrative that develops a unified impression of life, a consistent theme, consistently presented. He would say that *Moll Flanders* is a string of episodes bound together only by Moll's life.

<u>Van Ghent</u>. Dorothy Van Ghent in *The English Novel: Form and Function* treats *Pilgrim's Progress* before *Moll Flanders* but regards *Moll Flanders* as unified through conscious irony and therefore a unified work of art.

She agrees with Schorer that Moll's morality is vicious but thinks that Defoe is aware of her inner corruption and that Defoe is presenting her with ironic detachment.

Allen. Walter Allen in *The English Novel* calls Defoe the "archetypal novelist."

To try to settle whether Defoe is the first English novelist or not is to labor over an irrelevant question. But it is important to consider what qualities of *Moll Flanders* make it a novel or not a novel. It has been a cliché in the study of English literature to call Richardson's *Pamela* the first English novel. Some say Bunyan's *Pilgrim's Progress*; some say Defoe's *Robinson Crusoe* or his *Moll Flanders*. Some point further back to Thomas Nashe's *The Unfortunate Traveler, or The Life of Jack Wilton,* and some point a bit ahead to Fielding's *Tom Jones.* Personally, I think Defoe's genius merits the distinction of "father of the English novel," although I agree with Schorer's estimate of him and *Moll Flanders*: the novel does lack moral integrity and artistic unity.

But granting these defects does not for me exclude *Moll Flanders* from classification as a novel, albeit a poor prototype—and certainly *Moll Flanders* contains both the realistic mode and the concern for practical life (the world of middle-class society) that characterize the emergence of the novel as an art form. When, after vernacular languages (English in this instance) were all established and great numbers of people were educated to read them, then the old world views—the idealistic philosophies—clashed with realistic thinking, the rising secular materialism, and a new art form was born from the existing prose romance and elements of other literary types. Defoe was a first citizen of this modern world. Cervantes was "the first," so far as the novel is concerned. *Moll Flanders* is a good place to begin the study of the English novel.

DEFOE'S RELATION TO THE DEVELOPMENT OF FICTION (see Schorer's introduction in your text)

Moll Flanders' Middle-Class Appeal. *Moll Flanders* is the first English work of fiction to take the reader into the very heart of the English middle class, even as that class was coming into a position to dominate English society. *Moll Flanders* concerns a middle-class heroine seen through the eyes of a middle-class author, revealing middle-class standards of morality. As I stated before, the rise of the novel is a cultural development that parallels the rise of the middle class, the rise of economic realism and Puritan utilitarian morality.

Moll Flanders Is Built on the Existing Rogue Biography. The rogue biography had been a conventional and low form of literary expression since Elizabethan times. Rogue biographies were usually shortened and sensational biographies of real criminals. Their ostensible purpose was to expose and warn against vice (see Defoe's Preface); their real purpose (like "true confessions") was to thrill an undiscriminating audience with melodrama. To this conventional type Defoe added the quality of what we call "circumstantial realism."

Moll Flanders' Relation to the "Picaresque." I hope to

touch on this later in relation to Roger Alter's *Rogue's Progress: Studies in the Picaresque Novel.* Chapter III, on *Moll Flanders,* is titled "A Bourgeois Picaroon" and treats Moll as a quasi-picaresque heroine. You ought to read Ian Watt's *The Rise of the Novel,* by far the best book on the beginnings of English fiction, or at least read the early chapters of Walter Allen.

DEFOE'S CONTRIBUTION TO THE NOVEL: CIRCUMSTANTIAL REALISM

In general, Defoe's method is to create the impression of factual reality. I would note particularly three ways in which this impression is achieved (see Schorer):

The Use of Documentary Detail. A piling up of external facts, even to bolts of goods, inventories, itemized accounts, landlady's bills, lists, ledgers, etc.

The Use of a Sustained Point of View. By point of view I mean the eyes, the mind through which the story is revealed. Moll's story is consistently revealed in the first person, through the main character, through Moll herself.

The Use of a Matter-of-Fact Tone. Defoe levels all incidents out on a straight narrative plane. Every incident seems so guilelessly without emphasis that the illusion of truth is created. Moll seems so innocently imperceptive, so uncomprehending of deeper moral issues, so blandly matter-of-fact that we have the illusion of reality; we think her story must be true. Of course, the story is actually fantastic, and that raises some questions about her and Defoe's perceptivity, about her and Defoe's character.

THE DOMINANT MEANING, MORAL DIRECTION OF THE NOVEL

Let me suggest some possibilities:

The Shocking Results of a Life of Vice. Defoe's expressed moral direction in his Preface is the shocking results of a life of vice. But one asks, what shocking result? Material or spiritual loss? Moll, at the end, is very well off. Vice and crime have paid off handsomely. And she seems to be not aware of any spiritual loss, any hypocrisy, any irony in her situation.

Surviving According to the Standards and Values Society Sets. Moll herself seems to emphasize the moral direction that heredity and environment makes the criminal. This is her repeated excuse for depravity and extends to the judgment that crimes, her crimes, are the product of a heartless and improvident society. She is merely surviving according to the standards and values society sets. But prostitution and thievery and viciousness were not necessary to her survival, as she herself admits. Ultimately, she blames the devil.

Corrupt Social Values. It could be that the moral direction of the novel is contrary to Defoe's stated purpose in his Preface: that is, in Moll's society crime does pay. It could be (as Van Ghent believes) that Defoe is using Moll through a system of ironies to show the corruption of Moll's middle-class society and its material values. Moll is really the representative of her society. The irony and hypocrisy are in the very maxim that "crime does not pay." Why *pay*? The corollary is that virtue should pay, as Moll insists, which leads to the middle-class emphasis that material success, no matter how achieved, is the equivalent of virtue. If you have it, God must be on your side. Moll and the values of the society she accepts are corrupt, criminal, vicious. Moll is a criminal only when she is on the wrong side of the law that protects those values. The very language of middle-class maxims ironically exposes the corrupt values: crime does not pay; virtue pays. *Payment* is the language of material values, material remuneration. And some critics say that in the novel Defoe is consciously exposing, artistically directing exposure, through a system of ironies in Moll's point of view—exposing the corruption of Moll and her society and its values of material success that deny humanity and the feelings of the heart.

The Critics' Views. Both Schorer and Van Ghent believe that Moll is the representative of her middle-class society and its values, and those values are criminal, corrupt, vicious. Moll, they think, is no more criminal than her society: both she and her society have the same criterion for acceptance in all things, including the spiritual: material success. There indeed is poverty of spirit! But whereas Schorer thinks Defoe is in agreement with Moll's values, is Moll himself, and practiced her values—is unaware of any irony in Moll's situation and professions, and couldn't be—Van Ghent thinks Defoe is exposing the corruption of a society, consciously and artistically, through point of view and irony and tone—through Moll. And therefore Schorer thinks the novel (which he thinks is not a novel) lacks moral integrity and artistic unity, and Van Ghent thinks it has both (and is therefore a novel).

What do you think? What do you think the point of view and irony and tone of *Moll Flanders* reveal about the meaning of the novel? How do they shape, form its content? I tend to agree with Schorer that Defoe is unconsciously revealing his own morality of worldly success, Puritan-Calvinistic middle-class success.

MOLL FLANDERS IS THOROUGHLY A WORLD OF SOCIETY, NOT SELF

Whatever you decide, I think you will agree that the world of *Moll Flanders* is thoroughly a world of society, not of self. Despite the first-person point of view, Moll completely lacks depth, conscience, imagination, feeling, sensitivity, color. She is a bland-surface reflection of society. She *is* society. She is a grotesque monster, a calculating machine that sums up husbands and children in terms of pounds and pence. And Moll sees everything in terms of her society's values, without spiritual insight: her surroundings, the setting of the novel, do not come alive—the novel has no sense of place. Even the presence of London is not felt because Moll does not feel it in any depth (compare to Dickens in *Great Expectations*); the novel lacks atmosphere, emotional background—and the tone is throughout almost impossibly matter-of-fact, without feeling, without variety of mood. The imagery is quantitative rather than qualitative—descriptive of things, objects; the style is that of reporting in the language of the counting

house. All this, of course, may be purposeful art consistent with the point of view of Moll—the ironic genius
of Defoe.

Henry Fielding, *Tom Jones*
(1970)

THE MOVIE AND THE NOVEL

It is not necessary that you have seen the movie. If you have, all the better. The movie presents in its version of *Tom Jones* quite rightly an emphasis on the natural lust for life, but also it presents a cruel irrationality in the natural lust for life which is so exaggerated and so grotesque that the story becomes, subtly, not comic but sick. In the movie, Fielding's balance of common sense and the lust for life is obliterated by a cruel animality. For example, the hunt scene, which is central to the action of the movie, is a terrible and bloody ritual. The bloody victim of the hunt is a doe, not a fox as it is in the novel, symbolizing, I suppose, animal viciousness in sexual pursuit. In the novel, this hunt scene is much more minor in significance, with no such suggestion. It is as though Albee had written the movie script. Another instance of changed emphasis is the sexual animalism suggested by the movie in the eating scene (with Mrs. Waters and Tom at Upton): eating becomes a sexual exercise. The novel does point up sexual spirits in this scene but not to the point of the horribly grotesque, inhuman. If you have observed the movie, you were also impressed by the lust for murder exhibited by the spectators who come near the end of the novel to see Tom hanged. They have a sexual appetite for death. Nothing like this occurs in the novel: there is no hanging scene. To sum up, the movie tries to point up the absurdity, the sickness of life, whereas the novel, I believe, points up good health and good nature.

Now, my purpose is not to attack the movie but to get a perspective on the novel. I have enjoyed the movie three times now; the photography is a wonderful evocation of eighteenth-century life. What I do think is that the spirit of the movie, at bottom, is not a comic spirit at all (nor tragic), and the spirit of Fielding's novel is comic. To me, *Tom Jones* is a comedy of manners that balances a joyous lust for life and assumptions of natural innocence with the need for social prudence, rational discretion. That is, the comic spirit of Fielding is to temper the lust for life with common sense (although there is a latent irony in his words that assists the movie interpretation). Fielding, I believe, satirizes human frailty for the very purpose of asserting the dignity of man and human society. He does not mean to exaggerate man's (and woman's) natural appetites to the point of grotesque horror and revulsion (ask why, at the moment, the hunt scene, and the eating scene, and the hanging scene in the movie excited you).

To Fielding, life is uproariously funny, basically good, and wonderfully joyous, despite human faults, which are redeemable by reason and common sense. This is the comic spirit. Life, to Fielding, is not an irrational and horrible joke, not cruel, or dirty, or absurdly meaningless. To Fielding, life is comic in a healthy way; his humor is never sick.

All this is said so you may look more closely at the novel to see if I lie—and at the movie if you get the chance again. As I said, there is irony in the novel: what we must do is to try to discover, as with *Moll Flanders*, the "implicit author" (a term of Wayne Booth) in *Tom Jones*. What manner of man speaks behind the mask the author puts on, and with what tone?

COMPARISON BETWEEN DEFOE AND FIELDING

Before I go on to talk more particularly about the theme and method of *Tom Jones*, let me make two points of comparison between Defoe and Fielding:

Moral Significance. The first point concerns moral significance. There is plenty of moral statement and pretense of seriousness in *Moll Flanders*, but its moral consistency, its artistic unity, is questionable. The same cannot be said of *Tom Jones*, despite its comic tone. Fielding is perfectly aware that he is writing in a new literary genre. He purposefully uses the elements of that new type of literature, the novel, consistently to express a theme, a view of life. In fact, Fielding, in *Tom Jones*, helps to define the new genre of the novel; his prefaces to the sections of *Tom Jones* are the first criticism in English of the novel as a literary type.

Novel of Character. My second point of comparison is that neither *Moll Flanders* nor *Tom Jones* is truly a novel of character in any deep psychological sense, even though their titles are the names of their heroes.

The focus in *Moll Flanders* is on unplotted social action; the focus of *Tom Jones* is on the manipulation of social action, on the manipulation of manners—that is, on plotting. In *Moll Flanders*, character subserves circumstantial detail; in *Tom Jones*, character subserves social manners. The English novel of character, in the psychological sense, is yet to be born, when the subject is the self of the hero in Conrad, Joyce, or Lawrence, with their special techniques to aid that penetration.

THEME IN *TOM JONES*

Now for a few statements concerning what *Tom Jones* is about, the view of life in the novel. My terms are pretty much those of George Sherburn in the introduction to the Modern Library edition.

Subject. The subject, most broadly, of *Tom Jones* is "human nature." Tom is, of course, a representative man. In his first pages, Fielding introduces his repast of human nature with a banquet metaphor.

Thematic Design. Fielding's consistent thematic design is a contest between instinctive feeling in human nature and formalized appearance (that is, outward show) in social action. The core contest is between Tom, who errs in the direction of instinctive feeling, and Blifil, who errs in the direction of formalized appearance.

Thesis. Fielding's thesis, if I may use that horrid term, seems to be that the best "human nature" is a balance of instinctive feeling and social intelligence. Neither emotional license nor formal rigidity will do. Social intelligence must be a check to the fundamental rightness of spontaneous feeling. Obviously, Fielding is optimistic about instinctive feeling in the person of Tom, optimistic about basic human nature. But instinctive nature is capable of indiscretion; Tom must learn discretion. Tom must not only be good, but act good, without becoming false, rigidly formal.

TECHNIQUE IN *TOM JONES*

Now to Fielding's art, his craft, his way of writing. My main point here is that contrast is the basic technique in *Tom Jones*, fundamental to the novel's form. Every element in the novel (point of view, narrative structure, characters, setting, etc.) is used in this comedy of manners to contrast instinctive feeling with formalized appearance to make Fielding's point about "human nature."

Point of View. Fielding is the first English novelist to use the point of view of the omniscient author. His scope, his world, in *Tom Jones*, is too populous and extensive in space for the survey of one character within the book. But Fielding does not merely write in the third person, objectively, playing the omniscient God; he frankly intrudes, usually in his prefatory essays, to talk familiarly with the reader. He comments on the story he has created, thus giving the reader the double perspective of the author's critical intelligence commenting on his materials and his creative intelligence working within his materials. The omniscient author is a traditional narrative technique, deriving from the epic; frank intrusion by the author derives from the familiar essay (Addison's *Spectator Papers*). In your reading of *Tom Jones*, does Fielding's intrusion spoil the illusion of reality for you? Do you get too much the feeling that Fielding is telling you about something that has happened, rather than the feeling of something immediately happening?

Narrative Structure. Narrative structure is the author's arrangements of the elements of the story. On the level of external action, *Tom Jones* has one of the most intricate, complicated, and cleverly manipulated plots of any English novel. There is hardly a single circumstance that does not contribute to the final outcome. The superficial structure of the novel is three equal parts which carry Tom at an accelerating tempo through the settings of eighteenth-century English country, highway, and city, revealing the manners of each, toward the suspenseful resolution of Tom's conflict (his instinctive feeling *versus* Blifil's formalized appearance). Innocence *versus* evil?

Formal Structure. More subtly, the formal structure of *Tom Jones* is a careful juxtaposition by Fielding of contrasting elements (as I said, point of view against point of view, act against act, scene against scene, setting against setting, character against character, oneself against another, mood against mood, tone against tone). Fielding's basic method of comic revelation.

The Comic Epic. Fielding calls *Tom Jones* a comic epic. The novel does contain characteristic techniques derived from the epic (e.g., epic sweep, epic battles, epic invocations, epic similes, etc.). It also contains techniques derived from the essay and the drama (Fielding had a thorough knowledge of each form, including Cervantes' comic-epic novel of Don Quixote's adventures). Fielding's prefaces are familiar essays, comic-epic invocations. The narrative story itself is a balanced brand of summarized narrative and dramatic scenes. The handling of dramatic scenes shows Fielding's experience in the theater.

ℒ

Jane Austen, *Emma*
(1965)

GENERAL POINT ABOUT THE NOVEL

<u>Technique and Structural Principles</u>. Like *Tom Jones* (and perhaps unlike *Moll Flanders*), *Emma* is a very well-constructed novel. All its elements are bound closely to a central theme. Like *Tom Jones*, too, its central organizing principle is a system (or fabric) of ironies. But unlike *Tom Jones*, *Emma* is a much more concentrated artistic effort. It is a wonderful example of the use of artistic means for greatest effect. Austen, for instance, uses point of view much more organically for calculated ironic effect than does Fielding. Austen has been called the first artist in English fiction.

<u>Subject Matter</u>. Like *Tom Jones*, *Emma* concerns society, manners, though its social focus is much more concentrated than that of *Tom Jones*. Though *Emma* could be called a novel of character, and though its plot grows much more organically out of character than that of *Tom Jones*, Austen's subject (like Fielding's) is still more society and English manners than individual character (titles notwithstanding). Emma's story (like all of Austen's stories) is about marriage,

and restricted to a certain genteel class of Englishmen in a certain locality of Hampshire, England.

Tone. Like *Tom Jones*, the tone of *Emma* is comic—it is a comedy of manners, humane, satirical, rational, common-sensical, and essentially optimistic. But whereas Fielding's tone is inclined to be urbane and gentle and light and mild, Austen is more ironically sharp, witty, cutting, biting, caustic.

Before getting to the theme of *Emma*, I confess I am not one of Jane Austen's greatest admirers. Like D. W. Harding, Marvin Mudrick, and, I think, Lionel Trilling, I much respect Jane Austen but cannot like her, much less love her. And I cannot get deeply interested in her repeated subject of good sense to be used in solving the problem of the marriage of girls in a certain class of English society. And I have never yet been able to like an Austen heroine, be it Elizabeth Bennet or Emma Woodhouse. But within Austen's subject, she has no peer as an accomplished novelist until Henry James, whom she resembles, or *vice versa*. I agree with the critics that *Emma* is Austen's best novel. Its ironic form is beautifully developed, and in the growth of Emma, the heroine, there is an implicit self-knowledge on the part of Austen herself that she does not exhibit in other novels. I do like Emma better than I do other Austen heroines.

THEME OF THE NOVEL

Practicality *versus* Fancy. *Emma* is typical of Austen's novels in that it pits common sense practicality against misleading fancies in the realm of marriage. Emma is a girl who practices her romantic fancies on others. Emma's basic fault is too much respect for her own judgment; she has a misleading fancy through which she fabricates an imaginary reality that she tries to impose on others, by constructing one marriage match after another. Emma is young, rich, intelligent in a dabbling way, beautiful, charming, perceptive, and gay. She is also a snob, domineering, rash, and selfish. She has had her own way too much, and she thinks too well of herself. Emma's worst fault is that she is so selfishly wrapped up in herself that she cultivates a detachment from others to the extent that she believes she could have no desire to marry any man. She is never personally involved with anybody; she cannot commit herself humanly; she is incapable of tenderness, as one critic puts it. Therefore, she does not arrange other people's lives because of kindness or sympathy, but because she is a selfish meddler.

Development. The development of the novel lies in the series (3) of progressively ironic disintegrations of the fancied realities Emma creates—a series that brings her eventually to a kind of honest self-knowledge and also to the realization of how much she wants and needs the man who has been all along her warmest friend and critic: Mr. Knightley. Mr. Knightley is, in a sense, Emma's antithesis and complement, in that he stands for common sense against fancy.

The Character of Emma. The questions I would leave with you today are all about the character of Emma. This is a very complex novel, one about which you will change your mind at every reading. To be sure, Emma learns common sense and self-knowledge and a kind of honesty. But, as the critic I mentioned says, does she ever learn tenderness, the capacity to share feelings with others? This is a lack in all Austen's novels, to my mind, and the reason I dislike her and her heroines. But you must decide for yourselves, because I am soft-boiled.

BIBLIOGRAPHY (important because *Emma* is a much more complex novel than you might imagine and because I am prejudiced): Howard S. Babb, *Jane Austen's Novels: The Fabric of Her Dialogue* (1962); Andrew Wright, *Jane Austen's Novels: A Study in Structure* (1953); Mary Lascelles, *Jane Austen and Her Art* (1939); Sheila Kaye Smith and G. B. Stern, *Speaking of Jane Austen* (1944); Robert Liddell, *The Novels of Jane Austen* (1963); A. Walton Litz, *Jane Austen: A Study of Her Artistic Development* (1965); Marvin Mudrick, *Jane Austen: Irony as Defense and Discovery* (1952); Ian Watt, ed., *Jane Austen*, 20th Century Views; a chapter on *Emma* in Elizabeth's Drew's *The Novel: A Modern Guide to 15 English Masterpieces*, 60 cents Dell pb; good chapter in Arnold Kettle, *An Introduction to the English Novel*; good chapter in Bruce McCullough, *Representative English Novelists, Defoe to Conrad*. The introduction by Lionel Trilling in your Riverside text is the best you can get.

𝒮

Emily Brontë, *Wuthering Heights*

THE POSSIBILITY OF CONTRADICTORY THEMES
IN *WUTHERING HEIGHTS*

<u>The Moral Magnificence of Unmoral Passion</u>. ("Unmoral" to be taken in the sense of defiance of social convention.)

<u>The Futility of Unmoral Passion</u>. (The vanity of rebellion against social convention.)

Neither of these themes is necessarily correct. But they are antithetical. The job is to discover which theme is fulfilled by the various elements in *Wuthering Heights*.

ELEMENTS OF TECHNIQUE

Suggestive questions:

<u>Point of View</u>. What does point of view contribute to the meaning of *Wuthering Heights*? Who tells the story of Heathcliff and Catherine? Why Lockwood? Why Nelly Dean? Is it significant that there is a contrast between the conventional attitudes of the storytellers

(Lockwood and Dean) and the rebellious attitudes of the main characters in the story they tell (Catherine and Heathcliff)? What does the attitude of Joseph contribute to the theme?

Structure-Plot. What does the arrangement of elements in the novel contribute to the theme? In the narrower sense of plot-pattern, what is the structure of the action in the Heathcliff-Catherine story? The action has four stages:

- Establishment of a special relationship between Heathcliff and Catherine and their common rebellion. This stage ends with their visit to Thrushcross Grange.

- Catherine's betrayal of her relationship with Heathcliff. This stage ends with Catherine's death.

- Heathcliff's revenge.

- Heathcliff's change and death.

In the larger sense of structure, every element in *Wuthering Heights* is used to create a tension between convention and rebellion. The conventional points of view of Lockwood and Nelly Dean conflict with the rebellious attitudes of Heathcliff and Catherine; the rebellious characters Heathcliff and Catherine conflict with such conventional characters as Hindley, Edgar, and Isabella to produce the action; Wuthering Heights contrasts with Thrushcross Grange; violent moods contrast with calm. Which way does the theme tend?

Characters and Characterization. What are the characteristics of Lockwood and Nelly Dean as opposed to those of Heathcliff and Catherine? Those of Heathcliff and Catherine as opposed to those of Hindley, Edgar, Isabella? Every character has a relevance to the theme. What is the relevance of young Catherine and Hareton at the end of the novel?

Setting. What does background contribute to the meaning of *Wuthering Heights*? Is there any significance in the time and place being Yorkshire, England, about 1847? Is social background, milieu, used to create social tensions? Is there an intended contrast, for instance, between the Liverpool slum origins of the orphan waif Heathcliff and the bourgeois luxury of the Lintons? (Actually, there is probably more significance in Heathcliff's being likened to a gypsy and his origins being mysterious.)

Atmosphere. Does setting exist in *Wuthering Heights* mainly for the creation of atmosphere, emotional tensions, moods? What does atmosphere contribute to the theme of the novel? What use do the opposing moods of storm and calm serve in relation to the theme, the explosive violence that flares up like fire and subsides into the tranquility of spring at the end?

Symbolism-Imagery. The question of atmosphere brings up the question of symbolic imagery. What do the opposing images of Wuthering Heights and Thrushcross Grange, and the atmospheres that surround them, represent in relation to the meaning of the novel? Does the author use names suggestively, symbolically? Explain the significance in the sound and meaning of *Wuthering* and *Heights, Thrushcross* and *Grange, Heathcliff,* etc.

RESEMBLANCES TO DICKENS

A Poetic Novel. Like *Great Expectations, Wuthering Heights* is impressionistic, imaginative, poetic. Meaning is emotionally suggested rather than rationally presented. Atmosphere, imagery, symbolism contribute more to meaning than does logical thought.

A Focus on the Inner Individual. Like *Great Expectations, Wuthering Heights* focuses on the inner individual. This statement, that Dickens focuses on the personal-private self rather than the public-social self, is overstatement. But the point can be made that Pip, Heathcliff, and Catherine all undergo moral development through inner suffering, though change of different kinds. Heathcliff and Catherine can hardly be said to be transformed in the manner Pip is. But their reactions, though more passive, are emotional reactions. *Great Expectations* and *Wuthering Heights* are both affairs of the heart, and tragic rather than comic, as no other novel we have studied thus far has been (though Emily Brontë surpasses Dickens in psychological penetration of character as she does in poetic imagination).

ℒ

Charles Dickens, *Great Expectations*
(1968)

In looking back, I remember that I placed Emily Brontë in contrast to Jane Austen as representative of a more suggestive, imaginative, poetic mode of expression than Austen's rational satire. I am reminded of one of Elizabeth's sentences from *Pride and Prejudice*: "I wonder who first discovered the efficacy of poetry in driving away love." Brontë explored more deeply the wilder emotional qualities of human nature; Austen stuck more closely to a narrow world of conventional society, and hers is an eighteenth-century rather than romantic sensibility. I would like to place Charles Dickens close to Emily Brontë in his poetic, imaginative mode of writing, though there is certainly a much greater social emphasis in his writing than there is in that of Brontë. In fact, there are two worlds in Dickens: the public and the private; he mediates the world of self and the world of society. Just a look at some of the important books on Dickens makes one realize that one can emphasize either of his worlds: the social world of Victorian England, or the world that explores the private self.

DICKENS AND *GREAT EXPECTATIONS*: TWO GENERAL BUT VERY IMPORTANT POINTS

The Values of Human Compassion and Feeling. These values rule Dickens' world. For Dickens, the greatest crimes are those against what he calls "natural love," crimes against the warm heart. This is Joe's virtue (that is, a compassionate heart) and Estella's vice (that is, her lack of heart). Pip's crime is his denial of heart for social expectations.

Attitudes Reflected in Technique. These attitudes of Dickens are reflected in his techniques. His language is highly colored by feeling; his meaning emerges from the imagery and symbolism of his language.

THEME, MEANING

Let me now make a few tentative passes at the subject of *Great Expectations*, its content.

Growth. On the psychological level, it concerns the growth of a young man from innocence, through disillusionment, to moral maturity and recognition. Thus, on this level, the novel concerns the growth of a young man from great expectations of selfish acquisition to a tragic recognition of warmly human values. The "tragic" depends much on which of the two endings of the novel you accept as suiting its form best.

Atonement. More deeply, more mythically and religiously, *Great Expectations* concerns a young man's atonement for the crime, or sin, of dehumanization;

that is, the denial of humane feeling, heart. Consider that Pip does more than straighten out his thinking: he endures an ordeal of fever and fire, emerging to accept Magwich as his "father."

Social Injustice. *Great Expectations* can be looked at as being primarily concerned with social injustice. The deformation of the heart, the denial of compassion, springs from social inequities, crimes committed by the paternal society upon their social children because of material values being placed higher than the human values (bourgeois luxury and snobbery).

TECHNIQUE IN *GREAT EXPECTATIONS*

Now let us look at a few technical aspects of *Great Expectations*, its form.

Point of View. Note that once again, as in *Moll Flanders*, we have first-person point of view. Can a person telling his own story be objective enough, perceptive enough, for a theme of moral growth, a theme of self-recognition?

Moral (Spiritual) Autobiography. *Great Expectations* is generally regarded as a kind of moral (spiritual) autobiography, Dickens coming to terms with his father, his heritage. *David Copperfield* is also autobiographical in an even more particular way. But in *Great Expectations* Dickens means to be more objective about his subject (that is, himself) and yet get deeper into him than in he did in *Copperfield*. *Great Expectations* belongs to Dickens' period of greater, though darker, novels, his later period of highest achievement in serious thinking and effective technique.

<u>Narrative Structure</u>. Dickens is not noted for well-made novels, tightly constructed plots. Often he worked very loosely, exploiting a character or situation for the interest of the moment, without regard to organic form or central purpose. *Great Expectations* is a notable exception to this looseness: it is very economically planned and about half the length of a typical Dickens novel. As I stated before, it can be regarded as a moral fable of innocence, fall, and regeneration, having a narrative structure that falls into three almost equal parts:

INNOCENCE. Part I is the story of Pip's natural condition in the country, responding and acting instinctively and therefore virtuously. Part I corresponds to the myth of Eden and has 162 pages in the Riverside edition (RE).

FALL. In Part II, Pip has his fall, acquires his "expectations." This corresponds to the myth of the fall from innocence. Pip renounces his simple origins, because of mistaken assumptions, and moves to the city. He now acts through selfish calculation rather than from natural love. This part has 165 pages in RE.

REGENERATION, REDEMPTION, RECOGNITION. In Part III, you wish to place or emphasize the religious or mythical aspects of this phase of Pip's development. Pip loses his "expectations" but grows morally. He abandons false values, returns to the simple ones of his childhood with a clearer though less optimistic view of the human situation. This happens after a purgation of fire and fever, a kind of death of his old self, and there is a renunciation, if one accepts the ending Dickens first intended. In RE, Part III covers 165 pages. Altogether, there is a nice tight structure for the narrative of the moral fable. (Note the resemblance to the progress of *Tom Jones*, the same romantic indictment of the city.)

Setting. The setting, that is social background or social milieu, is Victorian England about 1860. What does setting contribute to the total form and meaning of *Great Expectations*? Is Pip a product of his social environment? Are his "great expectations" of selfish luxury and social snobbery typical of his milieu? Is Dickens indicting the material values of his day? As I suggested before, should we say that the focus of the novel is on Victorian values rather than on Pip, on society rather than on self? At any rate, setting cannot be ignored as central to the total form and meaning of the novel.

Symbolic Imagery. My last point on Dickens' artistic techniques in this novel I want to consider under the term "symbolic imagery." This term includes imagery, atmosphere, and a kind of symbolism.

IMAGERY. By imagery, I mean the representation of sensuous experience, sense "pictures," through the language of the novel. E.g., the image of the Great Salt Marsh dominates the novel.

ATMOSPHERE. By atmosphere, I mean the mood, the emotional background, evoked by the elements of the novel, basically by its imagery. E.g., a mood of cold horror, a kind of death of the heart, is evoked by the imagery of the Great Salt Marsh.

SYMBOL. By a symbol, I mean something in the novel which stands for or suggests a different plane of meaning from the literal. E.g., the atmosphere, the mood and feeling evoked by the image of the marsh, becomes symbolic in suggesting the denial of warmth, that is coldness of heart in human affairs. It symbolizes the denial of "natural love."

To summarize this example of symbolic imagery central to the significance of *Great Expectations*: the image (sense impression) of the Great Salt Marsh evokes an atmosphere (a mood, a feeling) of cold horror that is symbolic in suggesting a kind of death of the heart. The death of the heart is related to both the condition of self and society, to the condition of Pip and Victorian England in their "great expectations." This mode of expressing meaning is imaginative, poetic.

SUMMARY

What Dickens expresses, ultimately in *Great Expectations*, and in many of his best novels, is the death and rebirth of love in Victorian England. There is a somber and important aspect in Dickens' later, so-called darker, best novels. There is the close association of his characters with the taint of guilt. There is a theme of crime and punishment, the crime being the dehumanization of life, the chilling of humane impulses in Victorian society, the punishment being the kind of alienation that Pip suffers through.

BIBLIOGRAPHY: Along the lines I have just been emphasizing, the very best thing on *Great Expectations* is Dorothy Van Ghent's piece in *The English Novel: Form and Function.* Also good is Mark Spilka's "Dickens' *Great Expectations*: A Kafkian Reading" in Shapiro's *Twelve Original Essays on* Great Expectations. My own prejudice. Note a few important books on Dickens: Humphrey House, *The Dickens World* (1941); J. Hillis Miller, *Charles Dickens, The World of His Novels* (1958); Earle Davis, *The Flint and the Flame, The Artistry of Charles Dickens* (1963).

∅

George Eliot, *Adam Bede*
(1968)

ELIOT'S MODERNITY

Eliot's lengthy intrusions and moral strenuousnes may seem old-fashioned and boring to present-day readers. Nevertheless, she is generally regarded as the first modern novelist writing in English. She is given credit for beginning a new phase in the English novel for two reasons:

Intellectual Approach. Eliot (Mary Ann Evans) did not write to lightly amuse or entertain, but to instruct. She was even more serious in purpose than Austen. She consciously planned her novels as serious criticisms of life, as dramatic presentations of moral philosophy and moral judgment. She was artistically concerned with the form, the shape, the structure of her novels. All the elements in them serve an intellectual idea.

Psychological Realism. Eliot penetrates, in a realistic sense, more deeply into the inner life of her characters than any novelist up to her time. Complex motivations and changes in character development are carefully traced and psychologically consistent. Psychological analysis is largely done undramatically by the omniscient author, but Eliot comes close to the modern stream of consciousness technique, even to unconscious motivations, in her handling and analysis of the moral conscience of Hetty Sorrel and Arthur Donnithorne.

ELIOT AS AN ETHICAL REALIST WHO IS IN TECHNIQUE A PSYCHOLOGICAL REALIST

Moral Position. Eliot's moral position is basic to the understanding of her novels. Eliot believed that human actions produce inevitable and inescapable consequences, for which the person who commits the action is responsible. Life, she thought, was just: the virtuous, in terms of natural morality, will be rewarded and the vicious punished, as the natural result of their deeds. Eliot was concerned with the problem of free ethical responsibility in an age (intellectual milieu) which increasingly stressed naturalistic conditioning and determination.

Doctrine of the Deed. The central theme of Eliot has been called the "doctrine of the deed": the idea that a man is morally responsible for the inescapable consequences of the acts he freely commits. There is a kind of paradox here, but the whole of *Adam Bede* can be regarded as an exposition of this central doctrine. E.g.,

- Rev. Irwine says to Arthur Donnithorne, "Consequences are unpitying. Our deeds carry their terrible consequences—consequences that are hardly ever confined to ourselves."

- Eliot on Arthur: "Our deeds determine us, as much as we determine our deeds."

Compare this ethical realism of Eliot with the later (next) amoral, though poetic, naturalism of Thomas Hardy in *Tess of the D'Urbervilles*. Both Eliot and Hardy, in the sexual lives of Hetty and Tess, show the natural consequences of human acts, but whereas Eliot, almost cruelly, makes Hetty morally responsible for her deeds, Hardy shows Tess to be a victim of heredity and her social environment. To Eliot, Hetty is guilty; to Hardy, Tess is innocent. To Eliot, life is just; to Hardy, life is unjust.

TECHNICAL CONSIDERATIONS

Point of View. Eliot is omniscient author and intrusive, according to the convention set by Fielding, but she does not use this point of view purposely to widen the time gap (spoil the illusion of immediacy) between reader and incident, as does Fielding, and the total effect of *Adam Bede* is probably more dramatic than that of *Tom Jones*. Eliot's intrusions, as with Fielding, support the moral emphasis of the novel. The intrusions are didactic; Eliot uses her omniscience to penetrate the moral consciences of her characters, as well as to make outside comments.

Form and Shape. The form and shape of *Adam Bede* spring from a reciprocity between certain key characters and the community. The form of the novel is shaped by the relations of an inner circle, a small group of characters (Adam, Hetty, Arthur, Seth,

Dinah), with an outer circle of characters who are the community, the social world in which the moral dilemma of the smaller circle must be resolved. The action of the novel depends upon the relation of the inner circle of central characters to the outer circle of the surrounding social community. As I said, the relation is reciprocal: the moral dilemma of the main characters cannot happen, cannot exist, without the traditional morality of the community; and the community is affected and changed by the actions of the main characters (Hetty's downfall does irreparable damage to the moral character of the community). Thus, the sequence of the actions is a pattern of individual-community relationships through which the meaning of the novel is released.

NARRATIVE STRUCTURE. This sequence of action (plot, narrative structure) which traces the moral dilemma of the main characters is simple and symmetrical. Note that three scenes join the inner and outer circles of the characters in the novel, and also divide it into almost equal parts: (1) the assembly of villagers on the green to hear the preaching in Book I; (2) their assembly at the birthday feast in Book III; and (3) their assembly at the harvest supper in Book VI.

ATMOSPHERE-TONE-TEMPO. The atmosphere of *Adam Bede* is that of rustic simplicity, a rural leisureliness, a pastoral quietness that is homey, Wordsworthian, Hayslopian—with, to suit the "doctrine of the deed," a hard core in it for consequences, symbolized by such place names as Stoniton and Snowfield in Hetty's journey. The tempo of the novel suits the pace of the rural community, usually slow-moving, leisurely.

A COMPLEMENTARY THEME IN THE NOVEL

Really, there are two movements in *Adam Bede*, and thus far I have stressed just one, the movement of natural justice, the "doctrine of the deed": "Our deeds determine us, as much as we determine our deeds."

Mercy and Compassion. There is a complementary, sometimes contrary movement in the novel. Without it, we cannot fully understand Adam's importance as the central, title character, or Dinah's significance, or the joining in marriage of Adam and Dinah, after the theme of consequences has been fulfilled in the tragedy of Arthur and Hetty: the movement of mercy and compassion, the idea that justice must be tempered by mercy in a world of hard consequences. Rather than an artificial appendage to the plot, the marriage of Adam and Dinah is a union that completes a total meaning of the novel, which is broader than the doctrine of moral consequences.

Pride Must Learn Humble Compassion. In judging on moral questions, pride must learn humble compassion through deep sorrow; feeling must inform the reason (common-sense). Dinah must be joined to Adam—for "in the midst of life we are in death," and during our short life there is little enough time to show mercy and tenderness to the frail companions (Hetty and Thias Bede) of our life's journey.

NOTE: I understand Eliot's intention in joining Adam and Dinah, but the marriage doesn't seem right to me. I suppose I can't credit Dinah's having compassion or Adam's gaining it.

⌀

Thomas Hardy, *Tess of the D'Urbervilles*

NATURAL FATALITY IN *TESS*

<u>Fatality in the Nature of Human Existence</u>. One way of stating the theme of *Tess* is to say that the novel expresses a fatality in the nature of human existence which works against human happiness—that caught between his hereditary instinctive nature and his developing social (moral) consciousness, man (woman, in the case of Tess—naturally) is doomed to frustration and despair. Looking back, we can see that there is in Hardy the same concern for the inevitable consequences of natural law that George Eliot had.

<u>Victimization by Natural and Human Laws</u>. However, unlike Eliot, Hardy does not stress man's (Tess') moral responsibility, but rather his (her) victimization by natural and social laws: Tess is a victim of her sexual development, the hereditary decay of her family (mother and father—what did she inherit from each?), and society's moral law (religious in the case of Angel Clare) which natural man cannot fulfill, in the present state of his development.

<u>Atmosphere of Magic and the Supernatural</u>. Further, Hardy does not fulfill his theme merely by plot development (narrative structure) or authorial comment (statement). There is, of course, plenty of both of these. The plot by a sequence of coincidences and accidents normally impossible emphasizes a natural fatality that dooms human beings; and Hardy over and over states this theme in his own voice. But, what is more significant, Hardy impregnates his novel with an atmosphere of magic and the supernatural (unnatural fatality) that gives the reader an emotional sense (feeling) of fatality and doom.

<u>Tess' Personal Dilemma</u>. One need not agree with the theme I have just stated: natural fatality in the conditions of human existence. It is possible to look at *Tess* as a personal rather than human dilemma, not symbolizing general human doom but Tess' personal problem—as she is caught between the biological circumstances of her growth into young womanhood and the Victorian sexual mores. Arnold Kettle (Introduction to *The English Novel*, II) says that Tess symbolizes the disintegration and destruction of the English peasantry, England's agricultural society, under the impact of capitalistic urbanization and mechanization; in other words, Tess symbolizes the victimized peasantry.

IDEAS

<u>A Sad Fatality</u> in the nature of things that works toward human misery.

<u>A Malevolent Providence</u> working evil in human life.

<u>An Impotent or Unconcerned Providence</u> unable or unwilling to prevent evil in the lives of men.

BIBLIOGRAPHY: Once again, I think the same of Van Ghent's analysis of *Tess* as of *Adam Bede* (she is not always best, but always good). Look into her essay if you wish. In general, Harvey Webster's *On a Darkling Plain* is the best book on Hardy. Webster traces Hardy's intellectual growth from religious faith, to fatalism, to naturalistic determinism, to finally meliorism. Each element is discernible in *Tess*.

ℒ

Joseph Conrad, *Lord Jim*

TRANSITION FROM ELIOT AND THEME

Inner Motivation of Character. The link between Eliot and Conrad is their common interest (a growing interest of novelists) in inner motivation of character. The problem of *Lord Jim* is approximately the same as that in *Adam Bede*, with a more penetrating psychological focus: the problem of moral will in man.

Conscious and Unconscious Will. The theme of Conrad's novel could be said to be the conflict between the conscious and unconscious will in any man (I realize that "unconscious will" might pose a contradiction to some minds; substitute "motivation" for "will"). The theme concerns not just Jim, or Marlow, or Stein, or the French lieutenant, or Captain Brierly—but all of us. Jim is "one of us," as the novel states.

Questions. The immediate questions to be asked when you read the novel are "Why did Jim jump from the *Patna*?" and "Why did he sacrifice himself in Patusan?" More important, the ultimate question to be asked is "Why do we do what we do?" "Are we (men) heroes or victims?" "Does the naked self reveal horror or glory?"

The Problem of Moral Will. The problem of moral will (possession or lack of it) is dramatized in *Lord Jim* as the conflict between illusion (a begging term) and reality (also a begging term) in one man's idea of himself, the difference between the idealistic, romantic dream of self and the world, the difference between his aspirations and his accomplishments. These antitheses can be taken tentatively as the theme of *Lord Jim*. In the probing of the moral will *Adam Bede* and *Lord Jim* have a similarity in significant meaning.

TECHNIQUE OF *LORD JIM*—GENERAL COMMENTS

Contrast between *Adam Bede* and *Lord Jim*. Whereas *Adam Bede* and *Lord Jim* have a similar psychological meaning, they differ greatly in technique whereby the meaning is released (and one should note that Conrad's method considerably modifies his meaning). Eliot uses the omniscient author to probe the minds of her characters. Conrad studies Lord Jim more objectively from many angles. The study of Jim is more external; he is studied more in his actions that in his thoughts.

Complexities. The problem and theme of *Lord Jim* are psychologically complex; so is the technique used by Conrad in telling the story of Jim. His use of the narrator Marlow is notorious for complication, some think unnecessary complication. But a complex theme demands a complex method to reveal it—or, rather, the complex technique creates the complex meaning. The extent of Marlow's and our human involvement with Jim and the complexity of the problem of self give us the key to the complex point of view and structure

used in *Lord Jim*; or, rather, again, the point of view
and structure reveal the tenuous theme—and pose, if
not answer, the ultimate question: Why do we do what
we do? Can we follow our ideals?

<u>Special Elements of Technique in *Lord Jim*</u>. Conrad is
particularly noted for three techniques, which I shall
stress in relation to the theme of *Lord Jim*: (1) narrator
Marlow; (2) chronological involution of plot; and (3) illustrative episode.

POINT OF VIEW

<u>Omniscient Narrator</u>. Conrad is omniscient narrator of
the novel's first four chapters. These chapters outline
Jim's career and lead to the crucial scene aboard the
Patna. They also introduce Marlow, a spectator at the
Patna Inquiry, Jim' s trial for desertion of the ship.

<u>Marlow</u>. Marlow becomes the narrator at the beginning
of the fifth chapter. Through him are introduced many
points of view regarding Jim's character and career—
what may be called reflectors of a complex problem.

<u>Commentators</u>. The reader of *Lord Jim* depends for in-
formation and attitude upon the following commentators on Jim's character: the author (a character in the
novel, since Marlow writes him a letter), Jim himself,
Marlow, the chief engineer of the *Patna*, Brierly, the
two Malay quartermasters, the French lieutenant,
Chester, Jim's first employer (the owner of a rice mill),
his second employer (Egstrom), Stein, Jewel, Corne-
lius, Jim's father (in a letter given to Marlow), Gentle-

man Brown, and Tamb `Itam. The three most signifi-
cant points of view beside Marlow's are Brierly's, the
French lieutenant's, and Stein's (the first two are very
indirect).

<u>Advantages of Multiple Points of View</u>. For a complex
psychological problem, Conrad secured the advantage
of many points of view. The function of Marlow is to
synthesize the several angles of vision, the disparate
material of the novel. He is the witnesser of witnesses—the advocate and prosecutor—and perhaps
judge of Jim's character. Conrad's technical "device" in
the case of Marlow—and Conrad's other "devices"—
represents much more than a "device." It represents
extreme ethical scrupulosity, even anxiety; because
the truth about a man is at once too immense and too
delicate to allow failure of carefulness in the examiner
of his character. And Jim's case is not an absolute but
a relative; it has meaning only in relation to what
men's minds can make of it. Marlow provides the necessary medium of an intelligent and morally concerned
consciousness that recognizes the relativity and irony
of judging human motivations, since he himself, in his
conscious perplexity, is a concrete example of relativity.

CHRONOLOGICAL INVOLUTION OF PLOT

There is a close connection between point of view and
the structure of events in *Lord Jim*: (1) the author gives
a broad outline of Jim's career; (2) Marlow appears at
the crucial point in the story, the Inquiry into Jim's
desertion of the *Patna*; (3) and various commentators

are brought in through Marlow to cast light on the significance of this action, largely on Jim's subsequent behavior.

Two Parts. Basically, the novel is in two parts: (1) the *Patna* half with its exposure of Jim's limitations, the contrast between his social ideal desire to save others (savior role) and his actual abandonment of the *Patna* pilgrims (betrayer role); and (2) the Patusan half which amplifies the gulf between heroic thinking and heroic acting.

Violation of Chronology. This double story *seems* straight enough. But Lord Jim's story is not told straight. Conradian violation of chronology takes the reader not into the middle of things (as in the epic) but to a point after the fact, then before the fact, then around and around the fact—an artistic evasiveness that brings added perception to the complexity of the moral problem.

ILLUSTRATIVE EPISODE

An episode is defined as a sequence of actions that is (or seems to be) unrelated to the main course of events, a parenthetical byway from the main road of action. And here again Conrad's technique is closely related to the point of view. The illustrative episodes in *Lord Jim* concern characters who serve as commentators on Jim's character—particularly Brierly, the French lieutenant, and Stein. Their stories seem to have little or no connection with Jim's—yet they shed light on Jim's moral problem, usually by contrast of attitude. They give other possible reactions to the conflict between dream and reality (for instance, the French lieutenant plays a high-grade Sancho to Jim's Quixote) in order to deepen our sense of involvement in the moral dilemma. Conrad employs these illustrative episodes as though they were purely irrelevant— but they are far from that.

COMMENTS ON CHARACTERS

<u>Brierly</u>. When he faces the reality of evil in himself, he kills himself because his egoism cannot stand even a small blemish. He takes himself too seriously, as the French lieutenant would have it.

<u>French Lieutenant</u>. The French lieutenant lives with his knowledge, practically. One must make a face to the world; "you have got to live with the truth."

<u>Jim</u>. Jim follows his egoistic dream of self till it destroys him. He is true to his dream (but is the dream true to life?). Jim never admits guilt. He is only sorry to have missed a chance to be heroic, to fulfill his romantic sense of self. Jim will not admit the reality of evil—in the world, in Brown, in himself (though it baffles him) because of his egoistic dream. Therefore the tragic consequence. Marlow is afraid to admit the same thing, for Jim "is one of us."

<u>Stein</u>. Stein is also true to his dream, but life is kinder to his dream. Even so, he grows disillusioned.

Joseph Conrad, *Heart of Darkness*

APPROACH TO *HEART OF DARKNESS*

For content (meaning), *Heart of Darkness* has more than one connected level of experience in it, but I shall take a certain direction.

<u>Deadness of Heart</u>. Very generally, it is about deadness of heart, the loss of humanly responsible heart. Looking forward to *Women in Love*, and backward to *Great Expectations* and *Wuthering Heights*, what happens to Kurtz (and his society) is what will happen to Gerald Crich, the industrialist, in *Women in Love*: the heart, the inner Being, goes bad (think of Lockwood's nightmare). The conscious Will (to use Lawrence's dichotomy) becomes a lust for power in a mechanical world. And all this in the name of idealism. It is not the savages, in themselves, who are evil. In themselves, they are magnificent; they have their own splendor and integrity. It is what the instinctive force (the heart) has been harnessed to and for that is evil.

<u>The Modern World as Wasteland</u>. Conrad, in *Heart of Darkness*, is giving us a view of the modern world, as he saw it, a "wasteland" of wrong values: ferociously

acquisitive; predatory materialism and imperialism that sacrifice human bonds and sympathy for wealth. Think of all the unvoiced and voiced (from Holland's radio stations among other places) responses to Martin Luther King's assassination that echo Kurtz's words: "Exterminate the brutes." Note the picture on the cover of your text: Kurtz has become the dead ivory (bone) he covets.

A Process of Initiation. *Heart of Darkness* is early Conrad, and it has been said that *Heart of Darkness* marks Conrad's arrival at maturity of vision about human nature and the experience of life. For Marlow (as for Leggatt in *The Secret Sharer*) the content of the novel is a process of growing up—initiation, apprenticeship, education in the truth of life. I am leading to a few points on the form, the artistic method in *Heart of Darkness.*

TECHNIQUE

Point of View. Point of view (the mind through which we get the content of the novel) is typical Conrad: Marlow is in the foreground telling one of his stories. But behind Marlow is the prime narrator, somebody reporting Marlow's story (possibly Conrad)—and Kurtz is in the center of their interest. We are left with a question: Should Kurtz be our center of attention, or should it be Marlow, or should it be the narrator behind Marlow, or should it be ourselves? To whom does the moral problem belong?

<u>Narrative Structure</u>. The narrative structure of *Heart of Darkness* (the effective arrangement of events in the story) is a simple one. I shall concentrate on the progression of images in the novel.

JOURNEY DOWN THE RIVER. Like the narrative structure of *Huckleberry Finn*, the pattern of events is determined by a journey down a river, a journey which becomes a quest for knowledge. Events follow the course of the river into the heart of darkness, into the interior of Africa.

INNER JOURNEY. The narrative structure, the journey into the heart of darkness, becomes a symbol for an inner journey.

IMAGES. The most important point to make about the form of *Heart of Darkness* is the series of images along the course of the narrative structure, this journey down a river—images that finally focus on Kurtz. We begin with the Dantean image of a Stygian marsh and a river that leads to an Inferno. As with Dante's journey to the pit of Hell, the growing darkness is central to the imagery.

DISCOVERY OF A HORROR. The journey and the external structure correlate with an interior quest that culminates in the discovery of a horror ("The horror! The horror!"). The images along the way are images of the "wasteland" of the human heart, images of "hollow" men and a "hollow" society—as understood by T. S. Eliot (another user of Dante) when he used Conrad's story allusively in both *The Waste Land* and in

"The Hollow Men." "Mr. Kurtz—he dead" (the epigraph to "The Hollow Men") does not merely refer to physical death.

THE HEART IS LIFELESS. For society, the ideal has gone bad, evil.

BIBLIOGRAPHY: Leonard F. Dean, *Joseph Conrad's* Heart of Darkness: *Backgrounds and Criticisms*; Bruce Harkness, *Conrad's* Heart of Darkness *and the Critics*; Frederick R. Karl, *A Reader's Guide to Joseph Conrad*; F. R. Leavis, *The Great Tradition*; Marvin Mudrick, *Conrad* (Twentieth Century Views); Mark Schorer, *Modern British Fiction* (contains Guerard).

☙

D. H. Lawrence, *Women in Love*

LAWRENCE'S WORLD VIEW: TWO POLARITIES

There are for Lawrence two directions that men, mankind, can take, two polarities.

<u>Conscious Will</u>. At one extreme, conscious Will (by "conscious" I mean only to emphasize ego-oriented), if an unreversed direction, is bad.

<u>Unconscious Being</u>. The other, unconscious Being (by unconscious I mean only to emphasize not ego-oriented), is better, because, Lawrence thinks, human society (Western) has gone too far in the direction of conscious Will.

<u>*Persona* and *Anima*</u>. Roughly, Will and Being correspond to *persona* and *anima,* the primal powers: undercurrents of energy life principle (in Jungian terms), mind consciousness and blood consciousness (in Lawrentian terms), masculine and feminine properties. At either extreme is a kind of death; the extreme of conscious Will is death in life, the extreme of unconscious Being is life in death.

Perfection in Love. Perfection in love is harmony of counterpoint between the two, a balance in which the two lovers are separate, in being themselves, yet one in rapport, like two stars.

THEMES IN THE NOVEL

Lawrence illuminates the relations of his characters in the oscillations of sexual force between the two polarities, oscillations of attraction and repulsion in the operation of male and female wills, conscious and unconscious.

The Tension between Will and Being. If conscious Will, intellect, mind consciousness, as Lawrence calls it, uses the life force as a means of domination, exploitation, as a lust for power, the result will be death in life, turning the individual icy cold and turning the world into a sterile, mechanical wasteland. Note the images of coldness, frozen iciness, sterility, rigidity that cluster around the industrialist Gerald Crich. He is out to order life, mechanize society, subdue the life force to the uses of his conscious Will. Salvation, for Lawrence (usually too consciously preached by Birkin), lies in reversing the fatal direction of conscious Will that Lawrence thinks Western culture has taken.

Couples. Lawrence's characters must be viewed in terms of a tension between these polarities, conscious Will and unconscious Being; certainly the two central relationships of characters—Gudrun-Gerald and Ursula-Rupert—must be looked at this way. By and large and finally, in the progress of the novel, Gudrun and Gerald, as I have intimated, take the wrong direction (toward conscious Will) and Ursula and Rupert take the right direction.

GUDRUN-GERALD. Between Gudrun and Gerald there develops a struggle between two powerful wills in which Gudrun (in a sense) wins by destroying Gerald, as she knows she will—and is herself destroyed (that is, her Being, the life force in her is destroyed). Really, Gerald's death is a kind of suicide, for, to Lawrence, the conscious will to power is one sort of death wish (the death of Being). Gudrun's will, which Gerald wishes to subdue to his own, is a fatal attraction for him, and for Gudrun the attraction is the same. Gerald's direction toward death and Gudrun's victory—if you can call it that—is suggested over and over from the beginning of the novel as an operative fatality in the life force. Gerald is an industrialist and his ultimate direction represents the death that comes from the brutal suppression of life to a mechanical social order. Gudrun's conscious Will means death for Art, the suppression of Art to mechanics, for Gudrun is an artist.

Gerald Crich the industrialist and the colorful Gudrun the artist: they are both death in life, if one understands death (and life) to be the exercise of the conscious Will toward the exclusion of Being. Gudrun Brangwen and Gerald Crich are close to a state of balance in the canoe in the crucial chapter "Water-Party," but the drowning breaks the delicate balance of their relation and confirms (symbolized by Gerald's plunging to icy depths) their trend to a battle of conscious wills that ends in a frozen waste.

URSULA-RUPERT. Ursula Brangwen and Rupert Birkin (D. H. Lawrence and his wife Frieda) break in the other direction. Ursula and Rupert fumble their way in the direction of Being (not completely satisfactorily for most critics), each toward a freedom and love that do not violate the Being of the other. They are, at the extreme they never reach, life in death, if one understands death (and life) as the exclusion of the conscious Will in a state of complete Being. At the extreme, it is withdrawal from the world of human society. Short of this the ideal state (and it remains ideal, though sometimes felt) seems to be the tremulous and delicate balance of free and separate stars (beings) in the rapport, the oneness of mutual orbit, which Birkin refuses to call "love" because love signifies physical dependence or domination.

Sexual Forces. You must remember that I have simplified these directions, these polarities, for the sake of understanding.

ATTRACTION AND REPULSION. *All* characters are combinations of attractions and repulsions generated by conscious Will and unconscious Being in the operation of the life force, the sexual force. And in certain combinations, conscious Will can be either sexually attractive or repulsive, as can be unconscious Being in certain combinations. In the operation of the life force, sexual energy, there is both desire to dominate and to be dominated. Characters thrill to both impulses. And characters are torn by the polarities within themselves as they encounter combinations of polarities in other characters, man to man and woman to woman. Rupert

Birkin, who represents the tendency toward the extreme of unconscious Being, blood consciousness, is both attracted to and repulsed by Gerald Crich, who represents the extreme of conscious Will, mind consciousness—as Gerald is both attracted to and repulsed by him.

HOMOSEXUAL LOVE. Here is suggested a possibility of perfection in the love of male and male (e.g., as Rupert says to Gerald, in referring to their blood brotherhood, "you waste your best self"). Homosexual female love of this sort is also suggested in the novel. Ursula and Gudrun complement each other; they both hate and love each other. Gudrun, although her direction in the novel is toward conscious Will, has in her a good deal of unconscious Being (female, *anima*), and Rupert, whose direction is toward unconscious Being, has in him more than a good bit of conscious Will. His *Salvator Mundi* aspect, his preaching of ideas, is what Ursula dislikes about him, though she certainly has a conscious Will of her own. (Here is an irony that Lawrence recognized in himself: he knew that the structuring of ideas in words kills life, yet that he must preach ideas.)

DOMINATION AND SUBMISSION. These combinations of sexual attraction and repulsion, often seemingly paradoxical, must be kept in mind, otherwise scenes in the novel will be unnecessarily difficult to interpret. For example, in the important scene of Gerald's cruel exercise of his will over the mare at the railroad crossing, Gudrun is both attracted and repulsed by his domination. She is attracted to a struggle of strong wills, and she is attracted to submitting to a strong will. But she is also revolted by submission to a strong will and the annihilation of her own. The images are sexually suggestive. Dominantly, Gudrun is attracted to Gerald's will (see "Diver" and opening paragraphs of "Sketch-Book") and hates Ursula for her weakness, for the naked revelation of her being. The experience for Gudrun is orgasmic (she swoons). Gudrun and Gerald will be locked in a duel of wills to the death; Gudrun's will is a mare that Gerald cannot finally ride.

FORM IN *WOMEN IN LOVE*

What I am saying is very important, for Lawrence's concern is not with character revelation in relation to social activity; his interest is in the character's psychic center, which Lawrence saw in physical terms, terms of sexual forces, and imaged them that way. *Women in Love* does not have the plot structure of a typical novel. The novel is a series of scenes like the one at the railroad crossing, and the action and the images of these scenes symbolically reveal the tension of attraction and repulsion in the operation of the life force. It is this oscillation, this pulsation of forces in the scenes, that one follows in the novel, rather than plot in the ordinary sense.

Illustration. To illustrate, the chapter "Rabbit" symbolically extends the pulsating tension of attraction and repulsion that was earlier revealed in the scene at the railroad crossing, and before that in earlier contacts between the two. It is a horrid understanding they have reached of each other in "Rabbit." Theirs is a pact of death, and they will move on to death, in the sense that the direction of the conscious Will, in extremity, *is* the direction of death.

No Plot Resolution. But *Women in Love* has no resolution of plot in the conventional sense. There is only the oscillating movement, the extended pulsation of tension in the action and images of scenes that comes to a sort of climax in "Snowed Up." Ursula and Rupert move closer and closer together in the direction of unconscious Being, their separate entities presumably more and more in rapport, but free to be their own selves. Gudrun and Gerald move closer and closer together in their battle of conscious Wills till Gerald loses in the frozen waste when Gudrun's will is joined to Loerke—for death in Art.

Women in Love as Poetry. *Women in Love* is not an ordinary novel, but a kind of poetry, a symbolism of image and action, mixed with discursive statement, its pages frustratingly packed with action and image that dramatize the complications I have tried to explain, complications in the relations of the two sisters and their lovers (Ursula Brangwen and Rupert Birkin, Gudrun Brangwen and Gerald Crich). The former pair goes the right direction toward renewal of life, and the latter pair goes the wrong direction toward what Lawrence considers death. A good place to start is in "The Class-room" with the lesson of the catkins. In the opening chapters, the two sisters are seen groping toward love and the fulfillment of their beings. Now in this chapter Birkin illustrates, pictorially, with a natural image, what love and fulfillment of one's being should be: the yellow and red catkins, the male and female flowers, brightly colored and therefore singled out in their isolate loveliness with the pollen flying between them.

STAR EQUILIBRIUM AND THE LAWS OF ORGANIC LIFE

I know that I have not been very clear. Neither is D. H. Lawrence. The most important thing to remember in reading *Women in Love* is the idea imaged in the symbol of the stars. For the same idea, Lawrence, in *The Rainbow*, used the natural image of the rainbow, with its poles rooted in the earth. In *Women in Love,* it is star-equilibrium, the polarity of stars.

The Pure Balance of Single Beings. Men and women have been singled out, male and female, from an original mixture into what must become the pure individuality of the male and of the female; accordingly, they *must* polarize rather than merge in love (physically merged love, as we might understand it, is the emphasis on sex that Lawrence dislikes). Hence, star-equilibrium: "a pure balance of two single beings, consciously preserving their own beings [Lawrence does not reject the use of mind to preserve being; it is necessary]—as the stars balance each other." This relationship transcends physical love and preserves the sanctity of the individual being in something that is above mere sexual egotism. Yet the roots are in nature, in the physical, in the source of life, and the merging must occur for the replenishing of life.

The Central Law of Organic Life. The individual soul, Lawrence says, "submits to the yoke and leash of love, but never forfeits its own proud singleness, even while it loves and yields." The fulfillment of the individual is primary for Lawrence. He says in one of his writings that "the central law of all organic law is that each organism is intrinsically isolate and single in itself."

The Secondary Law of Organic Life. But "the secondary law of life" is that the individual can only be fulfilled through contact and communion with his fellow men and women. The most vital contact of all occurs between a man and a woman, so long as it preserves the intrinsic "otherness," male or female, of the other participant. "Men live by love, but die, or cause death, if they love too much." This is what Birkin-Lawrence is articulating through the whole of *Women in Love*.

The Meaning of Loerke. To Lawrence, Loerke, the "sewer rat," above all, represents the most evil direction of the conscious Will, the death in life of Western culture. Dirty, mental sensuality. Ego-centered, selfish, possessive. It is not that Gudrun rejects her will; she moves further than Gerald in the uses of it for sex. I am sure there is something anti-Semitic in Lawrence's treatment of Loerke, as in Ezra Pound and T. S. Eliot. Loerke is a German-Jewish name that suggests also Loki in the Volsung-Nibelung myth, the Evil One, an insidious and destructive underground force. I think he is meant to represent the Western Jew who has harnessed the deep mysteries of life to the mechanics of commerce, thus destroying life. In his crippledness he is almost a Pietà figure, to whom women rush in both pity and revulsion. Lawrence's antipathy for Christ is notorious.

∅

James Joyce, *A Portrait of the Artist as a Young Man*
(1968)

THE PSYCHOLOGICAL NOVEL

In taking up James Joyce's *Portrait of the Artist as a Young Man,* I want to note that in passing from Conrad's *Heart of Darkness* (1899) and *The Secret Sharer* (1912) to Joyce's *Portrait* (1916) and next to Lawrence's *Women in Love* (also 1916) we have penetrated well into the twentieth century and have come upon novels that can truly be called psychological in their use of techniques to probe the minds and feelings of their characters. We have also come upon World War I and upon the beginning of the modern consciousness, upon a time of crumbling traditional values, in which the artist no longer finds a correspondence between the social environment and his own thoughts and feelings. Consequently, his mind turns inward in search of personal values that would give significance to his own experience. *Portrait* and *Women in Love* are both autobiographical. Joyce found his values in a religion of art, in his recreation of the artist's intellectual consciousness; Lawrence found his in a religion of feeling (blood consciousness), of the unconscious life force.

SOME STATEMENTS ABOUT *PORTRAIT*

<u>Consciousness and Conscience</u>. The novel is about the growth of the artist's consciousness, or, perhaps, I should say the growth of his conscience, in which the hero rejects the traditional patterns of authority and relies on his own integrity as an artist.

<u>Renunciation of Church and Country</u>. It is about the artist's renunciation of the Church (perhaps symbolized by the hero's mother) and the artist's renunciation of his country, fatherland (perhaps symbolized by the hero's father). It is about the artist's self-exile from his own society. It is about the artist's resolve of *non serviam*: "I will not serve that in which I no longer believe, whether it call itself my home, my fatherland, or my church."

<u>God Within</u>. *Portrait of the Artist* is about a religious quest for worldly beauty through Art. The name of the hero, "Stephen," carries the suggestion of the mythic Christian Greek hero-seeker-martyr; "Dedalus" carries the suggestion of the mythic pagan Greek hero-seeker-fabricator. Stephen Hero, Stephen Dedalus, the martyr-maker hero. *Portrait* "depicts a young man emerging from an environmental shell of faith, family, and fatherland to fix his sights on the spirit of worldly beauty" (Thomas E. Connelly). The emphasis in this religious quest must be on the words "spirit" and "worldly." In this religious quest the artist is saved from, not by, the Church, saved from the temptations of the Church, which denies the world and the flesh which the artist affirms. Yet it is a spiritual quest:

Stephen's climactic epiphany, his revelation, is not the sacred otherworldly beauty of the Church's teachings, but the profane beauty of the world's body from which Art is created. In Art is the spirit defined. The artist finds not a God outside himself but a god within, the god of his artist's conscience, the artist as God, creator-fabricator.

TECHNIQUE IN *PORTRAIT*

<u>Point of View</u>. The point of view in *Portrait of the Artist* can be called stream of consciousness. The most important aid in understanding *Portrait* is to know that its unity is internal-psychological rather than external-social. It is not a chronological narration of objectively recorded events in time and place. The point of view, the mental perspective from which the reader gets the story (and "story" is much less important in this novel than "character"), is the highly sensitive and impressionable mind of the novel's hero, Stephen Dedalus, who is Joyce himself.

<u>Scene</u>. The novel is a series of impressions: the important thing is not the event taking place but the impact of that event in the mind of Stephen—the important thing is the series of impressions that forms the artist Stephen (James Joyce) and make his portrait, which is the novel. Unlike the traditional novel, the scene in *Portrait* is not a place in the outside world where events, in the social sense, take place; the scene of *Portrait*, its dramatic center of focus, is the consciousness, the mind, of the hero. The hero is living through a series of social events in the outside world, but the

reader gets those events as impressions in the hero's stream of consciousness.

Stream of Consciousness. *Portrait* is the first prominent and sustained use of the stream of consciousness technique in English fiction. Stream of consciousness point of view is a technique (and don't forget that it is a technique, a deliberately formulated artistic means) that attempts the illusion of spontaneous flow of thought through the mind of a character, a stream that is diverted constantly by a multitude of associations. In a stream of consciousness novel we approach identity of subject matter and technique, identity of content and form. They are both the mind of the hero, the flow of his thought—what that thought is, and the way it flows.

I am overstating now to make a point, because the form of *Portrait* is certainly not wholly determined by Stephen's spontaneous flow of thought. But it is true enough to say that whatever we learn of the characters in it, whatever we learn of a pattern of events in it, and whatever we learn of a social or physical background in it we learn from selected impressions that are filtered through the hero's mind—not told by the author as would be apparent in the syntax of the conventional third-person approach. That these impressions have been, of course, selected should emphasize my point that the form of *Portrait* is determined by something more than the spontaneous flow of thought in Stephen's mind, and that stream of consciousness is a technique, a deliberately formulated artistic means.

At any rate, *Portrait* is a complex of sense impressions, images that tend toward abstract articulation in the progress of the novel and mold Stephen's artist's conscience during his first twenty years of life. For example, as Stephen sits in his algebra class, his mind, partly occupied by the unfolding equations, ranges from Shelley, sin, and the Blessed Virgin to events of yesterday or the day before. Through memory and thought, the particular moment in class acquires levels and meanings and dimensions, concrete and abstract.

Narrative Structure

STEPHEN'S MIND. Very likely, unless you have read a study (such as Cliff Notes) which has abstracted the story, you are still very puzzled about what happens in *Portrait*. I mean that you are probably unsure of the narrative as a pattern of events that occurs in a social structure. That social structure is hard to pick out because the dramatic center of the novel is Stephen's mind, not his position in society.

THREE PHASES OF STEPHEN'S YOUTH. Nevertheless, the series of impressions that forms Stephen's conscience as an artist in his revolt against the authorities (Family, Fatherland, Church) does follow the center of Stephen's chronological development in his society. The novel is symmetrically constructed around three phases of Stephen's youth.

- First Phase. The awakening religious doubts and sexual instincts that lead to carnal sin (and other attendant deadly sins). The first two chapters trace this development to carnal sin and intense guilt feelings at the age of sixteen. The external setting in the first chapter is Clongowes Wood College, and in the second Belvedere College, Dublin.

- Second Phase. Repentance and purgation almost to the point of Stephen's taking up the priesthood. This central portion, in chapters three and four, continues the cycle of guilt and repentance at Belvedere College, Dublin, to the moment of Stephen's profane (by "profane" I mean worldly, fleshly, secular, as opposed to sacred) revelation, his epiphany of the wading girl, his vision of Art. This impression is the crisis point of the novel, Stephen's turning from the Church to Art, and follows immediately after the Director's suggestion that Stephen take up the priesthood.

- Third Phase. Stephen's assertion of independence in repudiating the Church (and Family and Country) for Art and exile in France. This fifth and final chapter, twice as long as the others, develops the theories and projects of Stephen's student days at University College, Dublin, and brings him to the verge of exiling himself. As the novel advances, Stephen becomes less impressionable to outside forces and more intent upon speculations of his own. Friends figure mainly as interlocutors to draw Stephen out on various themes. Each phase in Stephen's development increases the sense of isolation, till at the end of the third phase, the end of the novel, his self-exile (to Paris) is complete.

Devices for Psychological Cohesion. While this external structure, the pattern of Stephen's actions in society, might not have been clear to you, I am sure the inner life of Stephen was. *Portrait of the Artist* does have coherence, a psychological rather than a logical coherence. The coherence of the novel depends on emotionally suggestive (poetic) elements, what I shall call devices for psychological cohesion. These devices, though they do not violate the stream of Stephen's impressions, do provide the cohesion, continuity, and firmness in which the separate impressions merge to create the unifying theme of the novel. Closely related to each other in performing this function are three devices for psychological cohesion: *motif, epiphany,* and *symbolic dream.*

MOTIF. A motif is the expressive reiteration of a theme, in an action or statement or image, which eventuates in a significant pattern of meaning or feeling essential to the unity of the novel. Sometimes the motif is scarcely noticeable to the reader, operating below the level of his conscious awareness. At other times it may be insistently present in his consciousness. The powerful motifs in *Portrait,* its recurring themes, are Family authority, Church authority, State authority; revolt, flight, isolation, exile; the religion of Art, the dedication to Art; carnal love, spiritual love (various kinds of love are symbolized by Eileen, E.C., the Blessed Virgin, the prostitute, Mercedes, the wading girl). All these motifs run through *Portrait,* pulsating, receding and then expanding to a climax of recognition, giving the novel form and meaning.

EPIPHANY. Most of the novel's motifs are consummated in what Joyce termed "epiphanies." "Epiphany" means "an appearance" or "a manifestation." To the Christian Church it was the appearance of the star to the wise men of the East. The Feast of Epiphany (Twelfth Night) is celebrated on January 6. In *Stephen Hero* Joyce defines "epiphany" as "a sudden spiritual manifestation" and states that the artist should "record these epiphanies with extreme care, seeing that they are the most delicate and evanescent of moments." Epiphany is Joyce's artistic (profane, non-sacred) equivalent of divine inspiration, illumination, revelation. They are accompanied by powerfully evocative images. The whole of *Portrait* is crowded with these moments of mental vision; every significant impression of Stephen culminates in an inner revelation which is part of the development of the artist. The most crucial epiphanies occur climactically at the end of each chapter, the central epiphany being Stephen's vision of the wading girl.

SYMBOLIC DREAM. Symbolic dreams could be called unconscious epiphanies, although all epiphanies verge on the unconscious by their intuitive nature. Of the many dreams and waking visions in *Portrait of the Artist*, three stand out: that of the dead Parnell near the beginning; that of the wasteland of cans and goats in the middle; and that of the cave of fabulous kings and little people at the end. Functional in the structural pattern of revolt against country, religion, and family, they are pivotal to the form of the novel and the fulfillment of its theme.

Virginia Woolf, *To the Lighthouse*

"THE PERFECTED MOMENT IN LIFE AND ART":
THE SHAPE OF VIRGINIA WOOLF'S *TO THE
LIGHTHOUSE*

By and large, I am not particularly fond of the novels of Virginia Woolf, but she has a rather special technique which I think she uses very felicitously in *To the Lighthouse*. It is her one novel I enjoy reading—all in all, I believe, a little gem of form and content. My remarks about it will be quite obvious, quite simple, and quite short. We won't spend the usual length of time on this novel.

<u>Two Main Points</u> on *To the Lighthouse:* (1) fragments of consciousness (2) all pulled together into a shape.

REFLECTIONS OF CONSCIOUSNESS IN THE FLUX OF TIME. First, *To the Lighthouse* does not employ the conventional outside angle of narration (point of view). Virginia Woolf makes us look *inside* her characters, as does James Joyce. What we get in this novel is a multitude of impressions, reflections of the consciousness of the *dramatis personae*. So far as the main characters are concerned, these reflections of consciousness are associated with two locations in time and place, two occasions at the Ramsay house in the Hebrides, that are ten years apart. They are two Durations, short Durations, of human consciousness that are absorbed in what symbolizes the infinity of Time. *To the Lighthouse* presents reflections of consciousness in the flux of Time.

A SINGLE CONSCIOUSNESS. My second main preliminary point is that these reflections of consciousness make a total form or shape that is the novel; they do not remain disparate, isolated fragments, even though they do not emanate from a single consciousness.

MRS. RAMSAY AS A UNIFYING FORCE. The discordant fragments somehow are pulled together by the dominant consciousness in the novel, Mrs. Ramsay. Though Mrs. Ramsay has died before the end of Part II, the mood of her mind continues as a force till the end of Part III, and beyond. It is a force for unity and a more timeless triumph for Mrs. Ramsay than her victories at the dinner near the end of Part I. In a very true sense, Mrs. Ramsay—that is, what is her mind, her consciousness—does not die, but lives through Time to knit together into a form the disparate reflections of consciousness that exist in Duration, and to unify the novel.

It is very significant that as Mrs. Ramsay sits with her son James at the window in Part I (that is, at the first location in time from which reflections originate) she is knitting a reddish-brown heather mixture stocking. This is a homey posture. This image of Mrs. Ramsay is significant not only as a symbol of the knit strands of consciousness that are pulled together to make the novel but also a suggestion that the dominant consciousness that pulls them together is a maternal one—one that pulls a family together, one whose peculiar sensibility is not intellectual but an intelligent love and kindness that transcends hard facts, that pulls a green mantle over the cruelties and sadnesses that time brings into every life. It is significant that the stocking has not been finished by the end of Part I and that the image of the stocking is carried into Part III. Symbolically, the unifying force that gives some shape to the chaos of time continues.

FORM OF THE NOVEL

I suppose I ought now to do a bit of textual analysis, to unravel some of the strands that are knit together in a small part of the stocking. We may get to that but if not you can find an excellent job done on Chapter 5 of Part I by Erich Auerbach in *Mimesis*. I want now to comment briefly on the relation of the three parts in the shape of the novel.

Part I. In Part I, "The Window," Mrs. Ramsay is at the drawing-room window knitting, with James sitting on the floor cutting pictures from the Army and Navy Stores catalogue. It is the first location in time and place with which is associated a multiplicity of reflections of consciousness in random moments, shifting and swaying, back and forth in time: the consciousness of Mrs. Ramsay, of Mr. Ramsay, of James, of Mr. Bankes, of Lily Briscoe, and of others.

REFLECTIONS SEPARATE FROM THE EXTERNAL SCENE. These reflections are, of course, controlled in the form of the novel by the mind of Virginia Woolf, and the presence of Mrs. Ramsay does knit them together in the passage of time. They are random and free in the sense of separation from the external scene, though Mrs. Woolf does, with shifting consciousness, succeed in giving us a contrast between the depths of private illumination (a psychological focus) and the surface of events (the social scene in time and place)— a contrast which becomes a fusion of Art and Life.

MRS. RAMSAY'S ACHIEVEMENT. This fusion is precisely Mrs. Ramsay's achievement (as recognized by Lily Briscoe in Part III). In the accretion of random illuminations, we get a sense of Mrs. Ramsay's capacity for adjusting the multiplicity of discordant moments of consciousness toward completion and perfection, giving them a kind of permanence and stability that persist through the disintegration of Part II, "Time Passes."

But the permanence and stability are tenuous and accompanied by a brooding mood of sadness born from Mrs. Ramsay's sense of transience and decay, and the fundamental cruelty of life. Part I culminates in Mrs. Ramsay's maternal "triumph" in drawing together family and guests at the dinner table, and getting them off to bed—to make fragmented moments into the harmony of a day, or such harmony as can be achieved in the flux of time. "For she had triumphed again"—so Part I ends, with Mrs. Ramsay "holding her stocking" that is unfinished. She triumphs even as she communicates to Mr. Ramsay that he has been right about the weather, that there won't be a trip to the lighthouse tomorrow—without saying it.

Mrs. Ramsay's triumph is a triumph of wifely love and maternal care which gives her pleasure: "nothing on earth can equal this happiness." For, through the disintegration of time, maternal care will triumph over the central discord of Part I, which discord is Mrs. Ramsay's dread—summed up in two lines that run like a motif through Part I. These lines also sum up Mrs. Ramsay's special genius: "'But,'" said his father, stopping in front of the drawing-room window, 'it <u>won't</u> be fine.'" "'But it may be fine—I suspect it <u>will</u> be fine tomorrow,' said Mrs. Ramsay, <u>smoothing</u> James's hair." Underscore <u>won't</u> and <u>will</u> and <u>smoothing</u>. Mr. Ramsay stands for objective fact, whereas Mrs. Ramsay is striving for concord of feeling. Her attitude is more subjective, responsive: he reads the signs of the weather; she is reading the signs of the people about her.

<u>Part II</u>. Part II, "Time Passes," gives us the sense of the deterioration and disintegration which the passage of time brings—the chaos of ten years that lie between the two gatherings at the house in the Hebrides. This section is filled with a profusion of seasonal images that tend toward darkness and death and decay, toward chaos and oblivion. It suggests the dwindling spark of human consciousness in the house in the Hebrides, kept barely alive by the presence of Mrs. McNab and Mrs. Bast, then revived by the habitation of returning family and guests.

In Part II, Virginia Woolf beautifully merges the end of Part I with the beginning of Part III. The night at the end of Part I's day blends into the morning of another day, the day of Part III, ten years later. The long night, the long darkness, is the chaos of "Time Passes." The question that Part II, the middle portion of the novel, poses is, Does anything endure the passage of time? Part II opens with the words of Mr. Bankes that conclude the day of Part I: "Well, we must wait for the future to show." They point the direction to the lighthouse. Part II ends with Lily Briscoe's first reflection in the morning, but a morning ten years later: "Here she was again, she thought, sitting bolt upright in bed. Awake." It prepares us for the answer to the question, What endures? Awake Mrs. Ramsay. Awake Lily Briscoe.

Part III. In Part III, "To the Lighthouse," we get the fulfillment of Mrs. Ramsay's capacity to draw the discordant strands of life—the random impressions that make up the texture of the novel—into a unity, into a structure. It is a victory of human consciousness over disintegration by time. Mrs. Ramsay's capacity to knit discord into a unity, a shape, is what Lily Briscoe discovers she owes to Mrs. Ramsay—at the moment she completes her painting, just when the boat with Mr. Ramsay and James and Cam reaches the lighthouse. For it is the persisting genius, the presence, of Mrs. Ramsay that draws the boat to the lighthouse, to reconcile James and his father ("Well done!")—that gives Lily the moment of illumination in the completion of her painting, after ten years.

Thus, the moment of touching the lighthouse is the perfected moment for both Life and Art. Apparently, Art draws its inspiration from Life, from what Lily learns from Mrs. Ramsay, from Mrs. Ramsay's insights into life, from what the lighthouse symbolizes for Mrs. Ramsay, and must for us the reader: the alternating light and shadow of the lighthouse beam symbolizes the rhythm of joy and sorrow in human life and the alternating radiance and darkness of even the most intimate human relationships. This Mrs. Ramsay knew, and it was enough.

FINAL THOUGHTS

But though Art draws its inspiration from life, from Mrs. Ramsay, and even though Art is knit from the homely stuff of a reddish-brown stocking, there is a triumph for Art in Virginia Woolf's achievement of the perfected moment that completes the form of her novel. In deference to Virginia Woolf's art, consider finally that the structure of the book itself reproduces the effect of the lighthouse beam, the long flash represented by the first movement ("The Window"), the interval of darkness represented by the second movement ("Time Passes") and the second and shorter flash by the last movement ("To the Lighthouse"). When this aspect of the book is considered, its subject is not merely a particular group of human beings: it is life and death, joy and pain, and a woman who understood this rhythm. Incidentally, Mrs. Ramsay is Virginia Woolf's mother.

BIBLIOGRAPHY: Best critiques are Joan Bennett, *Virginia Woolf, Her Art as a Novelist;* Erich Auerbach, "The Brown Stocking," in *Mimesis.*

William Golding, *The Spire*

Golding's *The Spire* continues the twentieth-century tendency of Conrad, Lawrence, and Joyce toward concentration on the self, away from social emphasis to the study of character from within.

THE NOVEL'S VISION

Dean Jocelin's Vision. *The Spire* dramatizes Dean Jocelin's inner motivations for building a spire upon inadequate foundations, his aspiration to add a 400-foot spire to a medieval cathedral. Golding's Barchester very much resembles Salisbury Cathedral, which has the tallest spire of any cathedral in the world. Salisbury Cathedral is built on marshland, not far from Stonehenge, and modern engineers marvel that its soaring spire, slightly off the perpendicular, continues to stand.

What the Spire Means

AN ACT OF FAITH. The novel opens with Dean Jocelin's presumably innocent vision. To Jocelin the projected spire is a diagram of prayer, an act of faith, springing up to God.

SINS OF THE FLESH. Golding takes us through the gradual process of humbling and terrifying recognitions by Jocelin that his spire is far from a pure aspiration and not unmixed with evil, that it springs as much from the corruption of pride and sin within him as it does from divine aspiration, holy vision. At one stage he thinks, This I have done for my true love. Ironically considered, who was Jocelin's true love: God or Goody Pangall, the spirit or the flesh? What he thought was a good angel, leading him on, giving comfort, turned out to be a devil (in the form of Goody). What Dean Jocelin finally knows is the mysterious relation of good to evil in all the works of men and in the providence of God.

AN APPLE TREE. Yet the spire continues to stand as a testament to faith. The themes of the novel are underlined in Jocelin's last thoughts, his final recognitions: "There is no innocent work," "God knows where God may be," and "It's like the apple tree." Only God knows, man does not, where God may be, in things good and in things evil. The spire is like the apple tree, springing in leaf and blossom to the heavens, reaching, but with roots in the dark earth—like that ambiguous first tree, the tree of knowledge of good and evil, on which hung the fatal apple.

An Exercise in (Self) Revelation. From inside Jocelin, we follow his progress from blindness to sight, to seeing. *The Spire* is an exercise in seeing, a revelation. In a series of light images, Golding develops Jocelin's recognitions as ways of seeing, up to the window, "bright and open," at the end, through which Jocelin sees the spire as apple tree. Golding's main symbols are as ambiguous as the relation of good to evil in the ways of God and men. For Jocelin the spire is sometimes a diagram of prayer and an act of faith, sometimes the phallus of a man lying on his back, or a crooked and diseased spine. It is the mast of a ship, the Ark of God, a dunce's cap, and a stone hammer waiting to strike. It rises from darkness to light, and from its dizzying height Jocelin must look down, descend, to pierce and understand the cellar of his being.

The apple tree thrusts upward and downward; it touches Heaven and Hell. And it is counterpointed in the novel by the mysterious mistletoe and its red berry, associated with pagan rites and sacrificial killing, the murder of Pangall. The ambiguity of Goody Pangall is in her name: good and God, pan and gall, for what she was and what she represents. For Golding there is darkness in the heart of man, but there is also "grace," salvation to be found in self-awareness. Dean Jocelin finds it, and the spire remains standing, a testament to faith, a miracle beyond human comprehension.

♨♨♨

THE EUROPEAN NOVEL

❧❧❧

THE EUROPEAN NOVEL: BALZAC TO SOLZHENITSYN

English 334, Spring 1979

1. The Modern Novel in France

Balzac: *Père Goriot* (1834), New American Library. January 17, 19, 22, 24

Flaubert: *Madame Bovary* (1857), New American Library. January 26, 29, 31, February 2

Zola: *Germinal* (1885), New American Library. February 5, 7, 9, 12

Test: February 14

2. The Modern Novel in Russia

Turgenev: *Fathers and Sons* (1862), New American Library. February 16, 19, 21

Dostoevsky: *Crime and Punishment* (1875-1876), New American Library. February 26, 28, March 2, 5

Tolstoy: *Anna Karenina* (1875-1876), New American Library. March 7, 9, 12, 14

Test: March 16

3. 20th-Century Novels

Gide: *The Immoralist* (1902), Bantam. March 19, 21, 23

Mann: *Death in Venice* (1911) & *Seven Other Stories*, Random Vintage. March 26, 28, April 9

Kafka: *The Trial* (1924), Random Vintage. April 11, 13, 16

Hesse: *Steppenwolf* (1927), Bantam. April 18, 20, 23

Camus: *The Plague* (1947), Random Vintage. April 25, 27, 30

Solzhenitsyn: *One Day in the Life of Ivan Denisovich* (1961), New American Library. May 2, 4

YOU ARE EXPECTED TO ATTEND ALL CLASSES

(Editors' note: For discussions of novels by Turgenev, Dostoevsky, and Solzhenitsyn, see section on the Russian Novel, below.)

Introductory Lecture
(Spring 1969)

I want to open this course by making a few remarks on the words in its title: Modern & European & Novel. Really, no such separate entity exists as the European novel. Except for the English Channel and the Atlantic Ocean, it is not something totally distinct from the modern English novel and the modern American novel. But the title of this course is a good way to bring together and to group some (though not all) of the best Continental novelists who wrote over a century and a half. It is true, however, partially because I have had to be very selective, that these novelists do more intensively reflect the "modern" element in the consciousness of Western man than do my selections in the English novel and the American novel. Therefore, in this course I am likely to stress, at my peril, the intellectual rather than the artistic aspects of particular novels. So we ought to begin by asking, What do I mean by "modern novel," and, What do I mean by the "modern element" in it?

THE "MODERN" NOVEL

The term "modern novel" is redundant and repetitive. There is, really, no such thing as an unmodern novel. The novel as a literary form is itself a modern development. By "modern" I do not mean contemporary or current with our own times: I mean something that defines a period of recognizable shift, change, in the consciousness of Western man. The literary type (genre) of the novel—as distinct from the romance—is by definition modern (that is, post-Renaissance) because it is a literary form that developed out of, and concurrently with, the modern consciousness of Western man.

My emphasis is on the word "consciousness." It is usually said that Cervantes' *Don Quixote* (1605 & 1615) is the prototype of the modern novel because it artistically reveals this modern consciousness. In the realistic prose of a modern vernacular language, Cervantes develops in his plot a conflict, a disparity between two worlds: the world of the private self, the individual's inner world of imagination and idealization, and the so-called real world outside the self, the practical work-a-day world, the world of structured society that often seems antagonistic to the fulfillment of private desires. In the art of Cervantes the conflict between self and society is hard for the reader to resolve in terms of the author's intent. The art of Cervantes is ambivalent, balancing two worlds. Is the old man mad or is the world of society degenerate? Does the truth reside in him or in the world outside him? The drama for the reader is the conflict between the two worlds, a

conflict the reader consciously realizes, and, perhaps, so does Don Quixote.

TOWARD AN EXPRESSION OF THE PRIVATE SELF

This conscious recognition of disparity between self
and society is the modern element in the novel; the
whole history of the novel's development is modern
in the sense that in the novel self and society tend
to be polarized, stand apart from each other. The
very fact that the novel is ostensibly (that is, pretends to be) a story (that is, an abstraction from
human experience) in prose testifies that the artist
must work with a social language, a form of rational
communication that restricts his private insight.
Poetic imagination and prosaic reality are at odds.
The history of the novel, and of our Western society,
shows that the increasing difficulty of finding personal identity has forced a gap between the artist
(that is, novelist) and society, has produced revolt,
alienation, dis-affiliation.

In point of view, the novel has plunged further
and further inward to stream of consciousness, interior monologue, or lyrical-confessional forms, in
which, at the extreme, the relation between the private self (at the center of the novel and now the total subject of the novel) and any external structure
is completely lost. The social context, any rational
fabric of communal selves, is destroyed as irrelevant
to a private sensation that dwells on the very edge
of conscious expression. And so we have the anti-
novel; "anti" because, it must be remembered, the
novel, at its beginning, presumed to be a rational

reflection of a society very conscious of its material reality.

THE NOVEL AS MORAL AGENT

Destroy conscious awareness, and the identity of the self is lost. Today, the problem of the novel, despite its many variations in form, is still primarily the tension of self and society, the creation of some kind of viable relation between self and society. Even in rebellion, the self must, I believe, take a conscious stance in relation to the external world in which it has its conscious existence in time, that world which depends, in fact, on the conscious existence of the self. When Lionel Trilling said that the novel of the last two hundred years (roughly our period) has been the most effective moral agent for our time, he meant that the novel has been a means to the moral identity of the self in society, a means toward preserving individual integrity from the socializing-civilizing forces that threaten to obliterate it.

Here are a few definitions of the novel that emphasize the points I have been trying to make about the novel's modernity, its cultural emergence in modern times:

- The new literary genre in *Don Quixote* (later to be called the modern novel) arose out of a changed situation of man in history, one in which incongruities between individual intentions and individual capacity for realizing them became apparent, and in which truth becomes a problem—not in the abstract nor in relation to transcendental forces but relative to man's own existence. (Ángel del Río)

- The modern novel is the search for the expression of the irrational, the soul, in and through an alien and hostile reality; the principle of its form is derived from the *consciousness that inwardness* [my italics; inwardness is significant only when consciously considered] has its own independent value. (Georg Lukács)

- The problem of reality is central to that great forefather of the novel, *Don Quixote*. There are two movements of thought in *Don Quixote*, two different and opposed notions of reality. One is the notion which leads toward saying that the world of ordinary practicality is reality in its fullness. The other notion of reality is that of the conceptual, the ideal, the fanciful, with which the first notion conflicts. (Lionel Trilling)

- The problem of the novel has always been *to distinguish* between these two, the self and society, and at the same time to find suitable structures that will present them *together* [italics mine]. (Mark Schorer)

- The novel derives its being from character, action, and milieu. More often, it transforms these entities into a process. The process is complex, elusive, manifold. It can be described, nevertheless, as an encounter: the encounter of the self with the world, or the hero with experience. Form, we see, may be the pattern which a concrete and existential encounter traces in the imagination. (Ihab Hassan)

SELF AND SOCIETY IN THE EUROPEAN NOVEL

I do not expect that you follow all that I have said; I certainly do not expect you to remember it in the words I have used. But I am suggesting that in Balzac's *Père Goriot* you do see a conflict between Rastignac's inner aspirations and the French society in which he lives. The shape that Balzac gives to this existential encounter in our imaginations, the peculiar balance Balzac sets between Rastignac's self and his society, is the form of Balzac's novel. Emma Bovary cannot live in her society, nor, in the twentieth century, can Joseph K. and Ivan Denisovich live in theirs, though Kafka and Solzhenitsyn have very different attitudes toward society. Each novel is different: life is in each, in its complexity and peculiar form, for your imagination to discover. Each novelist has at his disposal certain novelistic techniques, certain artistic means: point of view, narrative structure, characterization, setting, atmosphere, tone, imagery, symbolism, myth. For each novel, I shall point out the novelist's characteristic means for expressing his meaning, his vision of life. Form and content, means and meaning, are not separable in the experience of reading a novel, but in the process of critical discussion my stress on the relation of a novel's means and meaning, its form and content, will be a kind of test of the novel's artistic unity, its coherent form.

✍

Honoré de Balzac, *Père Goriot*
(Spring 1969)

Balzac is called the father of the realistic novel in Europe, the realistic novel in the sense of accurate notation and documentary method. Edith Wharton says that he was

> the first novelist not only to see his people, physically and morally, in their habit as they lived, with all their hobbies and infirmities, and make the reader so see them, but also to draw his dramatic action as much from the relation of his characters to their houses, streets, towns, professions, inherited habits and opinions, as from their fortuitous contacts with each other.

Père Goriot is only a small part of a huge structure of fiction, *The Human Comedy* (*Comédie Humaine*), which Balzac intended to be a complete copy of society in his world, and which finally came to 95 novels, four million words, and 2000 characters (500 of whom are in more than one story). Rastignac appears in fifteen. Balzac's structure is in three parts:

- Studies in Manners (to which *Goriot* belongs). Studies the conditions of society.

- Philosophical Studies. Studies the causes of these conditions.

- Analytical Studies. Studies the principles of society.

This is a huge and imposing structure, but only apparently objective and realistic; it is highly colored by Balzac's intrusive sentimentality, melodramatics, and moralizing. At bottom, Balzac is a romantic, a poet of dark images, and the better for it. For that aspect of his art you should read the introduction to your text edition (Wallace Fowlie).

THE SUBJECT OF *PÈRE GORIOT*

Tentatively, we can say that the theme of *Père Goriot* is material greed; the whole novel is a huge image of devouring human greed. Fowlie calls it *intèret,* self-interest, the desire to rise in society, largely through the power of money. *Père Goriot* records the corruption of character by the selfish ways of the world; society seems to mold men and blight their decent, human feelings. Balzac does seem to blame society, and the outcome of the novel is cynical: Rastignac's youthful idealistic aspirations bow to the ways of the world, to the power of money. In disgust, he decides to beat society at its own game, so that he may rise in that society. Ultimately, he marries the daughter of his own mistress; Vautrin becomes chief of police. Balzac himself worshiped wealth.

TECHNIQUE

Point of View. The point of view (that is, the mind through which we get the story) is obviously Balzac's own. It is the author-omniscient device for recording the manners of society from outside the novel, ostensibly objectively. But it is highly colored by Balzac's feelings, and it does not probe the characters very deeply.

Plot. The plot or narrative structure (that is, Balzac's ordering of the events of his story for the special effect he desires) is the accumulation of incident upon incident, circumstance upon circumstance, step on step, tap on tap, to a consequence of selfish greed in Parisian society that would be tragic if it were not that characters are molded by social forces. The total narrative structure contains a rise plot and a fall plot: the rise of Rastignac and the fall of Goriot. The Goriot story has a resemblance to the story in Shakespeare's *King Lear*, and the theme of material greed in the main plot outline is reinforced in the Mlle. Michonneau subplot.

Characterization. As Wallace Fowlie says in the introduction to your text edition, a Balzac character can usually be analyzed in terms of his past history, his milieu, and his dominant passion. How do the dominant passions of Goriot, Rastignac, Vautrin, Anastasia, Delphine, Michonneau, Poiret, and the rest develop the theme of the novel? Self-interest, material greed operates on the dominant passions of them all.

<u>Setting</u>. Setting, that is, the social background, the milieu of the novel, is really the dominant moving force in the novel. Paris is more than mere backdrop for scenery; it moves the action of the novel and develops the theme of human greed from two points, places high and low: (1) The Latin Quarter, with its center in the Rue Neuve Sainte-Geneviève (Maison Vauquer is a microcosm of Parisian low society, a little Paris world in a boarding house); and (2) the Faubourg Saint-Germain, where reside the aristocracy of Paris and the newly rich bourgeoisie, the high society symbolized by the Beauséant mansion. Balzac is attacking what he considers the corrupt society of the restored monarchy in post-revolutionary France, after Waterloo, 1815-1848.

<u>Tone</u>. Tone, that is, the mood of the author's voice, is deeply cynical. There seems to be little doubt as to which way men will be bent, and women as well. Human greed, the power of money, rules the world. Tone is the writer's emotional attitude toward his material. A good question: Does Balzac approve the actions of Rastignac?

<u>Images</u>. The images are dark images of human greed, representing an avaricious society: Maison Vauquer, the Beauséant mansion, the locket, Goriot's death and burial. In fact, the whole of *Père Goriot* is a monstrous image of human nature, human society. Is it a true vision of life?

❧

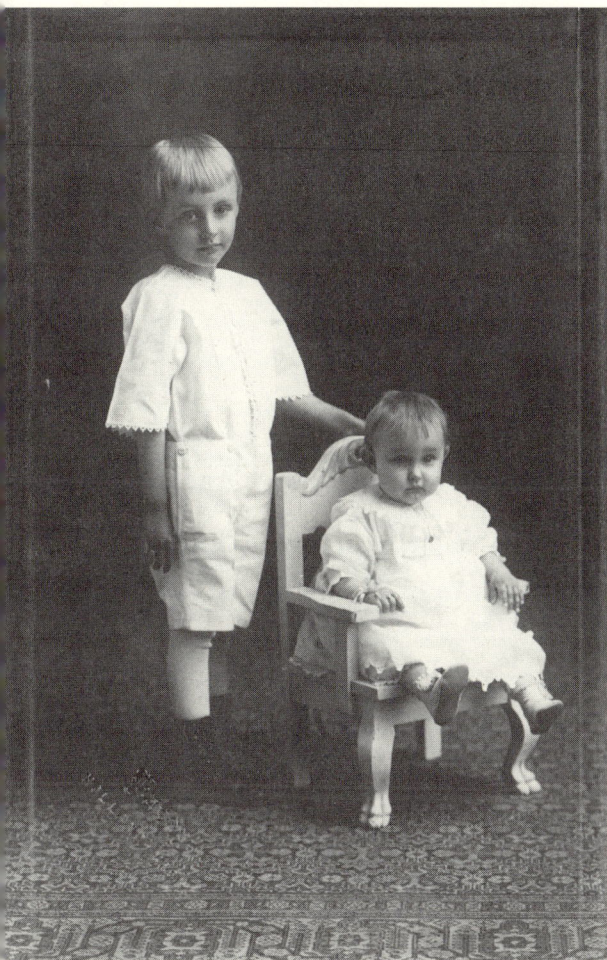

Prins as a boy, with his younger sister, Julia.

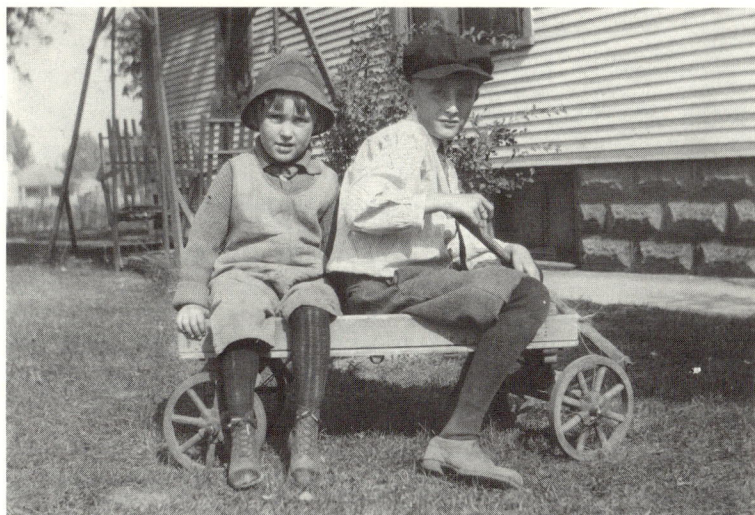

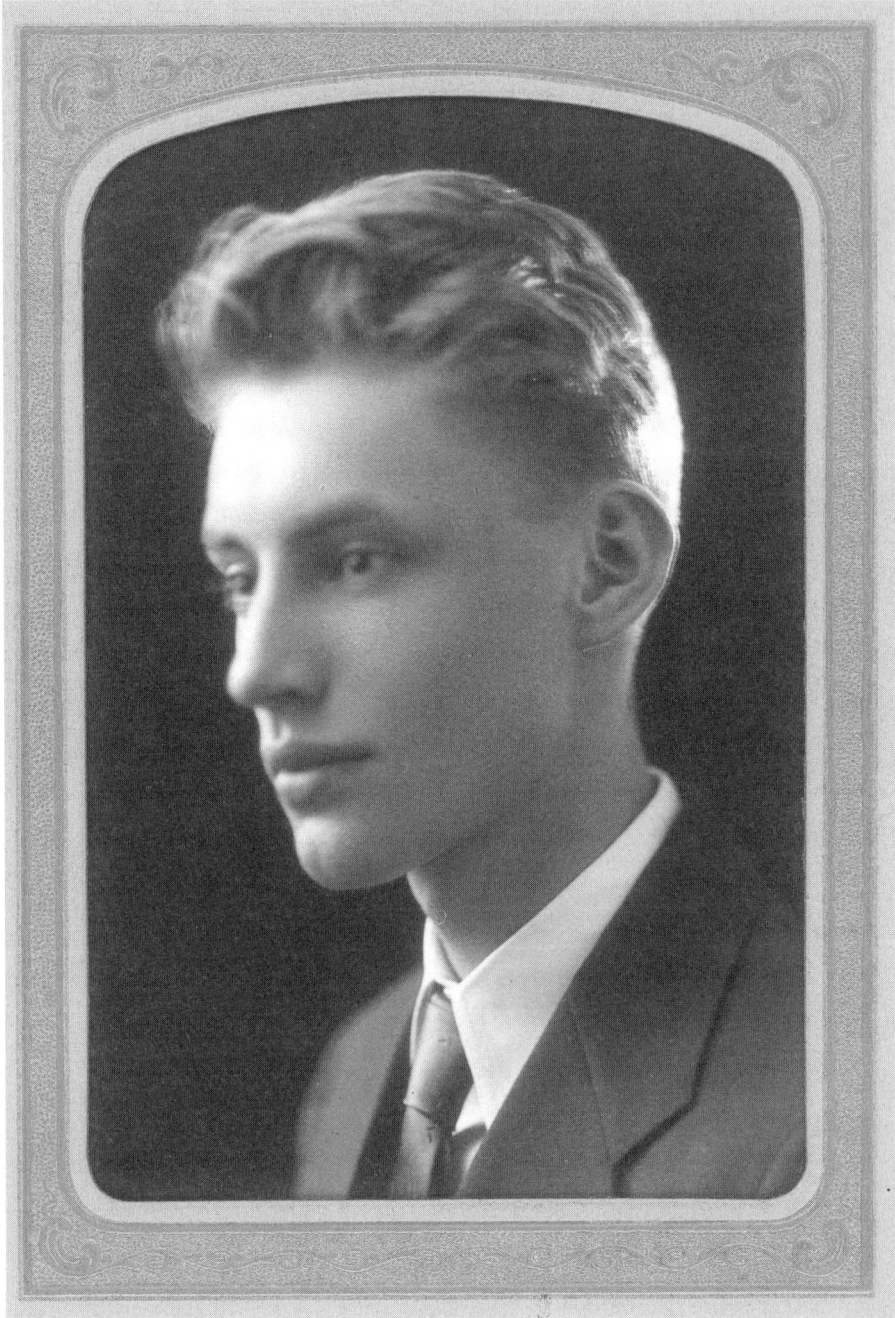

Graduation portrait, Holland Christian High School (1934).

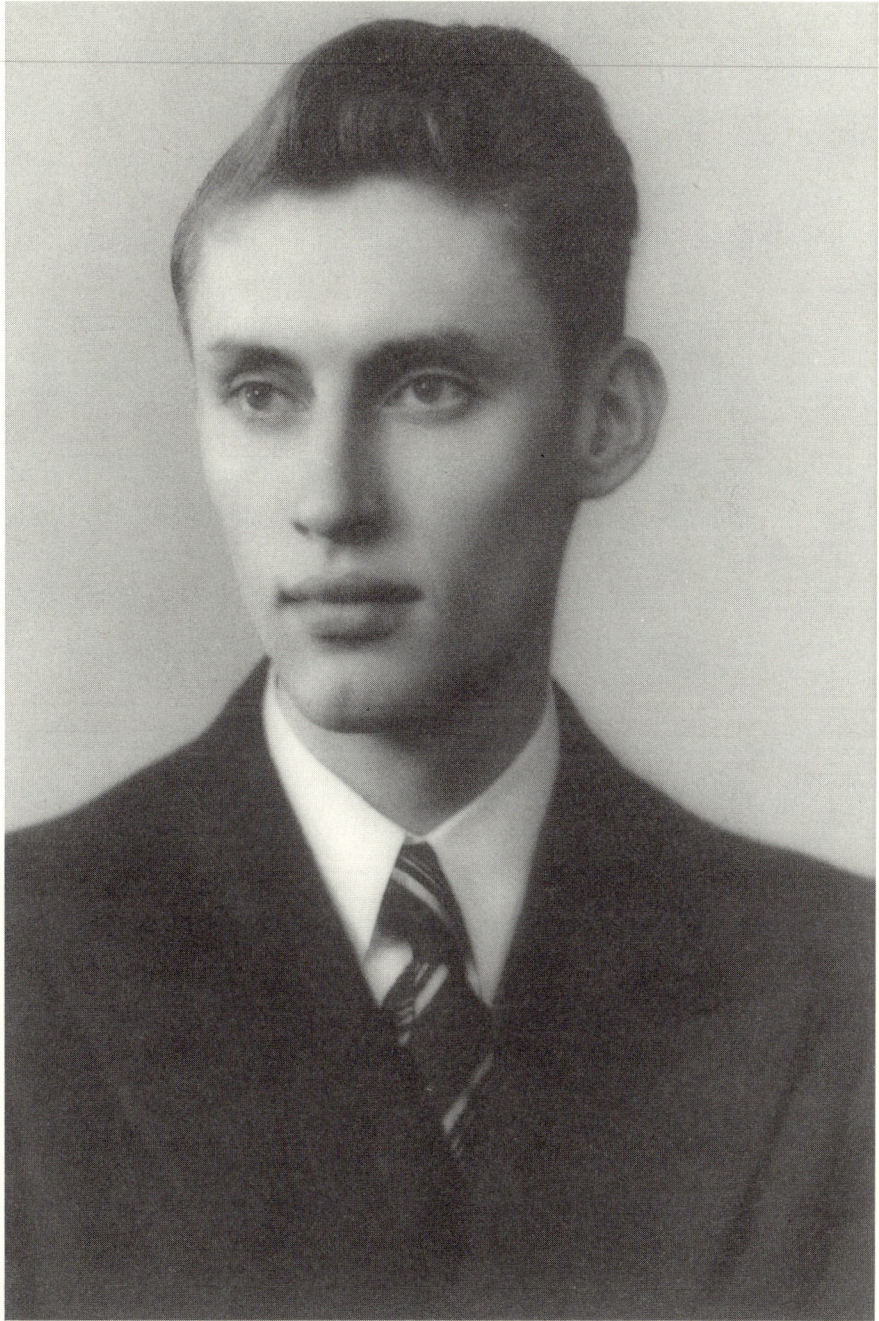

Graduation portrait, Hope College (1938).

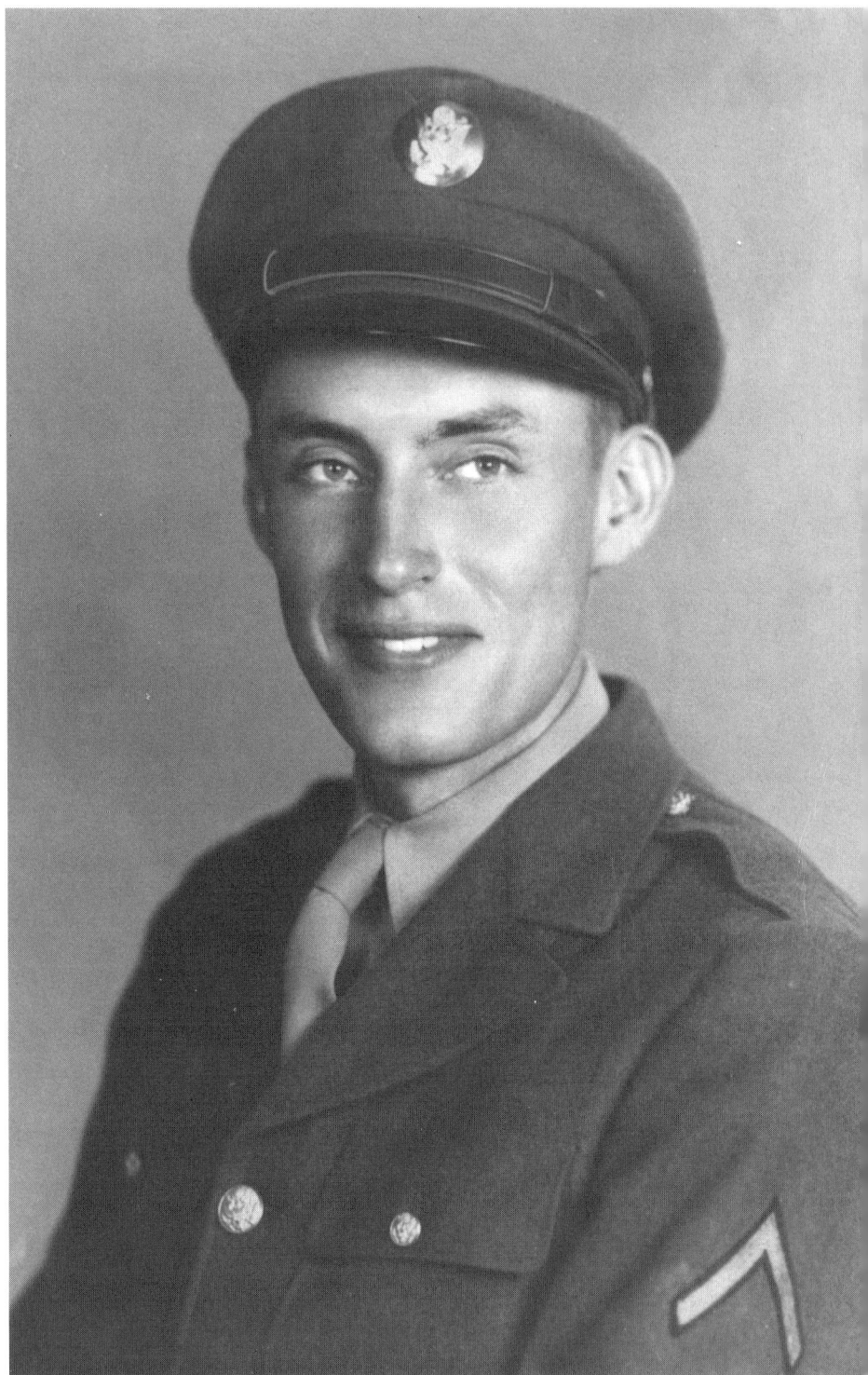

PFC A. James Prins, Second World War.

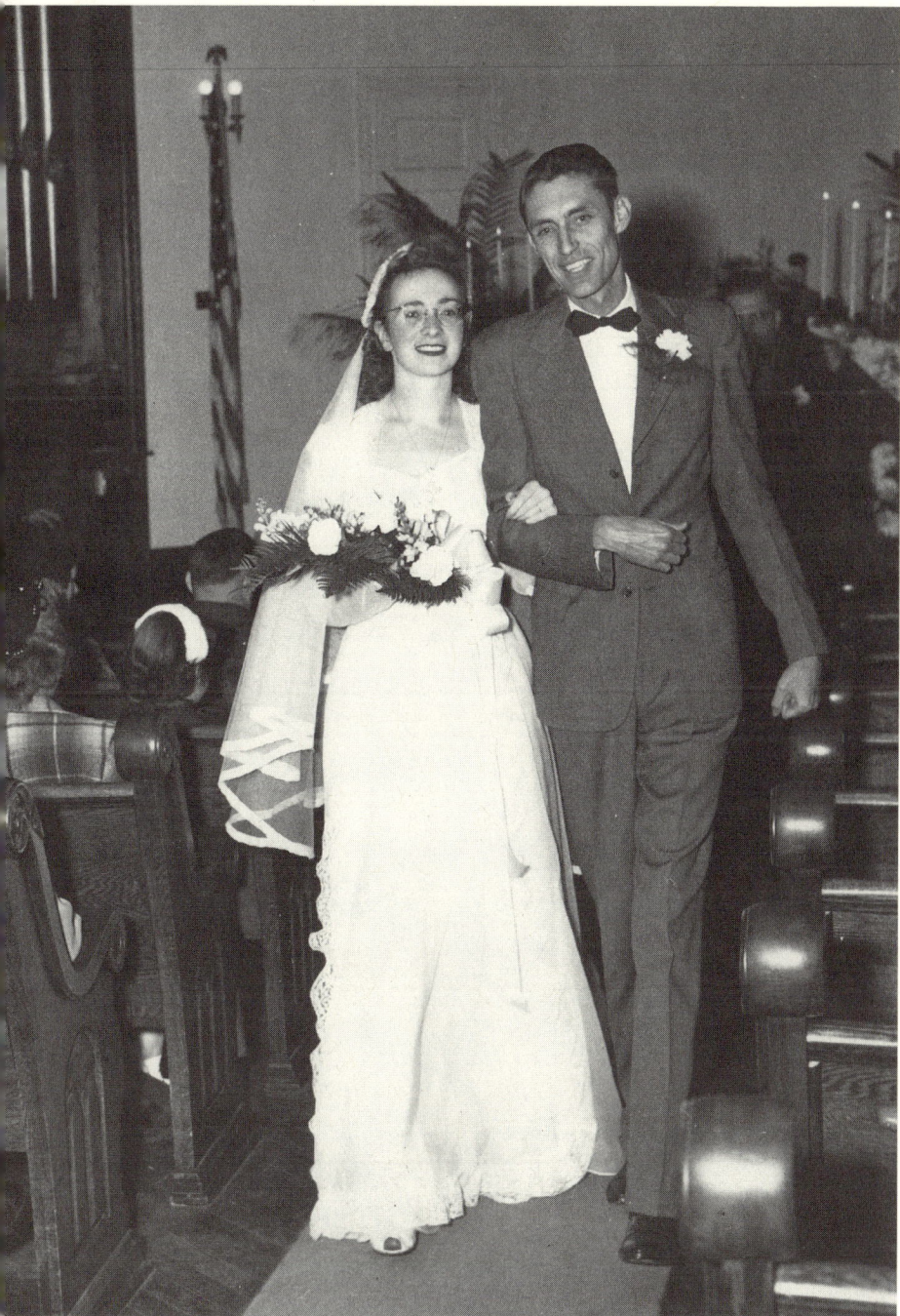

Prins with his new bride, Iris Bundy Prins (1949).

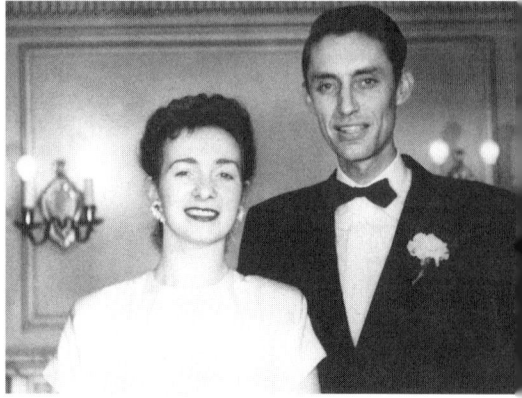

Jim and Iris Prins as chaperones for Hope College formals.

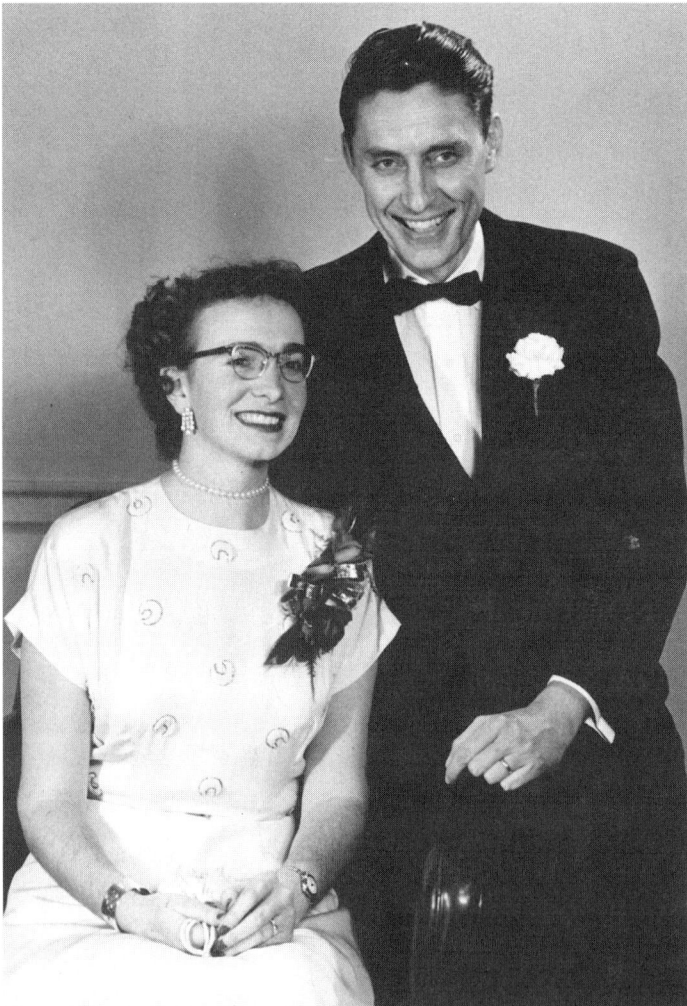

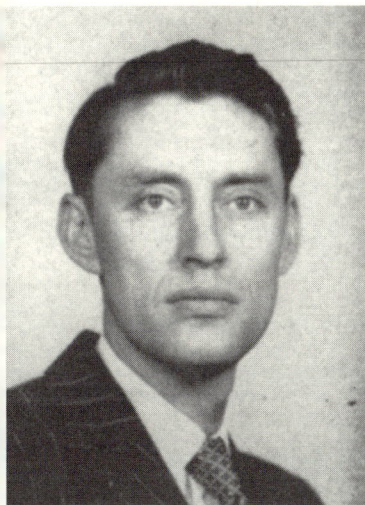

Hope College yearbook
portrait (1951).

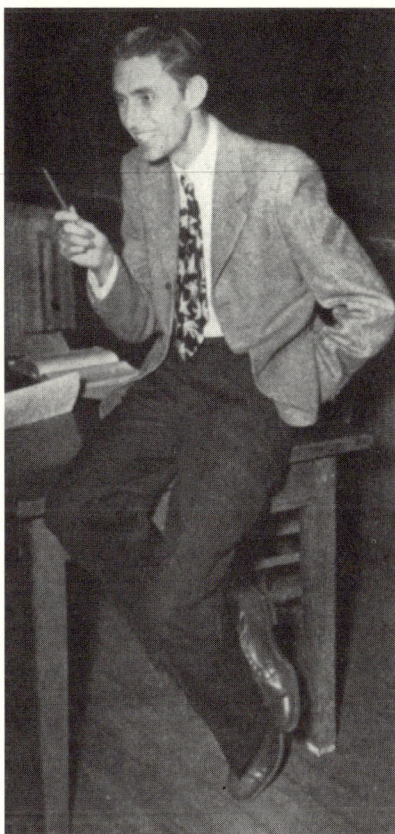

"Jim Prins, a popular English prof,
assumes a typical pose" (1948).

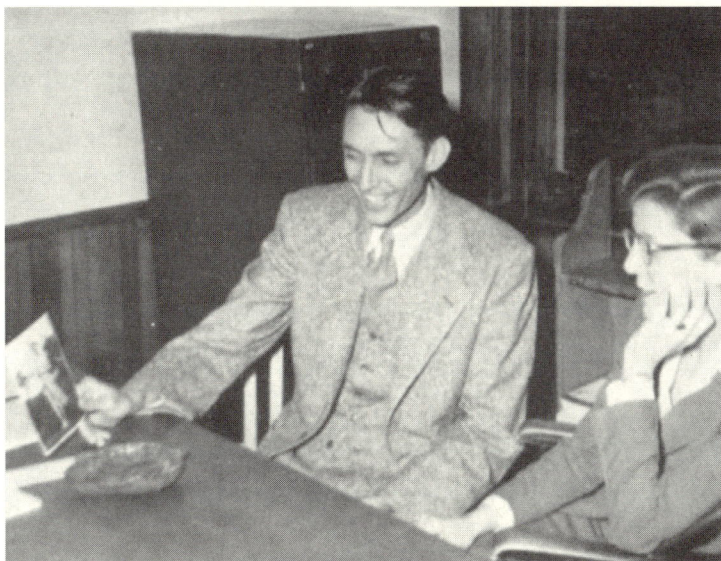

Prins showing a photograph of his wife
to colleague Lotus Snow (1950).

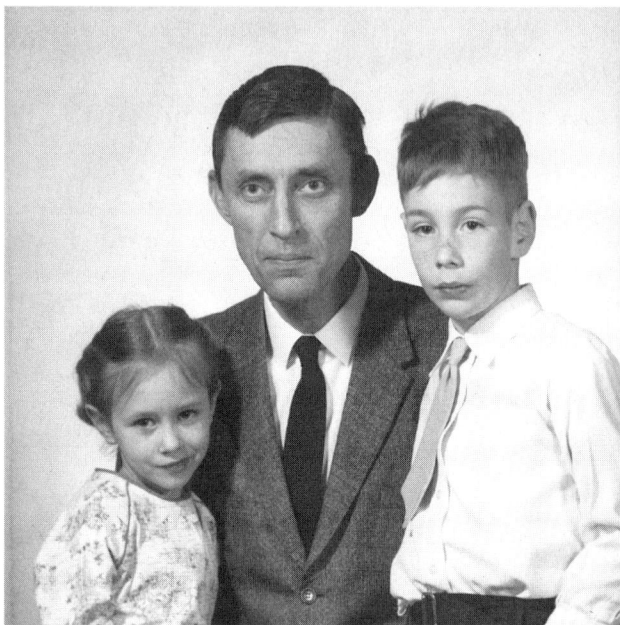

Prins with his children, Robin and Christopher (early 1960s).

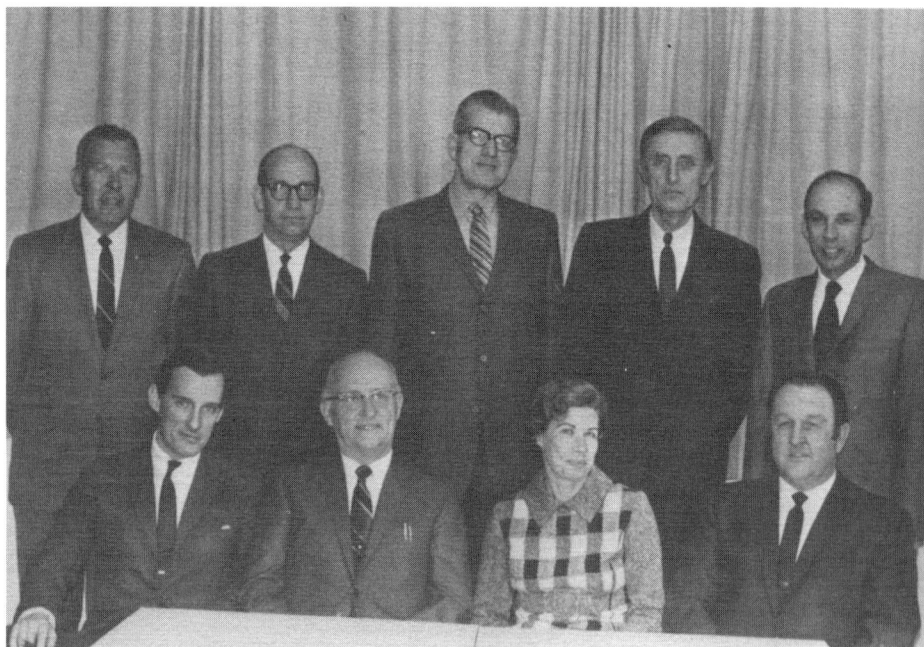

Holland Board of Education (1970).
Prins stands in the back row, second from right.

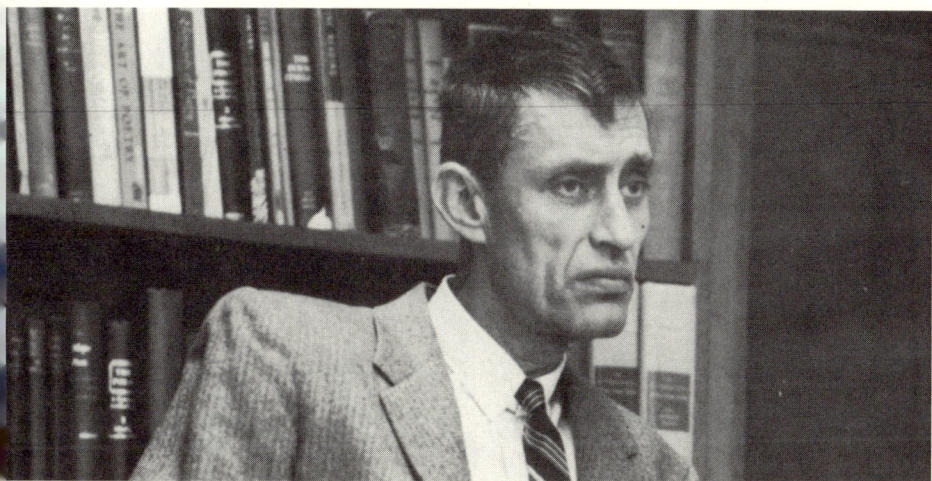

A sombre A. James Prins (1964).

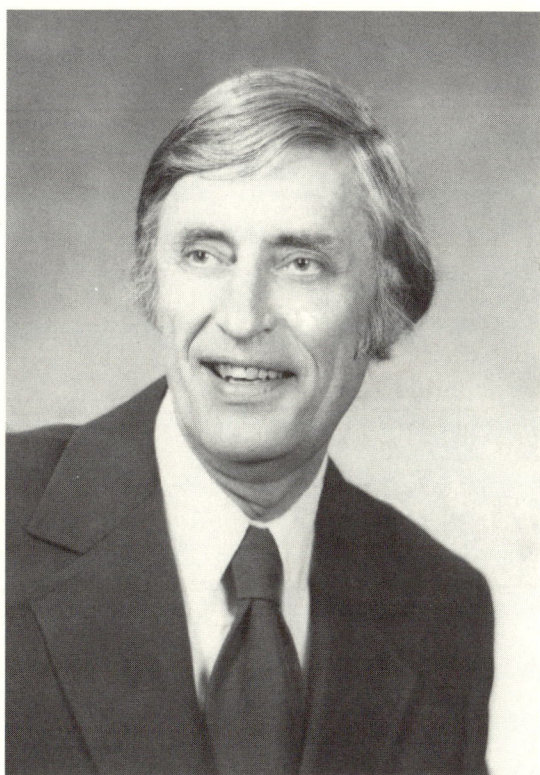

Hope College yearbook portrait (1973).

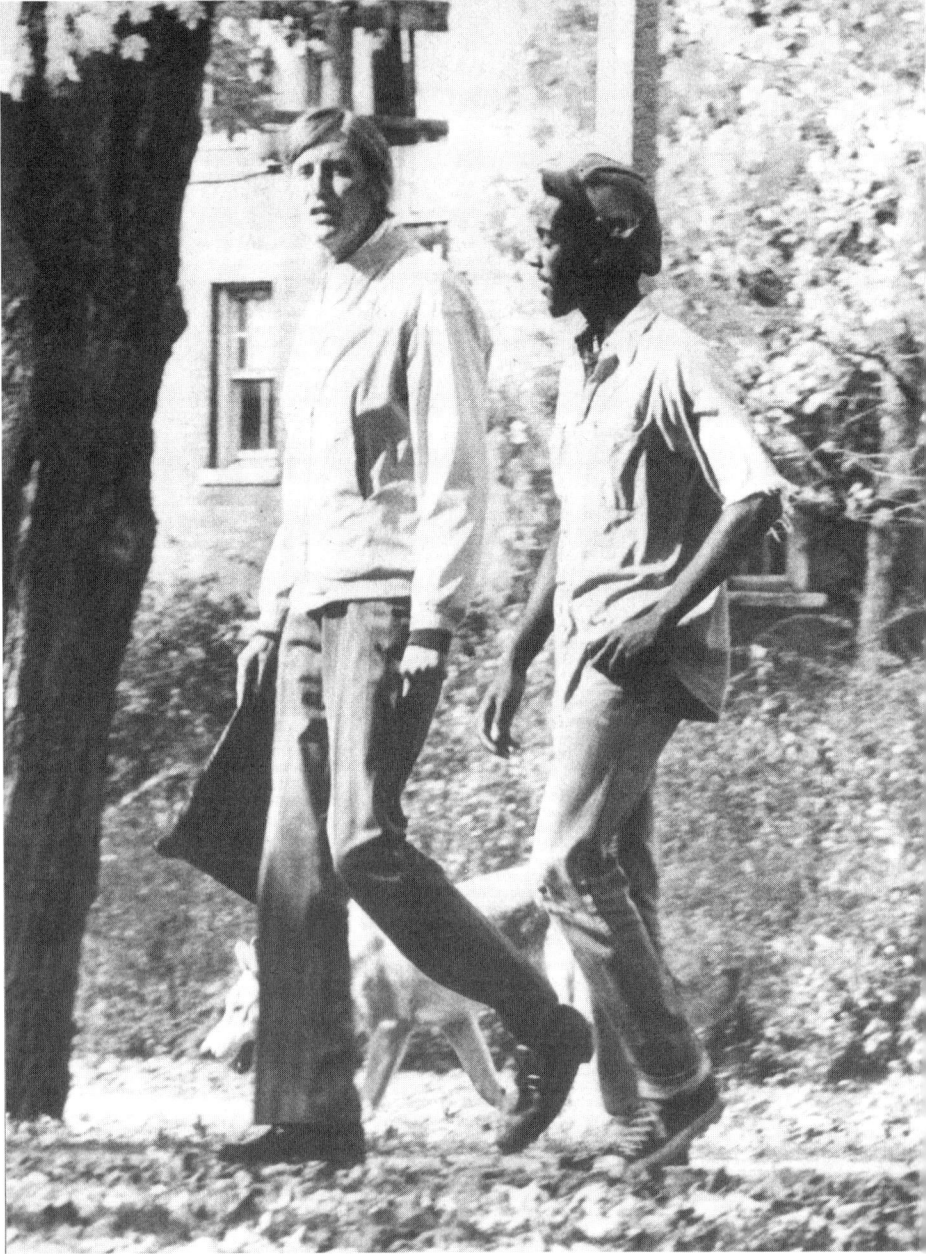

Prins with a Hope student (1975).

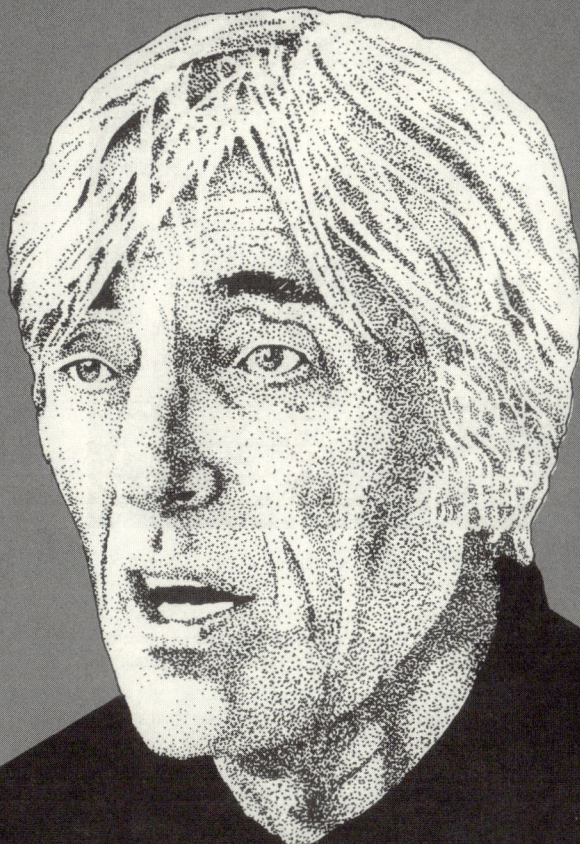

Cover portrait, *Hope College Magazine* (1975).

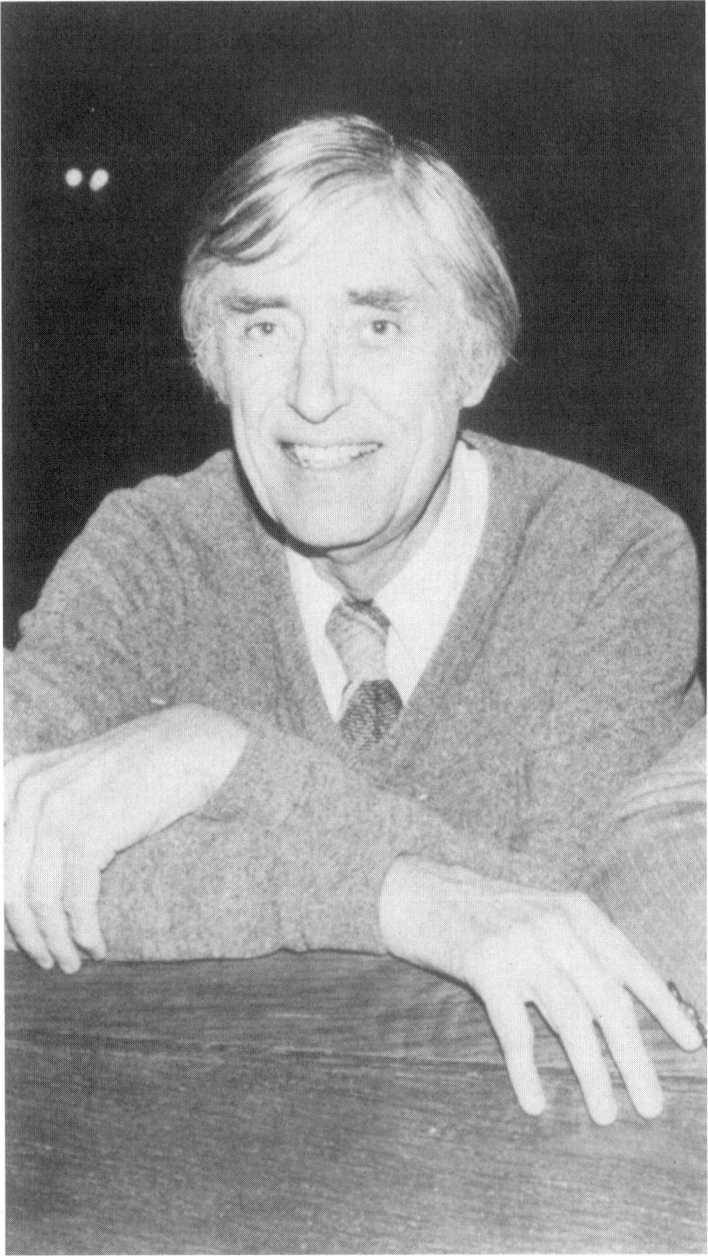

Prins in the year of his retirement (1981).

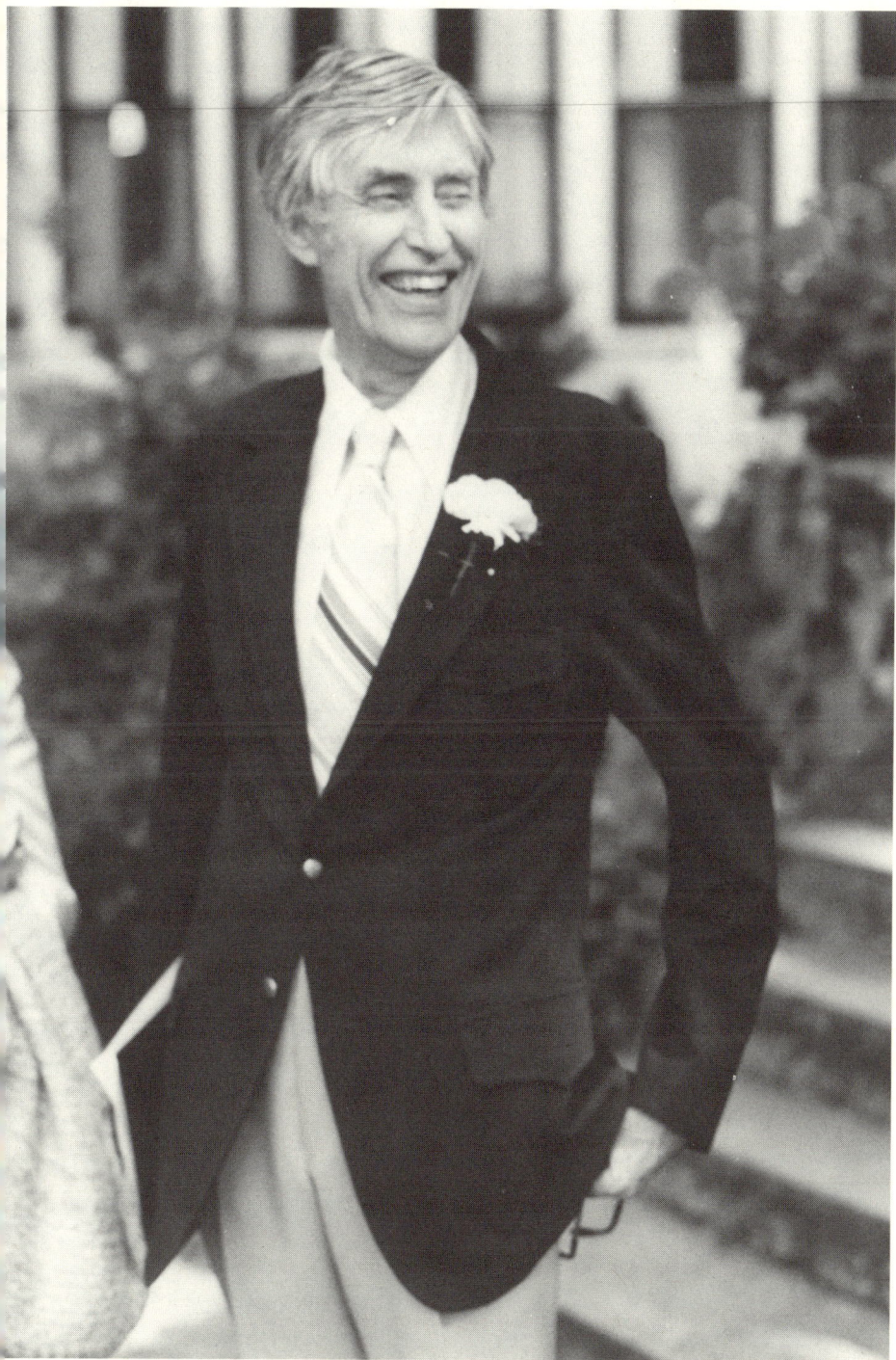

Prins enjoying his retirement celebration at the Castle (1981).

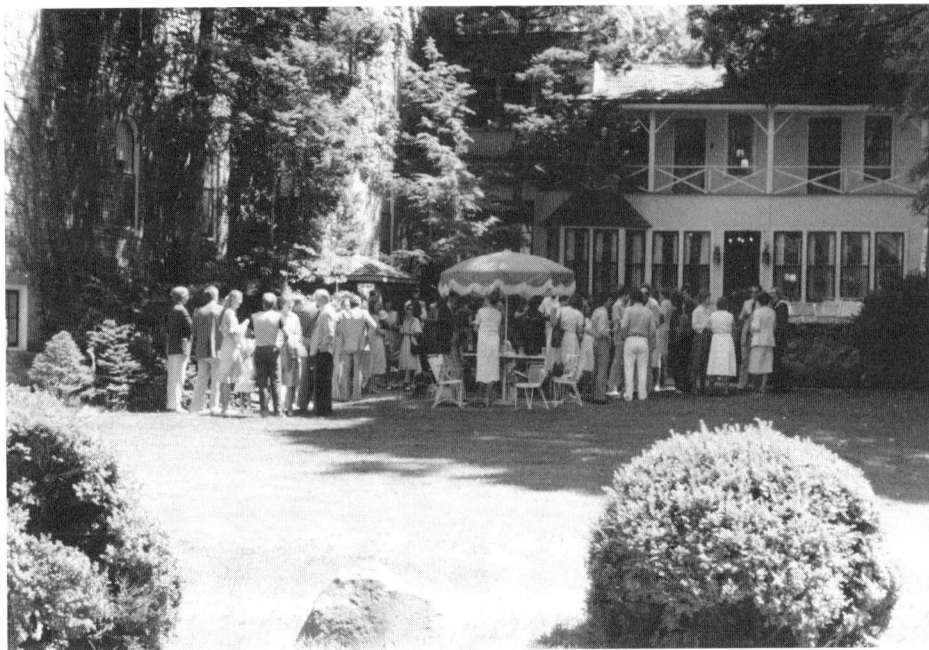

At the Castle (Castle Park, Michigan).

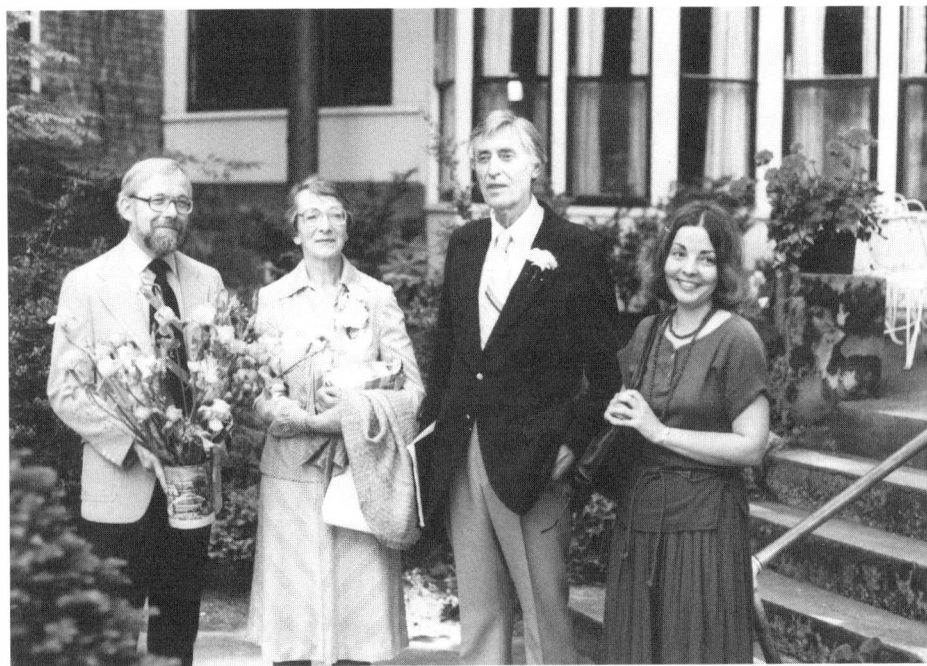

Prins with (*left to right*) Stuart Wilson,
Iris Prins, and Kathleen Verduin.

Sound and Fury Approach 1

Transition: In order to understand what Faulkner is trying to do
in S&F, we must think back to James' Ambassadors. In
that novel James limited the information of the novel
to the consciousness of a single character -- Strether.
The point of view is internal, psychological, but the
language used is the formal style of Henry James.
Faulkner goes the next step -- to what we call the
"stream of consciousness" PV -- in which the author
tries to render the continuous, unformalized flow of
thought of a character, according to the particular
psychology of that character. Faulkner tries to render
the mental impressions, without interference, of three
characters (first three sections) who have three greatly
different mental sets: the idiot Benjy, who mentally
cannot formalize thought, but only feels; the guilt-
ridden, introverted, and mentally sensitive Quentin;
and the materialist, realistic Jason. The fourth section is told from a more ordinary objective and omniscient PV. It draws together and concludes the decay
of the Compson family which the three minds have revealed.

Theme: 1. The decay of the Compson family -- an aristocratic family
of the Old South (read appendix).

2. The decay of the American South.

3. The decay and disintegration of modern society -- intellectual, moral, and spiritual decay -- in contrast
to the stable values of Dilsey.

4. The loss of innocence, of the South particularly, and
generally, the moral decay of the whole white culture.
All the characters are symbolic: the idiot and innocent
Benjy, whimpering after romantic firelight; the neuras-
thenic mother; the dipsomaniac and cynical father; the
guilt-ridden, introverted Quentin; the nymphomaniac
Candace; the greedy, prosaic, materialistic, selfish
Jason -- all are modern types. Candace, for instance,
to Benjy is the romantic dream of the South; to the
reader, she is the loss of sexual innocence. Faulkner
has said: "The story began with the impression of a little
girl playing in the branch and getting her panties wet.
The idea was attractive to me, and from it grew the novel."

5. The title is from Macbeth: "The Sound and the Fury" --
"/life/ is a tale told by an idiot, signifying nothing."
Nothing?

6. The novel unfolds the crumbling of the past into the
present to produce the present and future disintegration
of the Compson family (society) -- therefore the stream-

Lecture notes on William Faulkner, *The Sound and the Fury*.

APPROACH TO DARKNESS AT NOON

TRANSITION

Theme: the best way to get at the meaning of Darkness at Noon is to think back to Bazarov and Raskolnikov (similarity in sound). They and Rubashov are reasoning men. All three think that the logic of reason can place them beyond the moral law, that they can ignore immediate human feeling for ultimate human welfare, ignore particular men for mankind. Michel and Aschenbach are also rational men, but it is their sensual isolation that is emphasized. The isolation of Bazarov, Raskolnikov, and Rubashov is rational; they cut themselves off from human feeling by their rational, scientific approach to human affairs. Bazarov and Raskolnikov anticipate Rubashov, and eventually Gletkin with ice water in his veins. Koestler makes the same point with Rubashov that Dostoevsky makes with Raskolnikov: "man, man, one cannot quite live without pity" (opposite copyright page). One cannot ignore human feeling; conscience will accuse him (note the significance of Rubashov's broken tooth). Rubashov, like Raskolnikov, considers his logic correct almost to the end, but both are mentally bankrupt and compassionate insight is hinted at.

Technique: point of view. Crime and Punishment and Darkness at Noon are also handled similarly. Both are psycho-dramas: that is, the main action is the conflict of ideas taking place within the mind of the central character. This mental action is revealed in the 3rd p. from an omniscient-author point of view. Rubashov has day-dreams, induced by his toothache-conscience, that correspond to Raskolnikov's dreams (also induced by conscience) and emphasize his human position, the pricking of compassionate conscience (Richard, Loewy, Arlova). Both Dostoevsky and Koestler trace conflict of reason and conscience in the minds of their heroes through well defined stages up to the dead end of the bankruptcy of reason. Koestler's stages are more formally patterned than Dostoevsky's. In both cases, the recognition of compassionate insight is not achieved until an epilogue section, and reluctantly. Koestler's regeneration of Rubashov is achieved at the remove of the grammatical fiction—

MEANING

STATEMENT OF THEME (tentative)

The title is significant: it means that the socialist revolution has resulted in darkness rather than light at what should be the zenith of its progress. Rubashov's despair, mental bankruptcy, death are symbols of this darkness. Koestler is writing of darkness at what should be the full light of noon of the socialist revolution. The title is a reverse ironic twist of Joshua's commanding the sun to stand still. Koestler consistently uses the Biblical myth of the flight of children of Israel through the desert to the Promised Land as an analogy, usually ironic, to the progress of the socialist revolution toward the Earthly Paradise. Koestler is asking himself the question, what went wrong.

Possible theme 1: the darkness resulted not because the logic of the revolution was bad, but because of the corrupting effect that power put into individual hands. Men were led astray; but the logic of the the revolution was right.

Power corrupts

Gustave Flaubert, *Madame Bovary*
(1971)

APPROACH TO THE NOVEL

By way of general introduction, let me first make a couple points of comparison between Balzac and Flaubert with regard to their "realism."

Balzac has been called "the father of realism in the sense of accurate notation and documentary method" (Dargan). It is true that Balzac gives a thorough and detailed picture of his milieu, his society. Yet, finally, he is not realistic in that he is not truly objective in his observation. Balzac is morally involved in his situations, sometimes indignant, sometimes cynical. His image of life is often distorted, romantic, Gothic, melodramatic, impressionistic, grotesque (imaginative, poetic); the whole of *Père Goriot* can be said figuratively to symbolize a view of man in society. It is a poetic vision rather than a factual-realistic statement. In Balzac the distortions (exaggerated images) of money and manners (or money-manners) in a particular society symbolize the springs of greed and selfishness in human nature.

In contrast (by comparison), it can be said that Flaubert's portrayal of society is more realistic because Flaubert the author is more dispassionate, more detached from his story; in Flaubert's telling there is less sensationalism, distortion, exaggeration, melodrama, sentimentality, moralizing for imaginative effect. But Flaubert is not more objective for merely realistic purposes. The obvious difference between Balzac and Flaubert is best seen as an artistic one, even a technical one: the way in which Flaubert uses point of view (focus of narration) to put distance between himself and his characters and story. Where Balzac is emotionally involved, Flaubert manages to be intellectually detached, aloof from his characters and story, ironic in tone. About his art, Flaubert said,

The author in his work ought to be like God in the universe, present everywhere but visible nowhere. I do not believe the novelist should express his own opinions. According to the ideal of art I have, I think that the artist should not manifest anything of his own feeling, and that he should not appear any more in his own work than God in nature. The man [author] is nothing, the work everything.

THE SUBJECT OF *MADAME BOVARY*

Thematically, both *Père Goriot* and *Madame Bovary* concern the problem of self and society, the conflicts of the private individual with the world, with society. Both novels view society as an obstacle to the heart's desires. However, Balzac seems to think more in the direction of Rastignac's being corrupted by society, whereas Flaubert seems to present Emma more as a victim of her own romantic illusions, illusions that conflict sharply with reality. From where did Emma's illusions spring? From her inner spirit, from her sexual instinct, from a romantic view of society, from reading romantic books (as did Don Quixote)? Obscene students call her Madame Ovary, suggesting a certain source of her problem, and are at least partially correct. "Bovary" in the French suggests bovine, the oxlike, dull, stupid temperament.

The Critics on *Madame Bovary*. To get at Flaubert's subject broadly, and to get some bibliography by the way, I am going to read to you what a few critics say:

- "*Madame Bovary* is the story of a dissatisfied woman, bored with the tedium of everyday married life—the portrait of a woman's soul in revolt against conventional society." (Statement on the cover of the Pocketbook edition)

- "Emma has the romantic sickness, the need to live in dreams, the failure to accept life as it is, the longing for color, for miraculous loves in distant lands." (Alan Russell in the introduction to the Penguin edition)

- "The story of Madame Bovary symbolizes Flaubert's ironic yet pitying sense of the terrible inadequacy of human desire, and the difficulty with which that desire, tawdry and inadequate as it is, can be fulfilled." (Charles R. Weir in the introduction to the Rinehart edition)

- "Flaubert symbolized in Madame Bovary the malady of the modern soul: Bovaryism. An excessive development of our sensibility [meaning feeling, affections here] has made us too prone to suffering; we fret at our inability to satisfy our sensual and sentimental needs; our imagination sharpened by self-analysis, and by the reading of much romantic literature, anticipates and colors reality, and reality is in consequence disappointing to us. Instead of accepting others and ourselves as they are and we are, we are the objects of relentless self-deception, and are sincerely insincere. Then reality [society, the world outside] takes its revenge." (Henri Peyre in the introduction to the Modern Library edition we are using)

- "Flaubert's theme, that the quest for happiness cannot be realized in the world of everyday experience, is a theme of universal validity. Our world no less than Emma Bovary's world is split by the same tragic disparity between inner dream and external reality. We too are betrayed by reality at every turn." (West and Stallman in *The Art of Modern Fiction*)

- "Emma is the eternal, the universal, type of the amorous, romantic woman who mingles the vulgar and the humdrum with a touching need for love." (Pierre Mille in *The French Novel*)

Note how many critics (following Flaubert, of course) tend to identify Emma's peculiar sensibility (feeling) as typically part of womanhood—that is, as being typical of either the spiritually feminine or the sensually female (bitchishness), something intrinsic to women. Yet they acknowledge this sensibility to be universally human; the romantic aggravation (idealistic or sensual) is part of the masculine psyche too. Here is a question for Women's Lib to dig into.

- "The true subject of *Madame Bovary* is the increasingly great gap between circumstance and the dream. Always the dreamer's destiny goes awry because always external circumstances are hostile to the dream. Romanticism, though inevitable in every being, always fails because it pursues the inaccessible." (André Maurois in *The Seven Faces of Love*)

- "In *Madame Bovary* Flaubert is attacking the new world in which the moral sense is on the wane and in which meanness and mediocrity are triumphing. Emma is weak and silly, and a failure; but she is sincere and sensitive, and contrasted with those monsters of modern times, Homais and Lheureux, as Flaubert conceives them, she is almost a heroine." (Raymond Girard in *The Unheroic Hero in the Novels of Stendhal, Balzac, and Flaubert*)

- "*Madame Bovary* is a study of the Romantic outlook. Its principal theme is the Romantic longing for a happiness which the world of common experience can never satisfy, the disillusionment which springs from the clash between the inner dream and the empty, hostile universe. Emma's misfortunes are caused by her inability to adapt herself to the world of everyday life." (Martin Turnell in *The Novel in France*)

- "In *Madame Bovary,* the crux of the action lies in the contrast between Emma's sentimental illusions and the plain facts of reality. Flaubert encounters the main problem of realism, a problem that by its nature is imbedded in the very structure of realistic fiction, the novel. Could the symbolic values of poetry have any place at all in a type of literature founded on a realization of the difference between *objective* facts and *subjective* ideas? Flaubert's problem, you see, was how to write poetry in an age of prose. He said of *Madame Bovary* that 'it was in hatred of realism that I undertook this book'; and that though the story is one of romantic love, it is ultimately a denial of lyricism—that 'cancer of lyricism,' with which he thought himself consumed. Paradoxically and ironically, in the detached, impersonal freedom of his art, Flaubert destroys in Emma the very lyricism he loves by nihilistically denying the possibility of romantic freedom in the world of reality." (Anthony Thorlby in *Gustave Flaubert and the Art of Realism*; cf. Flaubert's claim, "Madame Bovary, c'est moi.")

- "Madame Bovary is the sister at three-centuries' remove of *Don Quixote*." (Lionel Trilling in "Manners, Morals, and the Novel," a chapter in *The Liberal Imagination*)

- In *The Gates of Horn* (a book on French realism that treats Stendhal, Balzac, Flaubert, Zola, Proust), Harry Levin has a chapter titled "The Female Don Quixote." He looks at *Don Quixote* as mock-heroic, a satire on the idealism of the intellectual, altruistic Don, and *Madame Bovary* as mock-romantic, a satire on the sentimentalism of the emotional-egotistic Emma.

- Ian Gregor says that Flaubert gives a false presentation of reality, narrows his vision to suit his artistic predilections. Not Emma or anybody has a chance; Flaubert uniformly devalues human beings and their minds to the status of indifferent material. His "apparent objectivity was the product not of scrupulous reporting but uniform condemnation; the book contains no positive values, makes no distinction between the intellectual and the moral, the imagination and the will; adultery is seen as a concomitant stupidity, and stupidity as the whole definition of human conduct." The book is not tragic or comic, it is nihilistic. What is the point of subjecting a woman empty of values to a society empty of values? (Ian Gregor and Brian Nicholas in *The Moral and the Story*)

Nihilism in *Madame Bovary*. What Gregor says is pertinent relative to what will later be called the anti-novel. There are critics who regard the nihilism in *Madame Bovary* as the beginning of the anti-novel. In my first lecture to you I argued that the very form of the novel as a genre grew out of a culturally generated tension between so-called illusion and so-called reality. The form of the novel held together self and society in tension as a moral comment on human experience. The nihilistic tendency of the anti-novel is to deny moral purpose, to destroy the form of tension between self and society which defines the novel, to destroy this form by retreat into self, the private world, and by minimizing the relevance of the external world (society), to the point that plot (narrative structure, events in time) ceases to exist in communication with the private self. Flaubert in *Madame Bovary,* by its nihilism, finally breaks down the form of tension between the real and romantic worlds, the public and private worlds. The ironic contradictions, the impossible polarities, leave the reader nothing—perhaps an intellectual structure, an author's triumph, but no existential form that we can live by.

THE ART OF *MADAME BOVARY*

Finally, as introduction to consideration of the text, let me say a few things about the art of *Madame Bovary*: about the point of view in it, about its narrative structure, about its aesthetic structure, and about the importance of setting.

Point of View. I have already implied a lot about the point of view (that is, the mind through which we get the content of the novel) in my first remarks about Flaubert's detachment. Though Flaubert's approach is a third-person, author-omniscient approach, Flaubert never intrudes (or, rather, he gives the illusion he never intrudes), like Balzac, his own voice, his own tone. The point of view is often very close to Emma's mind and feeling, but Flaubert manages to keep her at a distance from himself, apart from his personal attitudes. She is incapable of judging herself, and Flaubert does not intrude to do the judging himself, directly. The judgment of her is artistically accomplished by means of ironic juxtapositions of Emma's feelings with the real situation in which she actually lives.

Narrative Structure. Now a bit on the narrative structure of *Madame Bovary* (by narrative structure I mean much the same as plot, the way the author arranges the events of his story for a particular thematic effect). The chronological narrative of *Madame Bovary* is in three parts, which trace the gradual disintegration of Emma as her romantic sensibility comes into tragic conflict with the prosaic society (world) in which she lives:

- Part I of the novel covers Charles' early life and Emma's gradual discontent, and Charles' departure to Tostes.

- Part II covers Emma's romantic flirtation with Leon at Yonville, her actual adultery and partial degeneration through her sentimental seduction by the calculating Rodolphe, Rodophe's desertion of her, and Emma's prostration and illness, up to the second meeting with Leon in Rouen.

- Part III covers the complete degradation of

Emma in her relations with Leon, her deception of Charles and dissipation of his property, her virtual prostitution, and her suicide.

In this chronological development one ought to see, too, that Emma's life is framed and contrasted to the prosaic life of her husband Charles, who turns out to have had his own kind of impossible dream: the novel begins with him and ends with his total realization about Emma and death of a broken heart, all of which speaks something about human illusions.

Psychological Development. This three-part narrative structure of *Madame Bovary* in its chronological progression has a psychological correlative in the three stages of Emma's development:

- (1) From romantic dream to shock of disillusion, nervous collapse, and mystical relapse, after Rodolphe's desertion.

- (2) The mystical phase is followed by a phase of abandonment to sensuality with Leon, certainly more gross than her affair with Rodolphe.

- (3) The third and final phase of Emma's psychological development is her approach to prostitution, selling herself sexually, and the despair of suicide. The psychological center of the novel for Emma is Rodolphe's desertion. It tips her romantic illusions downward irrevocably.

Aesthetic Structure/Form. I come now to another kind of structure *Madame Bovary* has. By aesthetic structure, I mean form, a total structure in which all of the elements make the novel function to reveal its meaning. In this sense of structure, the basic structural principle of *Madame Bovary* is Flaubert's use of ironic contrasts for all elements: words contrasted to words, symbols contrasted to symbols, images contrasted to images, incidents contrasted to incidents, situations contrasted to situations, characters contrasted to characters, point of view contrasted to point of view, setting contrasted to setting, tone contrasted to tone—all done with irony. The basic contrast on which the novel is built centers on the fundamental opposition between illusory aspiration and the reality that is the social reality of Emma's world.

The pattern of ironic contrasts in *Madame Bovary* defines its structural form. There are contrasted moods of romantic illusion-elation and despair on the part of Emma that gradually build up to a high pitch of tension, then break; then another conflict of illusion and reality builds up to a greater tension and breaks in a greater despair on the part of Emma; this expansion-contraction process goes on till finally there is complete psychical breakdown, disintegration of Emma's character. Thus the novel's aesthetic structure, its form, is the counterpoint of illusion and reality in which they destroy each other.

Setting. It is not necessary to say much about the setting, the milieu, the social background of *Ma-*

dame Bovary. Although the novel has more psychological (inner) penetration of character than *Père Goriot*, it is easy to see that external forces of society organically move the plot in the ironic contrast between Emma's private experience, her inner expectations, and the reality in which she lives. So also for atmosphere and tone; a horrible and nihilistic irony pervades all elements of *Madame Bovary.*

ॐ

Émile Zola, *Germinal*
(1966)

APPROACH TO THE NOVEL

Naturalism. Zola's "naturalism" is our next step, the next step in the development of French realism. We ought to remember that Zola invented the term "naturalism," and that he is called the "father" of naturalism. Tentatively, for the moment, we shall say that naturalism is the application (theoretically, at least) of scientific method to the writing of fiction; that is, the novelist's observation of life becomes, ostensibly, the scientific study of natural phenomena.

Les Rougon-Macquart. Let us now turn to the outline I gave you. Incidentally, those pages may not be necessary to the study of *Germinal,* but their particular form cannot be duplicated from any book in our library. I handed them out (and a lot of work went into them) to show the relation of *Germinal* to Zola's grand scheme in *Les Rougon-Macquart.* *Germinal* is just one part of a cycle of 20 novels that traces the development of one family—or, rather, to put it in terms of the naturalistic novel, that traces the hereditary and environmental influences that mold two branches of one family.

LES ROUGON-MACQUART

The subtitle of it is "The Natural and Social History of a Family Under the Second Empire," and this history is an account of the careers of the legitimate and illegitimate branches of two families, and their evolution into various forms of disease, filth, vice, and crime—and occasionally success, or even something ideal. It, wrote Zola,

is a world, a whole society, a civilization, and all life is there with its good and evil manifestations, in the fire and forge that molds everything. Yes, our family may now suffice as an example for science whose hope it is to fix mathematically the laws of nervous and blood variations in race, as the result of an original organic lesion, thus determining, according to the social environment, the sentiments, desires, passions of its members, all the natural and instinctive manifestations whose products are called virtues and vices. It is also a historical document, covering the Second Empire from the *coup d'état* to Sedan; for our tribe, originating among the common people, invaded every station of contemporary society.

Now look at the pages I gave you. The scope of Zola's *Rougon-Macquart* gives a closely documented account of all the important trades and professions, and the manners and customs of every stratum of Zola's society, both urban and rural, in 20 volumes.

ZOLA'S THEORY OF ART

Science in Art. Let us now turn to something technical, Zola's theory of art: his definition of the "naturalistic" novel. Zola explained the term "naturalism" as a novelistic approach in a critical work titled *The Experimental Novel* (in our library). *The Experimental Novel* is patterned after the most famous scientific work of Zola's France, Claude Bernard's *Experimental Medicine,* and is a series of essays brought together in 1880.

By "experimental" Zola meant naturalistic in the sense of the methods of science. He defined "naturalism" this way: "Naturalism is realism held in the current of the progress of science; it is an attempt to assimilate the processes of realistic literature to the processes of science." Says Zola, "We should operate on the characters, the passions, the human social data, in the same way that the physicist operates on inanimate things." One can easily see, he boasts, "how little part in art imagination has" in his novels. Zola saw his business, the business of the artist, simply to collect the most complete and correct data attainable, arrange these data logically, and thus produce not guesswork but verifiable fact in his novels; not fiction but truth.

In *The Experimental Novel,* Zola writes, "Since medicine, which is an art, is becoming a science, why should not literature also become a science, by means of the experimental method. We naturalistic novelists submit each fact to the test of observation and experiment." The novelist should experiment on dangerous sores poisoning society in the same way as the "scientific" doctor should try to find initial material causes. By pursuing this method, the naturalists could construct what Zola called a "practical sociology," and their work would be an aid to political and social science; they would thus be "among the most useful and moral workers in the human workshop."

Zola's Scientific Intention Applied to the Novel. Zola was trying to do a new thing with the *Rougon-Macquart* series. In the series, he looked to materialistic, experimental science as the hope of mankind, and in his writing he applies a materialist-scientific interpretation of social phenomena. For Zola, the *Rougon-Macquart* series was a scientific study of the natural and social development of a family in which he applied the scientific theories of his times to its several generations. Zola believed that the scientist (and novelist) could not conceive of the universe as anything but matter and energy. He junked the ethical philosophy of the older order of morality and accepted a hard-boiled materialism. He was sure that there is no spiritual, no empirically unknowable. In these views, he believed he was following scientifically established truths. Zola's scientific doctrines have long been outmoded, but his attitude was valuable in that it emphasized that the literary mind must keep up with scientific progress.

THEME OF *GERMINAL*

For *Germinal,* Zola intended primarily a study of the working-class environment, the mining community, from the point of view of the miner (thus the proletarian novel prototype). Looked at this way, the mining community is the main character. The novel studies the social-economic and hereditary factors that shape this working-class mining community.

Evolution *versus* Revolution. Étienne is Zola's main instrument through which the novel becomes a critique of the revolutionary mind. As a social-reformer revolutionist, Étienne stands between Rasseneur, the conservative socialist, and Souveraine, the anarchist. *Germinal,* through Étienne and his tainted heredity (tendency to violence when drunk, and neurotic fantasies), is a sharp critique of revolution as a means of social progress: slow evolutionary development (Darwin) is pitted against sudden social and political change (Marx). Evolution, that is, *versus* revolution.

Zola, I think, favors Darwin and biological evolution, evolutionary development rather than violent change. He is critical of Étienne's early leadership, his neurotic revolutionary fervor and visionary zeal. Zola believes there is a natural fatality (determinism) in the very condition of human existence. Natural circumstances are responsible, not capitalist entrepreneurs or the workers; nobody is at fault but the nature of things, and this is developing and maybe controllable by scientific observation and experiment (here the naturalist rather illogically breaks his deterministic law of natural causation).

In reading, I ask you to note particularly the words of Deneulin (the small capitalist) and especially those of Maneude (the mother of slaves) to

Étienne as he leaves the mining country: what happens, she says, echoing Deneulin, must be; it is an age-long fault (both socially and biologically). Although Zola has great sympathy for human suffering, caught in the trap of deterministic natural forces, Étienne must learn patience. Nevertheless, there is hope: a new world of social justice is germinating, naturally developing (note the similarity in title, theme, and many other respects to Steinbeck's *The Grapes of Wrath*). Zola is primarily an evolutionary meliorist, tending to reconcile natural causation and political action, but mainly interested in natural forces and their social consequences.

Is *Germinal* a good novel if it is limited by Zola's naturalistic theories? I would argue that it is more, thank God. *Germinal* is an artist's powerful and imaginative expression of tragic human experience, and therefore moves us to one another.

☙

Leo Tolstoy, *Anna Karenina*
(1966)

THEMES OF THE NOVEL

Anna Karenina is the most balanced treatment of self and society that you have met in this course yet, or will meet. In the end, Levin finds in himself something greater than self: a love for God and man in the world. Tolstoy's emphasis is on the broadening of social sympathy through the moral effects of useful work on the individual (*Arbeitskur*). *Anna Karenina* stresses the self-rewarding principle of living for the good of others. Your final estimate may be that Anna has too much heart for this world; she is like the mare Frou-Frou ("rustling silk") who runs like the wind in natural grace and beauty, cannot bear a check in stride.

The Urges to Life and to Death. The novel balances the urge to life and the urge to death, the human impulse to life and the human impulse to death. In the end, Anna seeks death, in a kind of petty revenge, unfortunately, on life and the world. Levin rejects suicide to affirm life and love in the world. It is a calculated irony of the novel that Anna, whose natural impulse is as much to delight in life and love, should finally deny life, and that Levin, whose natural temperament is toward rational denial of the significance of life, should finally affirm life and love. Anna's tragedy is that the world cannot contain her in its forms—or that she cannot contain herself, be herself in the world.

<u>Balancing Feeling and Intellect</u>. The novel also balances feeling and intellect, heart and mind. Anna gives herself so completely to the personal demands of her feeling that not the world, nor any man (or child) in it, can accommodate her to it. Not Vronsky. His spirit is not equal to hers. His freedom from moral restraint is part of the gallant's code. He cannot give himself to her as she gives herself to him. When he checks her stride with what he is, he breaks her spirit. The episode of Frou-Frou symbolizes the whole story of Anna. Anna's spirit cannot be checked by any convention, moral or libertine, without damage: in balance, Levin's stumbling block is not heart or passion for life, but an intellectual pride, a kind of rational nihilism that tends to deny the importance of human life. Levin's mind eventually carries him to a faith that is beyond the reasonable—an affirmation of human existence that is beyond rational explanation.

THE IMPORTANCE OF HEART

In summary, what we must learn from Anna, and what Levin understands in Anna, though he does not learn it from her, is the importance of heart, the importance of what is natural to life and love. What Anna and Levin have in common is an unwillingness to institutionalize their love, their approach to life; they must be intrinsically true to the nature of life. By contrast, Vronsky institutionalizes love in the codes of the military gallant, to the end; Karenin institutionalizes love in the forms of moral duty, religious and civil; the Oblonskys institutionalize love (including adultery) in the *comme il faut* of conventional society; Varenka makes an institution of love in professional piety. Anna and Levin must be truer to self than these—and for one with the intellectual honesty of Levin-Tolstoy, the balance of self and society, life and death, feeling and intellect, meaning and meaninglessness, is very precarious.

NARRATIVE STRUCTURE

Tolstoy's main structural device is the balanced contrast (the double plot) between the stories of Anna Vronsky and Kitty Levin. The latter is a story of idealized passion and domestic felicity; the former is a story of selfish physical passion and adultery. Anna is an example of the wrong way to live. Levin's search for the meaning of life and the answers he finds are Tolstoy's.

André Gide, *The Immoralist*
(1967)

Looking back to Tolstoy, I called *Anna Karenina* the best balance of self and society, the best balance of feeling and reason, that we will encounter—or have encountered—in this course. Gide's *Immoralist* is our first twentieth-century novel and something quite different from *Anna Karenina*. It is a novel of extreme alienation, extreme separation of self from society, extreme separation of feeling (instinct) from intellect (although in this last separation there is an ironic subtlety we will have to discuss later).

THEME

As usual, let's first talk a bit around the theme, subject, idea of this novel. First note the title. Why *The Immoralist*? "Immoralist" implies a defiance of society's conventions and laws, a freedom from connections with any of society's bonds, a freedom from conscience and freedom from guilt. (Nietzsche used the term "immoralist" for the person who rejects social conventions.) In *The Immoralist* we have Michel's near-achievement of complete separation, a freedom achieved through withdrawal into the privacy of his own sensations. I mean his voluptuous feelings, the sensations of his own body. Since Gide is an ironist, I won't attempt to say at this point whether Michel's achievement is moral (in the sense of a kind of personal integrity) or immoral (in the sense of shirking social obligations). At any rate, Michel's "immoralism" is his attempt to divorce himself completely from social responsibilities, to achieve freedom of self. He defies traditions and the moral codes of society in order to withdraw into his own sensual self.

This is a good place for me to insert the point that I am perfectly aware that Michel exhibits signs of homosexuality. But I prefer to regard the novel, as Gide would have it himself, as a symbolic poem about an increasing twentieth-century phenomenon: retreat into the sensual self. I'll also let someone else say what else I think needs to be said, right or wrong, about the theme of *The Immoralist*. Justin O'Brien is one of the very best scholars of contemporary French literature, and one of the best translators of contemporary French fiction, Camus, for example. In *Portrait of André Gide*, he argues that on the most elementary plane the conflict between culture (society, civilization) and instinct (biological drives) can be translated into an opposition between mind and body, and *The Immoralist* treats their necessary equilibrium. The young historian who marries Marceline seems pure intellect, but his nearly fatal attack of tuberculosis can be cured only by an exclusive concern with the physical.

GIDE'S METHOD

Now a little about Gide's method, because behind its apparent simplicity there is a lot of technique.

Point of View. The point of view is more complicated than it seems. Here is the main character, telling in the first person—in retrospect, that is, after the story is finished, and also with rational, objective detachment—his story to an epistolary narrator who writes Michel's story in the form of a letter, a letter which is the form of the novel itself. Michel has been called an imperceptive narrator, a self-deceived narrator: that is, a narrator who is not aware of all he is revealing, or may be lying, consciously or unconsciously, about what he tells. One of the ironies in the point of view of this novel is that here is a man (Michel) who has abandoned himself to private sensation (even to the abolition of thought), but who narrates, in retrospect, with cold, rational detachment—rationalizing his actions.

The Epistolary Form. Why the epistolary frame of the novel, the letter form?

OBJECTIVITY. Perhaps to achieve greater objectivity, one remove away from Michel's imperceptivity of his true (homosexual) situation.

MORAL FOCUS. Perhaps to achieve moral focus: the letter narrator is less moral than Michel at the beginning of the novel, more moral, in the conventional sense, at the end.

SYMBOLIC EFFECT. Perhaps to achieve the symbolic effect of human involvement, a sense of universality (the letter narrator says at the end, "We felt, as it were, involved").

Narrative Structure. Let's move to the narrative structure of the novel, which is, of course, linked with the point of view, and very subtly and symbolically done. The main action covers about three years. Michel narrates the action of these three years during one night, between dusk and dawn, to three friends (these facts are significant). About three months elapse between Marceline's death and the visit of his three friends (compare the story of Job). These friends are with him twelve days. As I said, the form of the novel is epistolary, a letter written by one of the three friends to his brother. The main action is action that appears to be direct retrospective narration by Michel to his friends, but is actually secondhand, part of his friend's letter, which is plainly directed, in the prologue and the epilogue, to the friend's brother. The prologue and epilogue form a frame to Michel's narration of the body of the novel, the content of the three years during which he was separated from his friends.

Organic Structure of _The Immoralist_. First, just a few subtleties about the form, the organic structure of _The Immoralist_. The main three years, of course, cover the action of conflict within Michel between the sensual and intellectual, the body and the mind.

GEOGRAPHICALLY. The novel moves from south to north to south, from down to up to down, from Africa (Biskra) to Normandy, to Africa. The main action begins and ends in Africa (the center of the novel, of symbolic significance, is Biskra).

CHRONOLOGICALLY. The three parts of the novel approximately divide three main stages of action. The three stages (parts) are successive stages of Michel's moral degeneration, if you wish to look at it that way: (1) the conquest of physical death by Michel in Africa and the awakening of his sensual self; (2) the crisis, balance period, the conflict between the sensual and intellectual Michel in the colder climates of Normandy and Paris, ending with the balance tipped toward the sensual, and the abandonment by Michel of his social ties and family obligations; and (3) Michel's complete abandonment to anti-social sensation, degeneration and evil, if you will, his progress downward, southward, hotward, toward Africa, to near-complete freedom in withdrawal into private sensation, ending with Marceline's physical death and Michel's moral death, in the sense of his separation from society.

MORALLY. Note that Michel's progress toward physical health and spiritual decay is complemented and counterpointed by Marceline's progress toward physical decay and spiritual decay, an interrelated imbalance because she cannot live without the flesh of Michel outside herself and therefore before dying denies the spirit thrice. In a psychological sense, Michel murders Marceline by his denial of

reciprocal fleshly compassion, his complete intro-
version of sensual self, his denial of his body to her.
The most important idea in the novel, as O'Brien
said, is the human mystery of the close interrelation
of spirit and flesh.

To Summarize. Finally, to say some things about
the form of the novel over again, its direction is from
up to down, from north to south, from cold to hot,
from rational to sensual and objective to subjective
(which are symbolized by the novel's formal directions). Most of the novel is told in the past tense, to
signify Michel's rational control in the coldness of
the night during which he narrates, but in the last
few pages the past tense, as we go southward,
merges gradually with the present: the rational objectivity is eclipsed by Michel's abandonment to the
sensual intensity of the moment without regard to
the past or duty, as his tempter Menalque (Oscar
Wilde) advised: "Every joy is always awaiting us, but
it must always be the only one. Let every moment
carry with it all that it brought." One could say that
the theme of *The Immoralist* is in Gide's quotation
from Psalms which faces the beginning of his preface: "I will praise Thee, for I am fearfully and wonderfully made."

ℒ

Thomas Mann, *Death in Venice*

INTRODUCTION

<u>Art Is a Disease</u>. Let me return to a theme I introduced the first day of this course. We could say, particularly after Dostoevsky (cf. Gide), that the most persistent theme in the twentieth-century novel is the split between Self and Society (alienation) and that in Thomas Mann the problem centers in the artist himself. Mann is the perfect example of the artist with a guilty conscience (Brée), the artist who is alienated from the common enjoyments of life because of his peculiar sensibilities: to Mann, art is a disease that separates the artist from the healthy bourgeois world. Mann's works develop the split between the artist and society to the point of attacking the artist, attacking the artist who is the purveyor of aesthetic feeling. To study Mann is to study the artist as anti-artist: *Buddenbrooks* is an autobiographical novel-history of the development of the split between the artist Thomas Mann and society. *Felix Krull, Mario the Magician, Doctor Faustus, Death in Venice*—all suggest the artist as confidence man, deceiver, liar, misleader, imposter, magician, poseur, subtly seducing a healthy society.

In *Tonio Kroger* Lizabeta calls Tonio a bourgeois *manqué*, a split bourgeois, and Tonio, who is Mann the artist, at the end repudiates any aesthetics which would separate him from common healthy humanity.

The Extinction of Self-Consciousness. In *Death in Venice*, our immediate concern here, the moral will of the artist Aschenbach suffers a death of voluptuous self-relaxation (all done symbolically). What dies in Venice is Aschenbach's rational control (somewhat like Michel's). Aschenbach's final urge is to follow Tadzio (a symbol of art) to the extinction of his self-consciousness in the immensity of the sea, to return to the womb of unconscious life, which is a kind of death.

There is a difference between *The Immoralist* and *Death in Venice*. In Gide's story the focus is on point of view, on the rational consciousness (in fact, rationalization) of Michel. That consciousness is casuistic, ambiguous, self-deceived, deceptive. It becomes enervated, but it seems to retain enough conscious control to call for help. And it burns with the hot-dry brilliance of a flame, sharply. By contrast, the focus in *Death in Venice* is atmospheric, symbolically so; the focus in *Death in Venice* is on the insidious voluptuousness, almost criminal voluptuousness, of the stinking city, on the fetid, rank, rotten-rotting, sodden atmosphere of sickness, disease, death. The focus is not, as with *The Immoralist*, on the rational expression of the sensual but on the sensual itself, symbolized in erotic Venice. Venice symbolizes the artist's way to beauty through feeling, through the senses. Venice represents the sensual lure of the mortal flesh, Venus, the venereal, erotic love, that which is mortal and must decay and die and stink.

Aschenbach (who like Michel has homosexual tendencies which are again symbolic of the artist's way) falls in love with mortal beauty (as gods always do) in the shape of Tadzio, a Greek form of masculine beauty, tainted with mortal decay (suggested, as always in Mann, by carious teeth). Aschenbach's, the artist's, infatuation with classic form is ironically a sensual passion that destroys by corrupting, relaxing the moral will, the moral control. I say ironically because the artist's concern for form, for the control and discipline of form, is itself a sensual passion, an intense desire and rage for order that because of its impossible tension breaks down the moral balance, as with Aschenbach. The artist's basic impulse is primarily erotic love of mortal life: concern for artistic form becomes, or rather is, a sensual passion for erotic content. This infatuation of the artist (best presented through the pseudo-Platonic dialogues), is abnormally solipsistic, a deviation from the socially healthy (particularly in *Tonio*). Michel burns enervated at the disappearing edge of consciousness but Aschenbach's moral will rots, is damply drowned, in his desire to follow Tadzio into unconsciousness, the sea, womb of nothingness, the pleasure of perfect harmony in extinction.

Dionysus and Apollo. Perhaps the most important thing to read in connection with Mann would be two philosophers: Arthur Schopenhauer in *The World as Will and Idea* and Friedrich Nietzsche in *The Birth of Tragedy*. Schopenhauer's distinction between will and idea and Nietzsche's between Dionysus (the Dionysian movement corresponding to Schopenhauer's Will) and Apollo (the Apollonian somewhat corresponding to Schopenhauer's Idea) are very applicable to *Death in Venice*. Heraclitus remarked, "Are not Dionysus and Hades / that is, Hades, the dark world of instinctive impulse, libido / one." Apollo inhabited, by contrast, the sunny, rational heights of life, Mt. Olympus. The Apollonian forces are the control, the discipline of culture, civilization (which Michel sought to subvert) in the daylight world.

Whether Mann *in Death in Venice* is on the side of Dionysian life force, the primordial energy, the will to life, self, power, the dark underworld of the irrational self, Id (Lawrentian blood consciousness), or on the side of Apollonian form and ethical control, the world of rational idea, the higher (in the sense of abstracting mind, universals) world of individuating rational consciousness, I leave for you to decide. Certainly, (1) he seems to be against an excess of Dionysian frenzy, orgy, but (2) certainly also, Aschenbach's breakdown (like Michel's) is at least partially caused by too great a tension between mind and feeling, by the effect of Puritan or *Burger* (bourgeois) rigidity, a tension that a Northern artist like Mann or Gide seems peculiarly prone to (at least they write about it, and I feel it). *Death in Venice* shows, above all, that the artist's concern for Apollonian form and control is, as I said before, an ironic aspect of the sensual desire for beauty and life, as destructive as Dionysian passion (rooted together deep as shown in Dostoevsky's dreams).

The Tragic Allegory of an Artist. *Death in Venice*, then, is the tragic allegory of an artist, the ironic story of an artist who is so obsessed with imposing moral discipline and serenity on the dynamic and chaotic forces of life through objective rational detachment that his concern for form becomes itself a voluptuous sensual passion. Tadzio is, of course, the symbol of the passionate concern for form. In the artist's concern for aesthetic beauty, for the sensuous attraction of life, is the artist's hazard, the tragic lure of destructive forces that can lead to death, because the artist is in love with the sensations of mortal life; he is searching for beauty in that which because of its very nature must die, the flesh (an inherent corruption symbolized by Tadzio's rotten choppers).

℗

Franz Kafka, *Metamorphosis*

Metamorphosis is about a change of being. It is about a son's defeat by the world of human society, by the family, by the routine of human existence. The paralysis, the demoralization, the degradation of Gregor Samsa as a human being is consummated by the metamorphosis, the change into a dung beetle, which Kafka puts in shockingly literal terms: "As Gregor Samsa awoke one morning from uneasy dreams he found himself transformed in his bed into a gigantic insect." He is a dung beetle.

In this story, startlingly, the climax occurs in the very first sentence (a climax for Western man, as Kafka saw it). Then in three stages Gregor tries feebly to reestablish the human connection; he is still drawn to his human condition. But he fails, he dies. Finally the dung beetle is cast onto the garbage heap by the charwoman, and soon forgotten by his family.

The Condition of Our Human Existence. Like Dostoevsky's underground man, Gregor Samsa, the son, is an antihero who cannot bear the strain of being human in the mechanisms of modern society. Dostoevsky's character speaks from under the floorboards where cockroaches hide; Gregor Samsa turn into a dung beetle that at the beginning of his metamorphosis (first) thinks like a man, but the human links are broken in the progress of the story, the human being becomes more and more a dehumanized dung beetle, and he finally escapes into death. Death is the complete (the second) metamorphosis of the human being Samsa. The dung beetle is Kafka's grotesque image for the condition of our human existence. Some critics regard Gregor's metamorphoses as a kind of rebellion and "cop-out." The rebellion, in the extreme symbolic terms of Gregor's metamorphosis into dung beetle, is like that of a man who refuses to get up in the morning and says, "to hell with it all." This is the impossibility of transcendence, the complete meaningless of life, impossibility of communion.

An Alternate Interpretation. There is another way, not completely contradictory, of looking at the story of Gregor Samsa. The emphasis is philosophical rather than social. Almost too obviously, a parallel can be drawn between Gregor and Christ and His function in the transformations of man from the first Adam to the second. There is Gregor's deep feeling of guilt before his father, the figure of authority, and his great love for and sense of responsibility for his human family. There is the utter desolation and humiliation that Gregor suffers in his first metamorphosis into dung beetle (as did Christ), being rejected not only by the father as the figure of authority but also by the whole human family. And finally there is Gregor's complete metamorphosis in death (as with Christ) that in some strange (mysterious) way vindicates the father, relieves the family from guilt, and revives it for life. Gregor has born the burden in humiliation and rejection. This is the possibility of transcendence. The family, at the end, particularly the girl with her vitality, feels free of the mortal burden of Gregor.

How much irony there is in this parallel I will not venture to say. Kafka's writing is full not only of ambiguity but of ambivalence. Many critics of Kafka (including Camus, one of the best) think that Kafka pressed hard to rationalize the absurdity of life, the rational absurdity of our mortal condition, to the very brink of despair and into despair, then took a leap of faith. It is possible that Gregor's death is meant to signify a victory beyond death (like Christ's), an escape from our mortal condition in life. I do not know, but I do know that I am not easily comforted by apples, however you reckon them.

∅

Franz Kafka, *The Trial*
(1966)

INTRODUCTION

Kafka and Camus should be related. I am going to relate *The Trial* to the thinking of Camus and treat it on the metaphysical level Camus treats it in his *Myth of Sisyphus*, that is, as a novel concerned with Camus' conception of the Absurd. By the Absurd Camus means that the universe, when rationally considered, gives no evidence that human existence is meaningful and purposeful. The universe reveals to the mind no indication of a meaning or purpose for human life that transcends physical existence. It is in this sense of absence of meaning and purpose for human existence beyond death that Camus thinks of human existence as meaningless and purposeless, that is, Absurd to human comprehension. Death is the inevitable and Absurd end to human aspirations. There is a sense in which Camus thinks human existence does have meaning, but we will leave that till we come to *The Plague*. Camus thinks that Kafka rationally recognizes man's Absurd condition in a meaningless universe. Camus also thinks that man's response to the Absurd, to a meaningless universe, should be resistance and revolt. On the point of response, Camus is in disagreement with Kafka: he thinks Kafka's response to the Absurd condition of human existence is to make an irrational leap of faith, rather than rebelling. I am not sure that I agree with Camus on this reading of Kafka. *The Trial* is an ambiguous novel about which it is difficult to make definite conclusions.

The Trial as a Parable of Life. Anyway, I will focus on Kafka's *The Trial* as a parable of life, a fable, a myth, as a universal archetype, an image of the human condition, not peculiarly English or German or French or Russian. I am well aware that *The Trial* has several levels of meaning, but I shall not treat the particular psychological and social-political aspects of the novel as they relate to Kafka's family, his child-parent situation, his sexuality, his country, his economic and occupational position, his national status, his racial characteristics and heritage as a Jew. All this is pertinent to the meaning of *The Trial*, but I shall assume that its most important meaning is in its broadest relation to human experience, in the sense that Joseph K. is one of us and that we, like Michel's three friends, are, "as it were, involved," "accomplices" in life with him. This is an assumption that one should always, I believe, take for granted in the study of literature—one, I think, that too few students start with. The story of Joseph K. concerns everyone's experience of life.

The Absurd Truth of Death. So I say that on its most significant level *The Trial* is *Der Prozess*, the process of life, the trial of life, the ordeal of life; it concerns the act of living in the conscious knowledge that death is the inevitable and (perhaps) meaningless, Absurd (that is, from the rational standpoint) end of life. Joseph K.'s arrest is the moment, the arrested moment in consciousness, the point at which Ivan Ilyich (for those of you who have read about him) or Levin knows it is a lie to say that he is not going to die. It is the point at which, as Camus says in *The Myth of Sisyphus*, "the stage sets collapse," the social-historical-traditional moral conventions, the philosophical, political, religious props, buckle—and one is left only with the Absurd truth, with the fact of Death. It happens for Joseph K. when "one fine morning," on his thirtieth birthday, as he was about to eat his breakfast, he "was arrested." This arrest, this stop, this check, this pause, this halt is the shock of recognition, the bald moment of truth. Joseph K.'s trial is an ordeal of consciousness; it is Joseph K.'s attempt to find justice, to find justification for his arrest, justification for the execution he knows is at the end, the judgment of death that is pronounced when a man is born.

And note: the trial does not begin till this self-conscious shock of recognition and does not proceed unless the accused wants it to. The novel makes this plain. The trial is a self-trial; the arrest can come only to those who are sensitively self-conscious, who think past or behind or above or under the conventional props of life. The inspector and warders let Joseph K. go freely as he pleases, up to a point. Nobody carries on a trial or pleads a case except Joseph K. himself. There is no trial except the one Joseph K. (J. K.) makes. The priest says, near the end of the novel, "The LIFE Court makes no claims upon you. It receives you when you come and it relinquishes you when you go." The self-examination, the arrest, the trial, are free if you want to go through the ordeal of consciousness after the shock of recognition; the judgment, the execution are not free, not a matter of choice: that is what is so Absurd, so meaningless about the whole thing.

Camus and Kafka. To return to Camus, there are important differences between Kafka and Camus, at least according to Camus. As I said, Camus accuses Kafka of knuckling to authority, admitting guilt, making an irrational leap of faith to hope, like Job and Dostoevsky and Kierkegaard. Camus thinks Kafka accepts the Absurd condition of human existence rather than revolts against it—"wags his tail," as Bazarov would say. Many critics, though, contrary to Camus, don't think that Kafka appeals to the irrational; they think he resembles Camus, not Kierkegaard.

Certainly, so far as the Lower Courts of the Law are concerned, so far as the logic of the Bank and the secular structures is concerned, so far as empirical evidence is concerned, Joseph K. cannot be accused of any particular crime. Insofar as he is like any other man, like you and me, he is no more guilty before the lower courts than any other man.

Joseph K. refuses to admit guilt, even to the end, and makes his choice for "definite acquittal" a verdict, according to Titorelli, that cannot be rendered; that is, death cannot be suspended, the absurd condition of human existence cannot be suspended. On the other hand, though Joseph K. cannot find in rational logic a reason for his arrest, and though from what we can determine by observing the working of the Lower Courts (human institutions, that is, claiming to represent a Higher Court) he is falsely accused, Joseph K. does feel and act guilty from the beginning. He assumes that there is a capital offense and that he needs to justify himself, he acknowledges that there is a Higher Court of the Law, he acts inhumanely in relation to other human beings (that is, he is humanly inhumane, just as all of us are, and thus shares a kind of common guilt).

And Kafka seems to point to "a radiance that streams inextinguishably from the door of the Law" (grace?). This may be merely human delusion. At any rate, Kafka is ambiguous about Joseph K.'s (man's) guilt before any court of authority, any moral order. Camus is more clear in his own philosophy, though he may not be right about Kafka's: to Camus, man is not guilty, his weaknesses are not failures before a higher power; there is no other world, no higher power, no transcendence of human existence, no norm except individual existence—only the human condition and morally meaningless death; to Camus there is no afterlife, no radiance that shines from the door, nothing on the other side of the door.

Whether to Leap in Faith. Now I am inclined to disagree with Camus about Kafka and say that Kafka
is like Camus, not Kierkegaard—that Kafka does
not leap in faith, but resists, revolts, rebels in Joseph K. Despite the ambiguity in *The Trial*, my own
impression is that the doors remain forever closed,
the windows always look out onto nothing, the
hands are stretched out into a void (in fact, they do
not really reach out). The lines of communion, divine or human, are never open. This is what Joseph
K. learns from Fräulein Bürstner and in the Cathedral (from the prison chaplain). Nonetheless, he
does not revolt. (Whether this makes it easier to live
and die I leave to you.)

The question you must answer is whether the
representatives of the Court that Joseph K. meets in
his pursuit of Justice are bunglers who distort the
Higher Law and the intent of the Supreme Judge. Is
there a Higher Law, a Truth, a Meaning that Joseph
K. finally submits to, giving up his rational pride,
bowing to the irrational, in effect, committing what
Camus calls suicide in a leap of faith, committing
himself to the hands of the unknown?

Or are the representatives of the Court that Joseph K. meets accomplices of an Unjust Judge, false
representatives of a Justice that does not exist? If
so, there is no Higher Law, no Truth, no Meaning
that transcends human existence, and it is this absurd Nothing against which Joseph K. finally revolts
and rebels in the human dignity of his rational
pride. Then he does not give himself willingly to
death; he forces the assassins to murder him. So is
it suicide or murder?

A PSYCHOANALYTIC INTERPRETATION
OF *THE TRIAL*

As I stated last time, I have chosen to regard *The Trial* as a metaphysical parable, according to Camus; that is, as a human search for some purposive justice in human existence, a search for an answer to the verdict of "death" that an inscrutable destiny renders all of us.

Obviously, I have slighted a multitude of other approaches (and they are legion), the most popular of them being variations of psychoanalytic interpretations, for example, that of the romantic Paul Goodman. *The Trial* can be regarded as the son's search for a father, or, put another way, the ego's search for the super-ego. Quite evidently, this way of looking at *The Trial*, the psychoanalytic approach, does not contradict that of Camus. These are all quests for authority—and, ultimately, either submission to, or rebellion against, authority.

Obviously, too, Joseph K.'s search is concerned with a feeling of guilt—before the father figure, or the super-ego, or some metaphysical justice that lies beyond life. This is suggested from the beginning with the apple of Joseph K.'s missed breakfast. Obviously, once again, Joseph K.'s sense of guilt is much related to a sexual frustration or failure: before the authoritarian father figure, before the conventional taboos set up by the super-ego, before an Hebraic father-God who commanded Adam not to eat the apple (he followed the woman instead). Here is the Christian connection of Sex and Original Sin.

I am using *The Trial* to help explicate Camus' idea of
the Absurd. You choose the emphasis you wish. But
in the end you must answer: does Joseph K. embrace the Absurd or submit to it? Does he submit to
the authoritarian father figure or revolt? Does he
submit to the super-ego or revolt?

⚘

Hermann Hesse, *The Steppenwolf*
(1971)

THEME

<u>Summary of the Novel</u>. Harry Haller is a forty-eight-year-old intellectual who is able to bear his despair only because he has promised himself the luxury of suicide on his fiftieth birthday. Haller is Hesse, the modern novelist, without Hesse's sense of humor. The reasons for Haller's despondency are Hesse's own: separated from his wife, alienated from his friends for ideological reasons, suffering from poor eyesight and sciatica, and grievously alarmed by the discrepancy between the ideals of his library and the reality of daily life. Harry Haller, on the verge of suicide, sees himself as a Wolf of the Steppes, torn between the Spirit (his divine immortality) and Life (mundane reality). Harry, in the story, learns to discover the "golden trace" in the ordinary, learns to laugh about what is not worthy of Spirit in Life—though he does not completely succeed in the fusion of Life and Spirit, and is therefore condemned (quite properly) to live till the lesson is learned. Welcome Pablo, welcome Mozart, as one. The theme of *The Steppenwolf* can be tentatively stated as the at-

tempt to reconcile the polarities of Life (that is, everyday reality) and Spirit (that is, some state of ideal existence). Body and mind; Nature and a higher reality.

Haller's Spiritual Re-education. The fictitious biography begins at the nadir of Haller's despair and records the events of a crucial month in his life. Haller has devoted himself wholly to the Spirit, to the "Immortals" (Goethe, Novalis, Mozart), to the "golden trace" that gives life meaning for him. We meet him first at a time when certain incidents have raised grave doubts in his mind about the Spirit: "Were those things that we called 'Culture' that we called 'Spirit,' that we called 'Soul' and 'Sacred' and 'Beautiful'—were those things merely a spectre, already long dead and still considered genuine and alive only by a few fools like me?"

About this time of despair, Haller obtains a mysterious document entitled *Treatise of the Steppenwolf*, which throws a new light on his dilemma. Haller has prided himself on being an outsider, a wolf from the steppes, cut off from (and despising) bourgeois life and its values. The treatise suggests that his misery actually stems from his failure to overcome many bourgeois inhibitions. Far from being an objective and serene outsider, like the true Immortals, he is wholly bourgeois in his instinctive fear of prostitutes (Life), in his antipathy toward the jazz and culture of his times. The Immortals, suggests the *Treatise*, were by no means men who rejected ordinary reality: their vision incorporated and transcended it; Mozart and Goethe were not only sublime geniuses, but very much men of their times. Ordinary mortals like Haller, says the *Treatise*, who are incapable of sustaining the icy isolation of the Immortals, can contend with ordinary reality by learning to laugh at it and by striving to recognize the "golden trace" even in the most trivial events of ordinary life.

Quite by chance Haller is thrown into contact with this underworld (*demimonde*) that he has previously avoided. To his amazement he discovers that he is able to enjoy the dancing, the idle chatter, the love-making of the prostitute Hermine, the musician Pablo, and their friends. In their conversations he gradually begins to hear echoed voices and thoughts of the Immortals. But the line between reality and ideal becomes tenuous. It is by no means clear—to Haller or to the reader—whether this wisdom actually comes from Haller himself; whether he is projecting these thoughts into otherwise trivial conversations and occurrences. In any case, the result is the same: Haller begins to recapture, during the month of his sensual apprenticeship, a new sense of the values of life.

Haller's spiritual re-education culminates in the scenes of the Magic Theater, a narcotic fantasy induced by Pablo's drugs after a masquerade ball that Haller attends with Hermine. Here he visualizes himself in dozens of situations that he had previously rejected indignantly. He perceives with the vividness of reality, that his rigid categories have completely collapsed, for he is theoretically capable of committing—and enjoying!—every human act from the basest to the noblest. This total acceptance of being involves a dreadful freedom that Haller is unable to sustain without the stimulation of drugs. When he grows sober in the early hours of the morning, he slips back into his old dualistic patterns and displays a fit of murderous jealousy when he finds Hermine in Pablo's arms. In his final vision Harry is confronted with a jury of Immortals to whom he had aspired. For his failure, for his confusion of the Magic Theater with mundane reality, he is condemned to remain in the world until he learns to laugh at the discordant aspects of life, until he perceives—in other words—the symbolic identity of Mozart and Pablo.

NARRATIVE STRUCTURE

Overall Structure. *The Steppenwolf* falls naturally into three main sections: the preliminary material, the main action, and the so-called "Magic Theater." The preliminary material, in turn, has three subdivisions: the introduction, the opening passages of Haller's narrative, and the *Treatise*. These three subdivisions do not constitute part of the action or plot of the novel; they are all introductory in nature. This fact distinguishes them from the second and longest part of the book, which tells the story and which alone of the three main sections has a form roughly analogous to the structure of the conventional novel. It relates action covering roughly a month, and is essentially a straightforward narrative. The third section, finally, sets itself apart from the bulk of the novel by virtue of its fantastic elements: it belongs, properly speaking, to the action of the novel, for it depicts a situation that takes place in the early hours of the day following the final scene of the main action (plot), and there is no technical division whatsoever. But the conscious divorce from reality separates this section from the more realistic narrative of the second (middle) part.

Preliminary Material

THE INTRODUCTION (PRELIMINARY MATERIAL 1). The introduction is written by a young man who is revealed as a typical bourgeois both by his own words and by the brief mention that he receives in the book itself. The function of this introduction is twofold: to explain the circumstances regarding the publication of the book and to portray the central figure through the eyes of a typical *Burger*. The editor, by his own admission, is a "bourgeois, orderly person, accustomed to work and the precise disposition of times": he drinks nothing stronger than mineral water and abhors tobacco; he feels uncomfortable in the presence of illness, whether physical or mental; and he is inclined to be suspicious of anything that does not correspond to the facts of ordinary existence as he knows it.

Haller offends all these sensibilities and many others. The young man makes it clear that Haller was by no means a man congenial to his own temperament: "I feel myself deeply disturbed and disquieted by him, by the sheer existence of such a being, although I have become quite fond of him." Despite his bourgeois inhibitions, the young man is portrayed as an intelligent and reliable observer.

His affection and interest allow him to perceive the conflict that disturbs Haller, and he mentions for the first time in the book the arbitrary dichotomy—split—into *Burger* and Steppenwolf, by which Haller chooses to designate the two polar aspects of his personality: a quiet, civil tenant who makes every effort to adapt himself to the orderly routine of the house; and a tortured outsider who seems unable to take the values of everyday life seriously.

THE OPENING OF THE MANUSCRIPT (PRELIMINARY MATERIAL 2). The opening pages of the manuscript itself recount one typical evening in the life of the *littérateur* Harry Haller. His dilemma of the totally alienated intellect, at home in neither world (ideal or everyday), yet longing desperately for roots in one or the other, is brought out with many pertinent examples as Harry contemplates his existence and its value in the course of an evening walk. On this walk he acquires the *Treatise* and takes it home to read.

TREATISE ON THE STEPPENWOLF (PRELIMINARY MATERIAL 3). *The Treatise on the Steppenwolf,* as Haller reads to his astonishment, offers still another description of Harry Haller. Whereas our first view represented the objective but superficial impressions of a typical *Burger,* and the second the subjective interpretation of the subject, Harry, himself, this third view is the observation of a higher intelligence which is able to see Haller transcendently, under the aspect of eternity. If, says the *Treatise,* the Immortals and the *Burger* represent the two extremes in the scale of individuation, the Steppen-wolf occupies a tenuous and anomalous perch be-tween them. The fact that he belongs to neither realm completely accounts for the Steppenwolf's dissatisfaction with existence and demonstrates why Harry Haller, the case in point, can find no sat-isfactory solution to his dilemma and often contem-plates suicide. The *Treatise* goes on to point out that only humor can make it possible for the Steppen-wolf to exist peacefully in a world whose values he despises: "To live in the world as though it were not world, to heed the law and yet to stand above it."

But humor in this sense is possible only if the individual has resolved the conflicts in his own soul, and this resolution can come about only as the re-sult of self-recognition. To this end the *Treatise* mentions three possible courses for Haller: "By ob-taining one of our little mirrors, or by encountering the Immortals, or perhaps by finding in one our Magic Theaters whatever he needs for the liberation of his ravaged soul." It becomes clear that the *Trea-tise* must be understood as the work of the Immor-tals themselves, for no one else could have this lofty and all-encompassing view of the world.

POINT OF VIEW AND MUSICAL FORM. Thus, the three parts of the preliminary material (introduc-tion, the opening pages of the manuscript, and the *Treatise*) present three treatments of the conflicting themes of Haller's soul, as perceived respectively from the three points of view outlined in the theo-retical treatise: the *Burger* point of view (the young man who presents the manuscript); Steppenwolf (that is, Haller, who regards himself as a wolf of the Steppes); and the Immortals (the transcendent view of the *Treatise*). The introduction states the two themes; the second part of the preliminary material brings the development in which the significance of these themes for Haller's life is interpreted; and the *Treatise* recapitulates the themes theoretically and proposes a resolution to the conflict.

This scheme, this pattern of exposition, development, recapitulation, and resolution, is the classical structure for the opening of the sonata—in which the first movement states two themes, with one in the tonic, the other in the dominant; the development follows in which the potentialities of these themes are worked out; and the recapitulation restates the themes as they occurred in the exposition, but this time both are in the tonic, and the conflict has been resolved. The resolution in the recapitulation of the tonic and the dominant is an obvious parallel to the proposed reconciliation of Steppenwolf and *Burger* in Harry Haller's own nature, the reconciliation proposed by the *Treatise*.

In *Spa Visitor (At the Spa)*, 1924, which is close to *The Steppenwolf* in both date and mood, Hesse tells of his struggle to achieve a musical form in his writing, an invertible counterpoint, "this two-voicedness and eternally progressive antithesis," a form "where constantly melody and counter-melody should be simultaneously visible," a form which should give expression to his own experience of duality: "For life consists for me exclusively in the fluctuation between two poles, and back and forth between the two fundamental pillars of the world," the duality, moreover, of phenomena and noumenon, multiplicity and the One.

We see that the correspondence between the pattern of the preliminary material and the musical form in the opening of a sonata was intended by Hesse. It points to the way in which the reconciliation of Harry Haller's conflict is to be attempted. Terms like double perception, counterpoint, and "two-voiced melody" are very pertinent to the form of the second and third divisions of *The Steppenwolf*. The *Treatise* introduces a transcendent, a supernatural point of view, and the concept of double perception plays an increasingly important role in the novel, for it is necessary throughout the remaining two divisions of the book to make a sharp distinction between two levels of reality: the everyday plane of the *Burger*, and the exalted, supernatural plane of the Immortals.

Haller is an eidetic (capable of imagining-imaging visual pictures of realistic accuracy), an individual who can produce subjective images that in their vividness rival objective reality. Accordingly, his experiences on the upper level of reality assume fully as much intensity for him as the action on the level of mundane reality. In this novel, in other words, we are dealing with an externalization of Hesse's magical thinking, a concrete rendering in reality of the metaphors of his mind. This double perception corresponds closely to musical counterpoint.

THE STEPPENWOLF AND FAIRY TALE. A more literary model for double perception (a model that is also fully implicit in the preliminary material of *The Steppenwolf*) is the fairy tale in which the reader fuses realistic and fantastic (imaginative) modes of apprehension, particularly the fairy tale as practiced in the tales *(Märchen)* of E. T. A. Hoffmann, where inner vision exists on the same level of authenticity as everyday occurrences. The fairy-tale atmosphere is created technically by the fact that the inner vision is projected as though it were real in the ordinary sense of the word; the author identifies himself at crucial points with the hero's point of view, describing the world as fantastically as the hero sees it in his vision. The implications of the whole are broadened by reference to an interpolated myth (wolf myth, cf. St. Francis) which is fulfilled symbolically by the characters of the realistic framework story.

This description of fairy tale could describe Hesse's *The Steppenwolf*: we begin with a dualistic plane of reality. The myth of reunification is anticipated in an interpolated document. The setting is contemporary and realistic, but in the course of the story the inner vision assumes greater significance for Harry Haller than the external reality which surrounds him; he interacts more naturally with the figures of his imagination than with those of external reality.

The Main Action (The Second Movement). So the three parts of the preliminary material in the novel contain the whole and suggest the attempted reconciliation of conflict through fusion: double perception, counterpoint, "double-voiced melody." In the second section, to overcome his bourgeois inhibitions, Haller must expand his soul to the point of embracing every aspect of life. Hermine is a test case; on a higher level Haller's acceptance of her and her world—dancing and jazz, the love orgies of Pablo and Maria, narcotics and the elemental pleasures of life—is symbolic for his repudiation of the entire narrow world of the *Burger* and his new dimensions as an aspirant to the kingdom of the Immortals. It is the art of life in which Hermine is Haller's preceptress. All that Haller learns from Hermine on the level of mundane reality is symbolic of an entire new world of experience that rushes in upon him. At the same time, this new experience brings about a re-examination of his previous beliefs, and many of them, Haller finds, no longer stand up under close scrutiny.

The second section of the novel portrays the full course of Haller's development from a schizophrenic intellectual morosely contemplating suicide because of an imaginary conflict between two poles of his being, to a man with a healthy appreciation of the world around him. In the second section he becomes ready to plumb the very depths of the potentialities of his life and personality in the "Magic Theater" and symbolic marriage with Hermine, representing the complete welding of all aspects of his nature. In the second movement of this fictional sonata, then, we find an extended narrative that consciously exploits the technique of double perception, the literary equivalent of musical counterpoint. In this second section, the themes of the first movement, Haller's notion of the polarity between

Steppenwolf and *Burger,* as well as the broader view of reality and illusion, are skillfully developed with constant interplay and reciprocity.

Hermine, Pablo, the entire *demimonde* (underworld) of *The Steppenwolf* exist on a realistic plane consistently throughout the novel. Only Harry's sense of double perception bestows on them the added perception by which they assume symbolic proportions. The entire action of the second section, on both levels of reality, culminates in the experience of the "Magic Theater," which takes place a little less than four weeks after the initial encounter with Hermine. Haller is prepared for it on both levels; he has learned to dance and to love; by implication he has embraced and affirmed all aspects of life. Symbolic for this acceptance of the cosmos, including its most abysmal depths, is the fact that Haller must descend to the basement bar, called quite pointedly "Hell," in order to meet Hermine. From there they gradually ascend to a small room in the upper stories where Haller later experiences the "Magic Theater."

The "Magic Theater" (The Third Movement, Finale). The third section is a resolved theme with variations. The "Magic Theater," like every other incident in the novel, is open to interpretation on both levels. On the realistic plane it is nothing more than an opium fancy in which Haller indulges after the ball in the company of Pablo and Hermine. But everything Haller is to see in the "Magic Theater" is also a reflection of his own inner life and a product of his eidetic vision under the influence of narcotics. Pablo

makes this clear when he tells Haller that he can
give him nothing that does not already exist within
him. "I help you to make your own world visible,
that's all." Individually, each sideshow in the "Magic
Theater" recapitulates a motif that has developed in
the course of the novel, and each one can be analyzed separately in order to demonstrate how carefully Hesse has constructed his work. The symbolic
murder of Hermine marks the climax of the novel,
for the whole structure is calculated to bring Haller
to the consummation of his wedding with Hermine,
to the total acceptance of all that she represents to
him: namely, the opposite of every pole of his personality. He fails because he allows a touch of bourgeois reality to creep into the images of the "Magic
Theater." He allows pedestrian jealousy to destroy
the image of Hermine as the complement to his being.

CONCLUSION

Haller must learn to perceive the eternal spirit behind the spurious phenomena of external reality; he
must learn to take seriously only those things
which deserve it: the essence, not the appearance.
Mozart chastises Haller for the murder of the image
of Hermine, and it is stressed that the stabbing took
place only on the dream level. Before a jury of Immortals, Mozart accuses Haller of insulting art by
confusing the "Magic Theater" with so-called reality
and "by stabbing an imagined girl with an imagined
knife." For his crime against the higher reality of the
Immortals Haller is punished by being laughed at,

just as Goethe had laughed at him in his earlier dream. The only penalty imposed is that Haller must remain in the world and learn to laugh at it. "You shall learn to listen to the accursed radio music of life, to venerate the spirit behind it, to laugh at the nonsense of it."

At this point Haller begins to realize that the figure which he had taken for Mozart is actually none other than Pablo, reproaching him for his previous outburst against Hermine. He comprehends that he was too weak to sustain the rarified atmosphere of the Immortals; he has confused the two levels of reality and taken seriously the prostitute Hermine of the first level, whereas he should merely have laughed at her. Thus, the novel ends on an optimistic note, for Haller now understands his situation and his shortcomings. He knows now that Mozart and Pablo are only two aspects of the same person: between the two of them they represent a complete union of the poles of spirit and nature, of life and the eternal. Haller's last words, with their tacit understanding and affirmation of this metaphysical union, indicate that he, too, may hope to learn magical thinking and to enter sometime the ranks of the Immortals. He has experienced it briefly, but must transcend himself (as in the *Treatise*) in order to maintain constantly this new view of life. "Someday I would play the game of figures better. Someday I would learn how to laugh. Pablo was waiting for me. Mozart was waiting for me."

BIBLIOGRAPHY: See the bibliography in our text. My approach is much indebted to Theodore Ziolkowski: *The Novels of Hermann Hesse, A Study in Theme and Structure.*

Albert Camus, *The Plague*

TRANSITION

Note that all of our twentieth-century novels treat variations of the theme of *The Steppenwolf*: attempted reconciliation of the polarities of Life and Spirit. From it springs a peculiarly twentieth-century question about the very importance of life, about the importance of conscious existence in the society of this world: whether this life should be affirmed or not. Would it be better to voluntarily give up life, conscious existence (like Christ) for a transcendent idea? Would it be better to commit suicide, rather than to cling to this life?

A quote from *The Trial* will point up this question: "K. was surprised, at least he was surprised considering the warder's point of view, that they had sent him to his room and left him alone there, where he had abundant opportunity to take his own life. Though at the same time he also asked himself, looking at it from his own point of view, what possible ground could he have to do so." Yes, what possible ground exists for giving up conscious existence in the society of this world? What possible ground for rejecting life?

Remember, the question with Michel is whether he should lapse to sensuous oblivion in the hot sun or be pulled back to usefulness in society. Aschenbach does lapse to sensuous (sensual) oblivion, nothingness in the womb of the sea; Tonio affirms the importance of conscious existence in the ordinary (blue-eyed) society of this world. Joseph K. at the end acts ambiguously: does he resist the sentence of death, or does he submit to it? Is it murder or a kind of suicide that affirms some meaning beyond life? Harry Haller looks forward to suicide on his 50th birthday to release him from the bourgeois society he despises, but finds he must accept his conscious existence in the society of this world as a part of his multiple essence, identity. The heroes of Camus, Dr. Rieux and Tarrou, emphatically affirm life in this world, vigorously revolt against embracing death in any form (including Christianity's Heaven, death transcending to a higher reality).

Bluntly, the twentieth-century hero has the temptation to cut off his head, in one way or another, and the temptation is very strong today. That is, the temptation is great to obliterate conscious existence in the society of this world. The twentieth-century hero, a culture hero, cannot bear the fragmentation of his self, the responsibility, the guilt, the tension that conscious existence brings and demands; he romantically yearns for perfect form, for the years of his innocence, his childhood; for absolute perfection, the simplicity, the oneness, the nothingness of death—a kind of immortality, where there is no consciousness of mortality, imperfection.

CAMUS' PHILOSOPHY OF THE ABSURD

As a preface to Kafka, I attempted to explain to you Camus' concept of the Absurd. By the Absurd, Camus means that the universe, when rationally considered (Camus would say, "confronted with lucidity"), gives no evidence that human existence is meaningful or purposeful in any transcendent sense. The universe, according to Camus, reveals to the mind no indication of a meaning or purpose for human life beyond physical existence. Death is the inevitable and Absurd end to human aspirations.

But though Camus thinks there is no transcendent meaning in the universe, no purpose beyond death, he does not think human existence must be (is) meaningless. In fact, Camus believes that a clear confrontation of the Absurd—that is, a clear confrontation of the idea that death is the logical end to human existence—gives meaning to human existence. He says (in *Noces)*, "There is only one sin against life, and that is not so much to despair of it as to set one's hope on another life and to blind oneself to the implacable greatness of this one." Here is the core of Camus' philosophy. As I told you in treating Kafka, for Camus, the great error is to submit to the Absurd—that is, to build from hopelessness a hope for something beyond life, whether that be the Christian heaven or Socialist Paradise on Earth. One must rebel against the Absurd, revolt against and resist the idea that death is good; Camus thinks that a clear understanding of death as the end of human existence gives one a greater appreciation of the only life there is, and the courage for communal effort to resist whatever threatens this life—to fight death in any form it takes.

Camus thinks that Nature is not amenable to human reason; in fact, Nature is inimical to the interests of human reason. To logical thought, Nature reveals only the inevitable end of natural death: this is the clear, the lucid conclusion of logical thought. Therefore, reason (human reason) must be used to fight against (to revolt, to rebel), to alleviate as much as possible, the suffering resulting from man's mortal condition. To clearly understand one's absurd fate, according to Camus, is to see the importance of our mortal existence, the only life we have. To place one's goals in a Christian afterlife or Socialist Utopia is to deprecate the significance of life, even to make one heedless of present human needs in the struggle with Nature. Dr. Rieux pretty much represents Camus' attitude.

Epigraph to *The Myth of Sisyphus*, from Pindar: "My soul, do not aspire to immortal life, but exhaust the limits of the possible."

CAMUS AND THE EXISTENTIAL PROTAGONIST

I quote from the first two paragraphs of an article by M. M. Madison in *Modern Fiction Studies* (1964):

The writers of contemporary existential literature portray man and the universe as odd-shaped pieces in some gigantic, meaningless puzzle. Deprived of teleological significance, the human creature is condemned, without hope of escape, to a barren and aimless existence. And the universe, devoid of cosmological design, is but a spinning mass of confusion. Hence, the existential protagonist is a metaphysical misfit, groping blindly in a black world.

Albert Camus, though included in the school of contemporary existentialism, differs radically from his colleagues who equate the irrational character of the universe with the character of man. Camus agrees that the universe is irrational, but that is as far as he is willing to go. Man, he discovers, is both rational and meaningful, manifesting the qualities of a benevolent human nature. Separating man from his universe by virtue of this rationality, Camus argues that human life can have value and purpose, though the chaotic universe stands in powerful refutation. In reality, then, man and the universe are antithetically related, giving the age-worn struggle between good and evil the form of rational man *versus* irrational nature; and the good life must be lived not in harmony with but in defiance of the natural order of things.

THE MEANING OF *THE PLAGUE*

Let me take off just a bit from what Madison says, to explore the meaning of *The Plague (La Peste)*. Camus' universe in *The Plague* is a meaningless universe, an Absurd universe, where death is the ultimate consequence of living. But though the universe gives no sign that it has rational purpose, man's life in it is not meaningless, and man is not meaningless.

Political and Metaphysical Parable. So, I will look at *The Plague* as a political and metaphysical parable, at one and the same time. The plague-ridden city of Oran represents not only the invasion of the forces of Death in the Nazi occupation of France, but also a universe wherein the plague—the Black Death—has exiled man from a purposeful universe. Key words to describe Camus' response to the condition of man in an Absurd universe are *suffering, exile,* and *revolt*. In our novel, certain exiles—Rieux, Tarrou, Grand, and others—find a meaning for man in facing the Absurdity of the human situation with solidarity and sympathy in the alleviation of human suffering. They revolt in organized resistance against Death; they fight the void, the Absurd, the meaninglessness of human existence.

The Camusian Hero. Rieux, Tarrou, and Grand all possess the two important qualities of the Camusian hero: the capacity to feel and the capacity to think. They are able to respond immediately to the sensuous touch of life, to the love and the beauty in life, and therefore to suffer when the forces of death exile them from life; they are also capable of abstracting ideas from their experience with life, capable of rationally, clearly and lucidly confronting the condition of the Absurd. All three have personal and abstract dimensions in the novel: Rieux, the scientific thinker, is separated (exiled) from his wife; Tarrou, the philosophic thinker, is estranged (exiled) from his father and authoritarian society; Grand, the statistician, who has perfectionist ideas on art, has lost (is exiled from) his sweetheart-wife. But note the hard core of rationalism. And see how Camus slights female characters. Remember how women have been used in our novels to represent seduction away from lucidity.

The Plague: Political-Social and Metaphysical Levels. The plague (*la peste*), then, very generally, is Death; man's mortal condition, the extinction of personal existence that awaits everyone—and Oran is the prison-house of our exile in the world. But the plague is also the forces organized for death in the German occupation of France. And it is important to see the plague as both the German occupation of France and man's common Absurd fate of death; that is, to see the plague joined on the political-social level and the metaphysical level, to see the plague as representing both at the same time. For Camus is primarily interested in the attitudes that men take toward death, not only to the physical certainty that is one's own death but also the attitudes of men toward institutionalizing death in religious creeds and penal codes. Most of the people of Oran—as did most Frenchmen under the occupation, and I witnessed it in part—soon adjusted to the conditions of the plague, almost refused to acknowledge its existence, and life went on much as usual.

But men, thinking men like Rieux and Tarrou and the simple Grand, revolted against the plague, organized resistance to it. They are Camus' main point, on both the political-social and metaphysical levels. Camus is against any human attitude that accommodates or institutionalizes man's Absurd fate of death—as is done in war and religion and capital punishment. He is for lucid, rational confrontation of the fact of death for what Camus thinks it is: the end of personal existence. And he is against religious doctrines which blur this lucidity by celebrating death as an entrance to a heaven beyond this life, or explain plagues of suffering as part of transcendent purpose, or justify the horribly painful death of a little child as the penalty of God's righteous wrath; he is against political-social murders in wars and capital punishment that are institutionalized by religious-moral sanctions (as we do in our churches and halls of Congress).

Life on Earth. Camus has said that *The Plague* (and all of his works) is a very anti-Christian book. Christianity gives death purpose and meaning beyond life, gives it institutional sanction, blurs and confuses the Absurd reality that Camus thinks we must lucidly confront and resist unto death. Nevertheless, note when you read, or remember if you have read, that Father Paneloux carries his own transcendent doctrine to its logical limit: he refuses to call a doctor, and whether or not he dies of plague (or, transcendently speaking, whether he dies or not) is left in doubt. I think Camus respects Paneloux for his faith and for the chastisement of soul he comes to. But he disagrees with Paneloux; he is concerned with only what he can see and rationally know of human existence. One cannot know about transcendent matters.

Camus believes that Tarrou is wrong for wanting to transcend life in the idea of secular sainthood. That is why the central character of *The Plague* is a medical doctor with a very special name. Take the x from Rieux's name, substitute a D for the initial R, and you have the French word for God. Cross the front leg of the R to make a kind of x—that is, collapse the doctor's name to its first and last letters—and you have the medical sign for prescription, the symbol for "take"—something to take in place of

God. Ultimately, Camus' message in *The Plague* is that men reduce the sum total of human suffering by refusing to admit arguments that justify killing under any form. The doctor's job is to relieve pain and keep them alive.

It has been said that Camus' view of life, a view which he has claimed to be an affirmation of life, is, after all, a very unsatisfactory and negative affirmation because Camus refuses to take a transcendent view of human existence, refuses to give human existence a meaning that goes beyond the contingency of life and death. This is probably a right view of Camus. Rieux the scientist, one of the heroes of *The Plague*, is an objective observer and recorder of data who does not reveal a personal identity till the end of his story. Another hero, Grand, is the statistician whose ideal of art is simply to use words clearly (this is perhaps also Camus' honest view of art). Both Rieux and Grand have a sensuous appreciation of the pathos of human existence, but neither has a transcendent view of life. Both live, survive the plague (though Grand becomes deathly ill and Rieux loses his wife). On the other hand, Tarrou, who clings to a transcendent view of human existence—the idea of secular sainthood that gives life a meaning beyond the contingency of life and death—dies.

It must be remembered that Camus, although perhaps more Rieux than anybody else in *The Plague*, is also Tarrou and Grand: the medical doctor-scientist, the philosopher (Camus was trained in philosophy), and the artist. Tarrou is the part of Camus who knows that man won't give up a transcendent view of himself, cannot submit to the idea that human existence has no meaning beyond the contingency of life and death, cannot do so even when viewing human existence rationally and lucidly—to do so would be to invite nihilism. Camus knows what Tarrou knows, but Camus is a very tough-minded realist who cannot honestly leap in faith. His claim to optimism is clean but precarious.

One last thought for those of you who have some familiarity with the radical death-of-God theology now current. Thomas J. J. Altizer says a lot about Camus in one of his books. There is a similarity in the atheism of Camus and that of Altizer, which pronounces God dead and calls for the birth of a mortally living Christ. Camus also asks for what can be called a Christian conscience in this world, a Christian conscience completely unrelated to belief in a transcendent God. They both call for the spirit of a secular Christ whose message is "My kingdom is of this world"; it has nothing to do with meaning or purpose beyond mortal life. For some theologians this is the gospel of urban renewal (the humanization of the secular city).

$$\mathscr{SSS}$$

THE RUSSIAN NOVEL

SSS

THE RUSSIAN NOVEL:
PUSHKIN TO SOLZHENITSYN
English 295, Fall 1980

I. The Transition from Poetry to the Realistic Novel

September 3, 5, 8, 10: Pushkin, *Eugene Onegin, A Novel in Verse* (1831), Dutton Paperback

September 12, 15, 17: Lermontov, *A Hero of Our Time* (1840), Penguin

September 19, 22, 24: Gogol, *Dead Souls* (1842), New American Library

September 26, 29, October 1, 3: Goncharov, *Oblomov* (1859), Penguin

TEST: October 6

II. The Great Realists

October 8, 10, 15: Turgenev, *Fathers and Sons* (1862), New American Library

October 17, 20, 22, 24: Dostoevsky, *Crime and Punishment* (1862), New American Library

October 27, 29, 31: Tolstoy, *Resurrection* (1899), New American Library

TEST: November 3

III. Revolution, Soviet Realism, Dissent

November 5, 7, 10: Gorky, *Mother* (1907), Citadel

November 12, 14, 17: Bulgakov, *The White Guard* (1924), McGraw-Hill Paperback

November 19, 21, 24, 26: Sholokhov, *And Quiet Flows the Don* (1928-1934), Random Vintage

December 1, 3, 5, 8: Pasternak, *Doctor Zhivago* (1957), New American Library

December 10, 12: Solzhenitsyn, *One Day in the Life of Ivan Denisovich* (1962), New American Library

FINAL: December 16, 10:30 am.

YOU ARE EXPECTED TO ATTEND ALL CLASSES

Alexander Pushkin, *Eugene Onegin, A Novel in Verse*

INTRODUCTION: PUSHKIN'S CONTRIBUTIONS

The word "novel" in Pushkin's title (*A Novel in Verse)* does not mean the novel genre as we understand it today but refers to the narrative elements in poetry like Byron's *Don Juan.* Nevertheless, Pushkin is considered to be not only the father of Russian literature but also the father of the Russian novel. Consider now a few of his contributions to the novel:

Language. Pushkin established a Russian language with qualities suited to literature—and also founded a Russian literature (this was Turgenev's tribute to him in 1880). Pushkin's poetry has a particularity of detail that easily transfers to the realism of the Russian novel; it creates a sense of that which is particularly Russian and untranslatable into English.

Structure. Pushkin in *Onegin* gave a model for the structure of a novel. The first three chapters present the three principal characters each in turn: I, Onegin; II, Lensky; III, Tatyana. These chapters form the exposition. The next three chapters give the central action: IV, Tatyana's declaration of love for Onegin; V, the quarrel between Onegin and Lensky; VI, their duel and Lensky's death. The last two chapters provide the epilogue: VII, Tatyana's visit to Onegin's deserted house, after which she is taken to Moscow; VIII, Onegin's declaration of love for Tatyana in St. Petersburg (the scene at the beginning) and his rejection. Of course, Pushkin did write prose fiction (*The Captain's Daughter*), but *Onegin* is considered more important to the formal structure of the Russian novel than that.

The Heroine. Pushkin gave the Russian novel the heroine (Tatyana, Tanya, Larin) who represents the soul of Russia, who is the imaginative sense of Russia itself, whose heart responds to Russia's deepest values, who is bound to Russia's past and traditions (e.g., the family, which Dostoevsky considered the most important element in Russian literature), and who loves the Russian country (landscape), the Russian cities, and the Russian people. You'll find her (in various forms) in almost every Russian novel, all the way to Pasternak (Lara—Mother Russia), even in Gorki *(Mother)* and Solzhenitsyn (Matryona of Matryona's house, something Solzhenitsyn thinks has been lost).

The Split Hero. Pushkin gave the Russian novel the split hero (Eugene Onegin), the so-called "superfluous man," the alienated hero who is a divided personality, cut off from class, his society, at war with himself; who, for one reason or another, can not act positively, can find no constructive role to play in Russia's rapidly changing society that so desperately needs a positive hero to lead the country to a solution to its problems. You'll find something of Onegin in almost every Russian novel; he points immediately to Lermontov's Pechorin, and later to Turgenev's Bazarov and Dostoevsky's Raskolnikov (whose name means "divided"), and to many others. The conflict between Onegin and Tatyana, the crucial contrast between their values, could be said to be the major theme in *Eugene Onegin*, and basic to the Russian novels that follow. Or, the conflict is in, within, Eugene Onegin himself.

Social Urgency. Pushkin in *Eugene Onegin* points to the capacity of succeeding Russian novelists to view their society with a sense of urgency (almost a terrible sense of urgency) and yet with also an analytical calm (in Pushkin's *Eugene Onegin*, an ironic detachment). The latter detachment, restraint, is the classical element in Pushkin's *Eugene Onegin*, that which contributes to the term "classical realists" to designate Russia's great realistic novelists. The terrible social urgency has always been a mark of the Russian novel; the Russian novel has always been linked with the problems of the times, the country's upheavals. And therefore the Russian writer is much concerned with whether or not this commitment to social problems is artistically right. But there is almost a sense of guilt if the social commitment is lacking. So social commitment is one of the most important characteristics of the Russian novel; even in their dissent from the social goals of Soviet realism's positive hero, social urgency lies underneath *Doctor Zhivago* of Pasternak and *The Master and Margarita* of Bulgakov. Social urgency is the undivorceable milieu.

But I have almost lost my point for Pushkin here: that in *Eugene Onegin's* poetry there is not just the expression of a spontaneous, lyrical self but also a point of view which looks at the hero Onegin with critical detachment and self evaluation in relation to the times. There is a divided self.

BIBLIOGRAPHY: Alexander F. Boyd, *Aspects of the Russian Novel*; Ernest J. Simmons, *Introduction to Russian Realism.*

⬥

Mikhail Lermontov, *A Hero of Our Time*

INTRODUCTION

Henry Gifford, in *The Novel in Russia: From Pushkin to Pasternak,* says that Lermontov's *A Hero of Our Time* made the necessary link between *Eugene Onegin* and the Russian prose novel of the future. You will be better able to judge that when we get to the novels which follow *Hero.* Looking back, you can see the connection between Onegin and Pechorin, both "superfluous men" and representatives of their aristocratic class, though certainly not the same man. Certainly, too, *Onegin* and *Hero* have different themes. There is not in *Hero* the balanced thematic contrast of Onegin and Tatyana; *Hero* focuses on the psychological type Pechorin, for whatever he is in relation to his time. The closest we get to Tatyana in *Hero* is Princess Mary, whose role is to reveal the bad side of Pechorin. Pechorin is the sole center of *Hero.*

NARRATIVE STRUCTURE

The Five Parts of *Hero.* The whole of *A Hero of Our Time* is a study of Pechorin, or, rather, a group of studies, variously presented and complementary. First, the old staff-captain Maxim Maximych recounts (to a writer, the author Lermontov) an episode in the life of Pechorin: the abduction of a local chief's daughter (Bela, for whom the story is named), in the Caucasus. Next (in "Maxim Maximych") the author, who has become curious about Pechorin from his faithful but limited reflection in this narrative of Bela, meets the man Pechorin himself and witnesses his detached way with Maxim Maximych. Finally, from Pechorin's Journal (Diary), the author copies down three further episodes. The first ("Taman") amounts to little in itself but is beautifully (romantically) evocative. It tells how Pechorin was robbed by a blind boy and nearly drowned by a girl smuggler. The second ("Princess Mary") is the most complete revelation (confession) of Pechorin by himself and follows the day-by-day (diary, journal) ups and downs of a double love story. The third ("The Fatalist"), a mere appendage to the whole, yet necessary to an understanding of Pechorin, is an anecdote by Pechorin on the theme of fatality (determinism, predestination)—a theme very important to Pechorin's character (read Nabokov in your text's introduction on chance, coincidence [eavesdropping], circumstance, and accident). Pechorin thinks romantically of himself as a free spirit but blames fate. Thus, all five parts of *Hero* disclose the mind and heart of Pechorin.

Relationship between Point of View and Plot. What I have just been talking about is the artistic relation of point of view (that is, the mind through which you get the story) to narrative structure (the plot) to bring out a theme: the character of Pechorin. Lermontov has cleverly arranged his story from various mental perspectives at non-sequential points in time to give us a penetrating view of Pechorin, a hero of his time. Lermontov has arranged the stories consequentially according to the author's acquaintance with Pechorin, but that order is not the chronology of Pechorin's life. The order of time is:

- "Taman"
- "Princess Mary"
- "Bela"
- "The Fatalist"
- "Maxim Maximych" (five years later)
- Author's "Introduction to Pechorin's Journal" (upon Pechorin's death)

There are in the novel at least three important mental perspectives (points of view) on Pechorin: the author's, Maxim Maximych's, and Pechorin's. Again, Nabokov in the introduction to our text is very good on the chronological relationship and points of view in the various parts of *Hero*.

Narrative Structure and Perspective on Pechorin. In the narrative structure, the arrangement of the parts of *Hero* as we read them, Lermontov (who is Pechorin) is able to detach himself from his hero (from himself), to transcend him and to judge him. Consider the effect of our getting in sequence the puzzled view of Maxim Maximych on the demonic sexual heroics of Pechorin in "Bela," then his account of his silly romanticisms in "Taman," and his introspections on his mean adultery and cruelty in "Princess Mary." He is not the free-spirited romantic hero he imagines himself to be, disdainful of others, smothered in his own ego. Kazbich in "Bela" and Yanko in "Taman" are more heroic than Pechorin. Kazbich's horse and Yanko's boat are symbols of their freedom, their free spirits. They fly away. In contrast, Pechorin pushes his horse to death in pursuit of Vera, and almost drowns in "Taman" because he cannot swim.

Perhaps it would be more correct to put Pechorin's attitude to fate and his character this way: Pechorin is a very uncertain, divided man. He has an egotistic, narcissistic, selfish pride that likes to believe he is totally free to dominate the lives of others, even destroy them, without regret. But when his actions lead to suffering and disaster, he does not blame himself. He blames the fate he doesn't really believe in.

BIBLIOGRAPHY: Henry Gifford, *The Novel in Russia: From Pushkin to Pasternak*; John Mersereau, Jr., *Mikhail Lermontov*

✄

Nikolai Gogol, *Dead Souls*

INTRODUCTION

First, let me point to the Critical Foreword (by
Frank O'Connor) and Translator's Introduction (by
Andrew R. McAndrew) to your text. I find it delight-
ful that a great Irish writer of short stories should
comment on a book translated by a man with the
most Scottish of names. And I find nothing to disagree with in what they say.

The setting for *Dead Souls* is Russia in miniature. There is truth in this statement, but take it
with a grain of salt. The setting embraces various
classes and social strata, officials and civilians,
landowners and serfs, who pass before us in the
narrative sequence. These characters had their pro-
totypes in real life. *Dead Souls* may therefore be
termed the first genuinely realistic Russian novel,
because it deals with Russian life *per se* and a
burning issue which occupied the best minds of
Russia throughout the nineteenth century—the
problem of serfdom—a parallel to which, against a
different background, may be found at the same
time in the United States, though the Russian
serfs, unlike the American Blacks, were of the same
racial stock and the same religion as their masters.

THEMES OF THE NOVEL

Social Criticism and Symbolic Imagination. Again, take my last two statements with a grain of salt. Many critics have denied that *Dead Souls* is primarily a work of social realism. A long-time controversy between critics has been waged between those who see *Dead Souls* as an earnest social document and those equally or more positive that it came into being for no other reason than that the volcano of Gogol's creative imagination simply erupted in this form. The second position is that of Vladimir Nabokov, and, generally speaking, Frank O'Connor agrees with Nabokov. O'Connor says that Gogol was not seeking for specific truth about certain people, but, rather, he was seeking for the general truth about most people in most situations.

I do not find these two views incompatible. Gogol regarded himself as a mock-epic poet and *Dead Souls* a poem on the model of Dante's *Divine Comedy*. Gogol is a writer of fantastic, even mythic and religious imagination, but there is certainly much of the social reality of early nineteenth-century Russia in *Dead Souls*. I find both particular truths about nineteenth-century Russians in the novel and universal truths about human nature for all time. What I am saying is true for most literature, and surely very true for the novel. My dissertation on Dickens' *Bleak House* (close to the date of *Dead Souls*) concerned the mingling of symbolic imagination and social criticism. I suppose the critical danger for us is to regard *Dead Souls* as only real for Russia.

Anachronistic Feudal System. It is unthinkable and absurd to believe that *Dead Souls* has no reality of contemporary Russian in it (as absurd as to think Dickens' *Bleak House* has none of the reality of contemporary England in it). There can be little doubt that the book does accomplish two things with such impact that Gogol seems to have said all that needs to be said about either. In the first place, he establishes the predicament of the serfs. The book elucidates what serfdom in Russia really meant as scarcely any other single document does.

Second, Gogol defines the class against whom those in bondage had to struggle—a landowners' class (the gentry), holding frantically to privilege but doing nothing to deserve it, a class out of date, corrupt, effete, niggardly, shortsighted, irresponsible, and parasitic (a composite description of the landowners in *Dead Souls*), a class whose members became more despotic as they rose higher in the social and economic scale until the absolute symbol of despotism was reached in the Czar (though Gogol was not anti-Czar). *Dead Souls* is a black record of an anachronistic feudal system based on the assumption that human life has no meaning and no value, that the human being has neither dignity nor rights. It is full of disregard for both the physical and spiritual needs of human beings. Gogol would have had to be pretty stupid not to have been aware of the social criticism that the irony of his title carries (dead souls), applied to either serf or master.

But Nabokov and O'Connor are right in insisting that a novel, that *Dead Souls*, is an artistic creation, not merely a social record.

Resurrection of Dead Souls. It is said that Pushkin suggested the theme of *Dead Souls* to Gogol. It is true that when he first heard the book read to him he cried: "God, what a sad country Russia is!" Originally, Gogol intended to write a trilogy, entitled "The Adventures of Chichikov." All that remains for us is the first part (our text) and a few pieces of the second. In the second part Gogol intended to work out the moral regeneration of Chichikov—an idea which provided a pattern for subsequent Russian writers, particularly for Dostoevsky in *Crime and Punishment* (and *The Brothers Karamazov*) and Tolstoy's *Resurrection.* Completing *Dead Souls* posed a problem for Gogol; the regeneration of Chichikov would have been an indirect attack on the political and social structure of autocratic Russia, and that was not to his purpose. To understand Gogol, one must see that his purpose was constructive. He aimed at individuals—not at the body politic. He held up corruption to ridicule but did not question the divine authority of autocracy. He rather aimed at those (as Tolstoy later did) who by their very abuse of power undermined it, as subsequent events proved.

The change of title from "The Adventures of Chichikov" to *Dead Souls* was appropriately intended by Gogol. In the light of his constructive criticism and his deep knowledge of Russian institutions, *Dead Souls* represents the accurate diagnosis by a competent physician, for the title signifies not only the deceased serfs in the novel, but Russia as a whole. Dead souls are not only the spiritual condition of the serfs who are the property of their masters when alive but also the spiritual condition of their masters, "sub-human" personalities, "dead" creatures in that they are motivated by greed, avarice, and envy and inhabit a kind of inferno, a spiritual hell like the hell of Dante's *Inferno*. The literal meaning of dead souls is, of course, dead serfs. Gogol in his title may also have been suggesting that all fictional characters are dead in the sense of being only alive in their creator's imagination. Anyway, Gogol saw that a combination of ignorance, superstition, corruption, inefficiency, graft, and abuse of power produced an environment in Russia only for dead souls—not living ones, and Gogol's intention was to resurrect them, bring them to life.

Technically, *Dead Souls* is unfinished and plotless, but the character of Chichikov in his adventures binds it all together in a picaresque structure. And readers (Russian, anyway) probably preferred the immoral rogue Chichikov, quite likeable and not unlike themselves (ourselves), a man who is only imitating the greed of the ruling class, to a resurrected Chichikov in Gogol's intended moral divine comedy. Chichikov represents something central not only to the Russian character but to human nature. And Frank O'Connor in the introduction to your text says that is how we should read him.

Explanation of "Dead Souls". Landowners were required to pay a yearly poll-tax on all the serfs they owned, and even if serfs died the owner still had to pay the poll-tax on what has ceased to be productive labor. Once Chichikov has collected a long list of "souls," he plans to mortgage them, since serfs could be mortgaged like property or land, and abscond before the next census can disclose his fraud. This scheme is the basis for the first part of *Dead Souls* (our text) and the pretext under which Gogol introduces us to a series of landowners, while Chichikov links the scenes together and provides his own observations and opinions.

The Series of Characters. There is the slothful, sentimental, sugary Manilov, living in a fool's paradise that is completely unrelated to reality; the congenital liar Nozdrev whose gross fictions are psychological manifestations of his need to quarrel and bully; that epitome of self-sufficiency, the huge bear-like Sobakevich, who regards every endeavor as a challenge to self-aggrandizement and says a good word for no one; the greedy old widow Korobotchka in her tiny pumpkin-like coach, who must first find out the nonexistent going rate on dead serfs before she will sell hers; and finally, the miser Plushkin, a monster of avarice, who owns thousands of serfs, yet continues to cram his bulging storehouses with all the abortion of life and uses a yellowed toothbrush that has been in the family since the time of Napoleon.

∅

Ivan Goncharov, *Oblomov*

THE NATIONAL DISEASE OF RUSSIA

<u>Oblomovism</u>. More than one critic has suggested that *Oblomov* can be considered a continuation of, a sequel to, *Dead Souls*. Cut down, it could serve as another chapter of Gogol's plotless novel: Manilov, Nozdrev, Sobakevich, Oblomov, etc. Such a judgment might be putting too much emphasis on the social aspect of both novels, particularly *Dead Souls*, but it can be said that both Gogol and Goncharov diagnosed the national disease of Russia—one called it dead souls, the other Oblomovism. However, in spite of Goncharov's emphasis upon the negative side of human nature (is it, really, a negative side?), *Oblomov* is not so gloomy as *Dead Souls*; the atmosphere is fresher. The title alone of *Dead Souls* is a bit morbid. When Goncharov's novel first appeared it made a tremendous impression, for the Oblomovs were more familiar to the Russian reading public than the Chichikovs, and many a Russian landowner (gentry, gentleman) recognized himself in Oblomov as in a mirror. I have told you that Pushkin, when he first heard *Dead Souls* read to him, said, "God, what a sad country Russia is!" Turgenev (coming next) said,

"As long as there remains one Russian, Oblomov will be remembered."

Goncharov, in *Oblomov,* gives a picture of the idle-rich Russian nobility of the nineteenth century from the cradle to the grave (Oblomov never got out of the cradle; that's the point of the novel). No more vivid or faithful portrait of Russia's Oblomovs than that by Goncharov has ever been painted. Oblomov spends the better part of his life in dressing gown and slippers (important symbols in the novel of the mental and physical stagnation of the wearer), and, significantly, it took Goncharov a whole chapter to get his hero barely out of bed. Oblomov represents to the Russian mind the ideal qualities of repose, seclusion, and unruffled peace, for which Oblomov sacrifices everything. These words (not altogether unsympathetic in their serenity) are the key to Oblomov's character and to Oblomovism. I have read that Oblomov's traits are distinctly Slavic and particularly characteristic of those directly or indirectly attached to the land. I am not competent to judge the accuracy of that generalization. But Oblomov became a household word in Russia, just as Babbitt in America, Bovary and Tartuffe in France, Pecksniff in England; names suggesting both national and international characteristics.

After *Oblomov,* the idle-rich nobility of Russia became a legitimate target for attack, and many Russian authors were quick to attack. I am thinking particularly of Turgenev, and our next novel, *Fathers and Sons,* is a perfect point from which to look back on what we have read thus far, and from which to look towards a future for Russia, by now largely fulfilled. Having read the four novels you have (I trust, I trust), you are likely to be less sympathetic with the Russian gentry and more sympathetic with the crude Bazarov than you otherwise might have been.

SLAVOPHILES AND WESTERNERS

<u>Clash between Tradition and Innovation</u>. In *Oblomov,* Goncharov depicts the clash between tradition and innovation in nineteenth-century Russia—between the old patriarchal landowners and the new industrial bourgeoisie represented by the successful and enterprising businessman; between rural life and urbanization; between culture and what the West calls civilized progress. It is the struggle between what have been labeled Slavophiles (holding to what is supposed to be inherently Russian) and Westerners. It is a clash not only between authors but within authors, all the way to Solzhenitsyn: Turgenev and Chekhov and Dostoevsky and Tolstoy and all the rest were torn; Solzhenitsyn, educated as a scientist, a mathematician, an engineer, writes with the heart and soul of a Slavophile.

For those of you acquainted with Chekhov, you know that the same clash between old and new in Russia runs through all his plays. And in all is found Chekhov's own version of Oblomovism. Madame Ranevsky, for example, in *The Cherry Orchard* is Chekhov's version of Oblomov (remember how the play opens in the nursery), and Lopakhin Chekhov's version of Stolz. The problem of ruralism *versus* urbanization is at the very heart of this play and the new direction Russia must take. The cherry orchard must come down, the orchard representing Russia's sentimental past. Of course, there are those who will not allow a political interpretation of this play—and they may be right. But, at least, the human disorientation is there.

Oblomov at his best (and he has good qualities) is a true representation of a declining patriarchal society whose roots were firmly fixed in the past. It had taken many generations to achieve the society of which Oblomov was, perhaps, the last representative. Goncharov's novel and, in particular Oblomov's Dream, are monuments to the past. Until the dawn of a more "practical" age, Oblomov's repose, seclusion, peace were ideals devoutly to be wished, the highest good of life, but now rapidly vanishing. When the industrial age began to encroach on patriarchal society, the Oblomovs, in protest against the hustle-bustle of practical businessmen, turned their backs upon it all, and defied the new world in dressing gown and slippers. They clung till the last ditch to what they believed to be the true Russian heritage. (Whither goest thou, O troika?)

Purging and Remaking Oblomovism. You may be sure that Goncharov, himself a nobleman (as was Turgenev), is dealing with Oblomov sympathetically, although he makes Oblomov the "superfluous man" and knows that Stolz is the "positive hero" who will inherit the future, though only temporarily (something Goncharov doesn't know), just as Lopakhin in *The Cherry Orchard* is only temporary. Goncharov does not condemn everything in Oblomovism, and he gives Oblomov more positive than negative traits. It was not the purpose of Goncharov to deprive the Oblomovs entirely of their dream of repose, for he was never an enemy of the existing order, but to show the price that must be paid for it. Goncharov wants to purge Oblomovism of its less desirable attributes of laziness and neglect, and give it a new meaning: the dream of repose must be the reward of labor and the exercise of practical ability.

And in Stolz we have Goncharov's attempt to portray the practical and enterprising businessman—the antithesis of Oblomov—whom he prophetically recognizes as the leader of a new age. The metamorphosis of Oblomov would not be easy; Goncharov knows that it will take many Stolzes under Russian names to change the inherent characteristics of the Oblomovs. In the novel, we wonder why Oblomov will not cooperate with Stolz, but Goncharov knows Oblomov cannot bring himself to adopt a mode of life which necessitates work and action, as well as everyday contact with the seamy side of life from which he holds himself aloof. Oblomov turns a deaf ear to Stolz's dream, the dream of an age of industrialism. In the battle between the Oblomovs and the Stolzes, the Slavophiles and the Westerners, Goncharov is predicting the victory of the Stolzes, but he hopes the victory won't come at the expense of Oblomov's good qualities, the good qualities of Oblomov's generation. You will see this nation-wide controversy between Slavophiles and Westerners joined again in Turgenev's *Fathers and Sons*, and, since that is a very good novel, you will find it hard to take sides. Oblomov's better traits are at the root of Slavophilism (Arkady and his father in *Fathers and Sons*); Stolz's ideas are those of the Westerners (Bazarov in *Fathers and Sons*).

The New Russian Woman. In Olga, Goncharov gives us a picture of the new Russian woman who has begun to wrestle with Oblomovism and the problem of Russia's future. Though a member of the St. Petersburg nobility, she's ahead of her contemporaries. She combines action and persistence with a fine mind, yet deep, tender feelings. She is honest, decent, sincere, but in search of convictions, rather than sure of them. Because she loves Oblomov, she tries to expose his weak traits, to arouse him from his inertia, to induce him to assume his responsibilities. Like Goncharov, she believes that if Oblomov can be cured of his negative qualities, he can continue to play a leading role in Russian society, without resigning his place to the Stolzes, and without giving up his good qualities. Olga fails. Like Pushkin's Tatyana, she is meant to represent the best of Russian womanhood. Many of Turgenev's heroines resemble her, but none, I think, in *Fathers and Sons*. But her spirit will live on in future Russian novels you will read.

Serfdom as Relic of the Past. We must not forget Zahar, the eternal serf, loyal as a dog to his master, yet dishonest in trifles, terribly inefficient, and incurably lazy. Although he does not contribute much to the novel, he was, nevertheless, an indispensable feature in the structure of the society of his time. The portrayal of his entire career as a serf, from the time he began to put on his young master's stockings to his end as a beggar, shows Goncharov's intimate knowledge of the evolution of classes, the close relation between master and man. Think of Firs in Chekhov's *The Cherry Orchard*, like Zahar a relic of the past, left behind, lost without the system.

ℒ

Ivan Turgenev, *Fathers and Sons*

THEMES OF THE NOVEL

<u>A Changing Russia</u>. What is the theme of *Fathers and Sons*? What experience of life is Turgenev trying to express with his story? Is there a problem here? The theme is of course not only the clash of youth and age at a particular time in Russia, but the universal clash of fathers and children. Particularly, this novel concerns a changing Russia and the struggle between the generation of the '40s and the generation of the '60s, just before the emancipation of the serfs; a struggle between old ideas and new ones, between sentimental traditions and hard scientific realism. Bazarov represents the sons and new Western ideas. He is a Westerner, in opposition to the fathers, Old Russia, politically speaking, the Slavophiles. He calls himself a nihilist, insisting that all the old ideas and traditions must be swept aside, old institutions must be torn down, and a new Russia built from the very foundations, on scientific principles.

<u>Where Does Turgenev Stand</u>? The problem lies in the question of where Turgenev's sympathies lie. With Westerner or Slavophile? We know that Tur-

genev classed himself as a Westerner and expressed his sympathy with Bazarov. And so the Slavophile Dostoevsky thought him to be, and hated him for it. Is, then, Turgenev putting forth Bazarov as the strong man needed to save Russia, but come before his time, misunderstood, and therefore defeated?

Or is the novel a tissue of ironies that reveals a blind hubris of intellect in Bazarov, who in his pride believes that he can deny his heart, the nature within him, and that he can control with his mind forces outside him? In the end, he is defeated in both struggles. Not only does he fall prey to his feelings for Anna but also nature kills him in his fight against disease. One of the ironies of this man who claims scientific objectivity is that his is the most individualistic, the most destructive ego in the story. He will kill to have his way, as he proves to Arkady. Dostoevsky will contend that men like Bazarov, with their rational pretensions for a better society, are really driven by ego impulses. Is Turgenev, perhaps, revealing the foolishness of Bazarov, a universal foolishness in the idea that the head can deny the heart? Man only rationalizes his instincts.

Or is Turgenev neutral, merely presenting the struggle of his times, in which there is also a message for men of all times? Politically, Turgenev was condemned by both sides: Westerners thought he treated the ideas of Bazarov unfairly, Slavophiles thought he was too favorable to Bazarov. Certainly, there do seem to be opposing sympathies in the novel.

METHOD OF THE NOVEL

The method of Turgenev in *Fathers and Sons* is to take Bazarov through all the classes of contemporary Russia to show him in contrast with them: with the liberal aristocrat Nikolai, with the romantic traditionalist Pavel, with the pseudo intellectuals like Kokshina and Sitnikov, with the bourgeois wealth and luxury of Madama Odintsov (Anna), with his own plebeian parents, with the serfs. How does Bazarov come off in these encounters? Is he the man to lead Russia into the future? Does he, in fact? Well, whether or not Turgenev wants him to, he does lead, and not only in Russia.

∅

Fyodor Dostoevsky, *Crime and Punishment*
(1967)

TRANSITION IN RELATION TO TURGENEV

<u>Dostoevsky's Psychological Realism</u>. In Dostoevsky we have a new kind of realism. Realism generally has been defined thus far as the literary practice of presenting people and things as they are in real life, without idealization. In Turgenev (and in Balzac, Flaubert, and Zola) there was little depth penetration into the minds of the characters; characters in these novels are mostly studied in conflict with external social forces, environment, circumstances, or other characters. In Dostoevsky, however, the conflict is internal, within the mind of the character, and the character study is internal, e.g., the internal consciousness (or dream state) of Raskolnikov, in *Crime and Punishment*. The conflict has an important social orientation and significance (a very important political significance), of course, but it is a drama centered within Raskolnikov's mind.

<u>A Rebuttal to Bazarov</u>. The second point in relation to Turgenev is that *Crime and Punishment* can be considered a rebuttal to Bazarov; not a rebuttal to

Turgenev necessarily, but to the Western ideas of men like Bazarov. Dostoevsky's critique of Raskolnikov is the Slavophile answer to Western rationalism, what Bazarov called nihilism, intellectual science. In general, Russian realism (particularly Dostoevsky and Tolstoy) rejected the agnostic and atheistic naturalism of scientific materialism. Dostoevsky and Tolstoy are ethical in purpose, almost too bluntly so, and certainly not amoral; rather than favoring rationalism, they favor irrational, religious mysticism.

POSSIBLE STATEMENT OF THEME

"Happiness cannot be achieved by a reasoned plan of existence but must be earned by suffering," that is, by compassionate love rather than intellectual pride: Sonia's way rather than Raskolnikov's.

To expand upon this first statement: intellectual pride is a sin against humanity that is punished by spiritual isolation from humanity (the antidote, of course, is Sonia's humility, the suffering which brings fellow-feeling, compassion, regeneration, salvation).

The significance for society here is that Dostoevsky believed that the transformation of the individual must precede the transformation of society (and not as Bazarov stated to Anna); each individual must be morally purified by suffering for guilt and thereby come to know spiritual values.

Most generally, Dostoevsky believed Russian (Slavophile) culture to be superior to Western ideas: holy, spiritual Russia *versus* the rational, intellectual West.

SOME POINTS ON DOSTOEVSKY'S TECHNIQUE

Point of View. As already stated, in *Crime and Punishment* Dostoevsky concentrates on the inner mental focus of Raskolnikov, on what he thinks about what happens, rather than on what happens. This we could call psycho-drama, a kind of forerunner to more artistically controlled stream of consciousness. Most (if not all) of the action of *Crime and Punishment* is seen through the mind of Raskolnikov. In fact, it would be better to say that the action of the novel is seen *from within* Raskolnikov's mind. The focus of the novel is on his mind, not on the external scene; the scene of the novel is his mind.

Narrative Structure. This concentration of point of view within the mind of Raskolnikov tends to tighten the narrative structure of the novel in the sense of limiting it in time and place, limiting it to where Raskolnikov can be and to a short time because of the great complexity of mental action. The place is limited to Petersburg, though a variety of sites within Petersburg. The time expended in the whole 500-page novel is only 15-16 days, not counting the epilogue. Only nine days of action are presented. Single days cover 92, 104, and 121 pages; a suite of three days covers 319 pages.

Psychological Modes of Characterization. My four points here are not mutually exclusive, but they do progress from simple to complex.

USE OF CONTRASTING CHARACTERS WITH DOMINANT CHARACTERISTICS. I have already mentioned Raskolnikov's intellectual pride, which is contrasted with Sonia's compassionate love and humility. This is the basic thematic contrast of the novel. There is also the voluptuous sensuality of Svidrigailov, which is used as ironic contrast to Raskolnikov's intellectual pride, of which I shall say more later. All these contrasts are expanded upon in *The Brothers Karamazov*.

USE OF SPLIT PERSONALITIES. Actually, Raskolnikov is split between intellectual pride and humane compassion, a conflict intensified by Sonia, who brings him (perhaps) to regeneration. Raskolnikov has a terrible inner conflict, a guilt feeling that later psychologists would call a neurosis. Svidrigailov is also split, but, as I said before, is dominated by sensuality rather than intellectual pride, though the difference between the two is an irony of the novel. For Dostoevsky, the root of Raskolnikov's intellectual pride and the root of Svidrigailov's voluptuous sensuality is the same, most deeply rooted in the libido and ego impulses that will brook no super-ego (as in Bazarov). My terms here, of course, are later than Dostoevsky, who himself anticipated much later thinking (Freud, Marx, etc.).

USE OF DOUBLES. This use of split personalities leads me to Dostoevsky's use of doubles for characterization. Dostoevsky creates doubles, alter egos, for his characters to objectify and dramatize their split personalities. Svidrigailov is Raskolnikov's double, his alter ego. He is a separate character, but objectifies one aspect of Raskolnikov's character in order for Raskolnikov and us to see it better.

Raskolnikov hates Svidrigailov for Svidrigailov's sensuality (particularly as that sensuality is directed toward Raskolnikov's sister, Dounia), yet Raskolnikov is forced to see that his rational pride and Svidrigailov's sensuality are part of the same entity, and equally destructive of others. They are both self-centered. Raskolnikov sees, and Svidrigailov knows, that Svidrigailov's cruel sensuality is no more ugly than Raskolnikov's rational motivation: they have the same source, the selfish lust for power or sex, the ego impulse, the passionate will. They both deny compassion and pity for what they destroy.

USE OF DREAMS FOR CHARACTERIZATION. Dreams in Dostoevsky always reveal something about the dreamer's split personality. Take the Raskolnikov dream of horse-beating, for example. On the rational, conscious level, Raskolnikov is planning to coldly and dispassionately murder, to scientifically and objectively for asserted humanitarian purposes take a human life; but on the subconscious level of his dream there is revealed his tendency toward human compassion and pity, which conflicts with his rational intention. In this dream, Raskolnikov's inner irrational self reveals the right path, Raskolnikov's true self, and Dostoevsky's intended truth.

Thus, Dostoevsky's dreams always have a latent content that stands in relation to the outer context and psychic conflicts of the character's life. The Freudian significance is that Raskolnikov's dreams reveal something of Raskolnikov's psychic conflicts, his neuroses, in the world in which he lives. But Dostoevsky's dreams also have another and perhaps more important symbol, that is, a universal and archetypal significance in regard to mankind and the human condition. This Jungian significance is that dreams reveal something about human nature, something archetypal in the collective unconscious. To use the horse-whipping dream again: it reveals not only Raskolnikov's personal psychic conflict of mind and heart, of reason and feeling, as he is about to murder the pawnbroker, but it also shows something about mankind, the combination of cruelty and pity, of good and evil closely coiled together in the self, in human nature, arising from a common unconscious source, an impulse toward self-expression.

SUMMARY

What are we to think of Raskolnikov at the end of *Crime and Punishment*? Raskolnikov is from the Russian "raskol," meaning schism, or cut off. Dostoevsky thinks of him, at least in the beginning, as an intellectual nihilist, an atheistic rationalist who rejects the authority of a supreme being, thus breaking with Russian tradition. One thing is sure: that if Raskolnikov does abandon his nihilistic theories of the Superman who puts himself above the moral law and denies Christian pity and compassion, this repentance is strongly resisted almost to the end. Another thing is equally true: that Dostoevsky intends Raskolnikov to be repentant, however artistically difficult it may be to accomplish that repentance.

Four Possibilities. At the end, there are three or four possibilities open:

FIRST. Raskolnikov, the intellectual nihilist, the atheistic rationalist, never repents. He never gets beyond the point of his reason for confessing to Porfiry, his confession of the murder. He confesses not because he thinks he is evil and the theory wrong but because, according to his own classification of human beings, he thinks he is a louse, not a Superman.

SECOND. The second possibility is that Raskolnikov never repents, but for another reason: in prison, in the extremity of his alienation from his fellow prisoners, in his lonely strength, he realizes, or at least believes, he is a Superman and that it is only a fate beyond his control that has thwarted him. In prison, he achieves complete separation from others; he has become a law unto himself, thrown completely upon his own resources, needing to follow no other imperative but his own existence (like Svidrigailov who makes the ultimate challenge to the absurd meaninglessness of existence in suicide). Raskolnikov is free—except, perhaps, for Sonia. Her compassion for him, her willingness to die for him, is an emotional hold on him which threatens his nihilism, his absurd existential freedom—therefore in unrepentant moods he hates her. The idea that Raskolnikov achieves the empty amoral freedom of the nihilistic Superman-hero is advanced by K. Mochulsky in a fine essay titled "The Five Acts of *Crime and Punishment*." Mochulsky considers the novel a tragedy: that is, in Dostoevsky's eyes, Raskolnikov is a tragic hero because he does *not* repent his nihilism.

THIRD. The third possibility, of course, and the one I accept, is that Dostoevsky intends to suggest that Raskolnikov repents, or certainly will go through a process of redemption to the end: that he submits his self-will, his proud ego, to the laws of God and God's nature, life, the fertile earth. He is thus converted, accepting Sonia's way of Christian compassion, self-sacrifice, and suffering for the burdens of all humanity (St. John 14:20, in Christ, all humanity is one man; "because I live," said Jesus, "you too will live; then you will know that I am in my father, and you in me and I in you").

FOURTH. The logical and artistic difficulty with Christian humility is that, when it consciously is practiced, it is just as ugly as the conscious rationalizations of Raskolnikov and Svidrigailov for intellect and sensuality and just as destructive of the life and freedom of others. Consciously practiced humility is sheer murder. It takes a Sonia or an idiot to pull off humility. That is why, I think, Raskolnikov's repentance must be suggested in the unconscious recognitions symbolized in his last dream. The redemption of Coleridge's Ancient Mariner is accomplished in the same unconscious way, when he blesses God's creatures, the water snakes: "O happy living things! I blessed them unaware." Dostoevsky consistently shows the right path for Raskolnikov on the irrational level of dreams.

Notes

- Raskolnikov's last dream is of a plague that infects humanity with intellectual self-will and leads to destructive violence. The world is saved by a chosen few. Or rather, only a few are left from the destruction to build a better world.

- Raskolnikov's dream is an Easter dream, a resurrection dream (cf. story of Lazarus).

- The microbes are abstract intelligences that destroy because of the extreme relativism of the separate egos that the virus develops.

- Now intelligence and will (pride) are diseases of mankind.

- The world is saved by the quiet people, like Sonia, who "renew the earth." "No one had heard their words or their voices."

∅

Leo Tolstoy, *The Death of Ivan Ilych*

APPROACH TO *IVAN ILYCH*

<u>In General</u>. Tolstoy's works make a good balance of self and society, of private and public experience. *Ivan Ilych* begins with the public reaction to Ivan's death, then shifts back in time to Ivan's private experience as he faced that death. The point is that Ivan was just like the selfish rest, until he faced his inner self (his true, existential self) in the experience of pain and suffering. The point is that there is a great difference to be discovered between the public self and the private self.

The Death of Ivan Ilych is the story of a plain, ordinary man (Mr. Everybody). His name in English would be something like John Smith. He is forced by his illness away from his public image of himself into the very depths of his private being; he is forced by the experience of Death to the place where he truly exists, his innermost private self. This happens when Death for Ivan changes from the conclusion of a logical syllogism to the felt catharsis of mortality, to the experienced-felt-in-the-blood truth of his basic existence. The recognition changes the whole meaning of life for Ivan.

<u>Idea, Theme</u>. As with all of Tolstoy's stories, the basic question behind it is, Why should a man live? And the answer in *Ivan Ilych*, as in the other stories, is: to love, to love God and one's fellow man, naturally, without the artificialities of social convention that separate us from love. The peasant Gerasim and the young son, both unaffected by the hypocrisies, the "lies," that society practices, point the way for Ivan to what is true, to love.

STRUCTURE

<u>Chapter One</u>. Structurally, it is important to look at the first chapter of *Ivan Ilych*. Time here is the dramatic present, after Ivan's death. In this chapter, we see Ivan in relation to the false conventional society that reacts to Ivan's death. This is the society to which Ivan belonged:

- There is the daughter who can only think of her delayed marriage.

- There is the wife who can only think, How *I* suffered and, after Ivan's death, What about the pension?

- There is Peter Ivanovich (note the patronymic), friend of the family, who cannot think Ivan's death is relevant to him, and who only wants to get to his card game, not to an inner recognition.

- And there, too, on the cover before them is the green dead face of Ivan, the face of Death.

<u>After Chapter One</u>. The novella proceeds after Chapter I to trace the steps of a psychological process, a development in Ivan. Looking back, the remainder of the story traces the growth in Ivan: from lies to truth; from public image to private being; from communication to communion; from indifference to love (physically speaking); from life to death and death to life (spiritually speaking). For, in truth, Ivan is reborn, he is regenerated, he finds out who Ivan is and what he should (have) live(d) for. And that makes suffering, and dying, much easier for Ivan, living better and more purposeful.

THE DESTINY OF IVAN'S SOUL

Finally, I want to bring up a problem as to the destiny of Ivan's soul. I once discounted the doctrinal implications of the last pages until I discovered that during the writing of this story Tolstoy was going through a very orthodox phase of belief. Still, whatever heaven Ivan goes to, the important thing, in the best and existential sense, is what Ivan discovers in the last refuge of his innermost being, where he faces the mortal human being for what he is. The torment of his agony and the love that he finds are Ivan's Hell and Heaven. Abstract Heavens and Hells are just that, abstract ideas, like Ivan's abstract idea of Death in the syllogism, in the public image. Abstract Heavens and Hells are only words until we find them in our private experience, just as Death is just a word until Ivan experiences its private reality.

✍

Leo Tolstoy, *Resurrection*
(Spring 1973)

THEMES OF THE NOVEL

<u>Two Levels</u>. *Resurrection* should be looked at on two levels:

SPIRITUAL REGENERATION. Like *Crime and Punishment*, it is a novel about the inner life of a man (and a woman), about his (their) spiritual regeneration and rebirth. Like *Crime and Punishment*, it is about the transformation of the private ego to unselfishness.

THE CONDITION OF RUSSIA. And, like *Crime and Punishment*, it also concerns the "condition of Russia" theme. Which direction should Russian society take? But, whereas the psychological element predominates in *Crime and Punishment*, the social aspect probably predominates in *Resurrection*—or at least more nearly balances the psychological aspect than it does in *Crime and Punishment*, despite the title of Tolstoy's novel. For, besides being a story of spiritual rebirth, *Resurrection* is very obviously a ringing indictment of the social and political crimes against humanity in pre-revolutionary Russia.

Guilt and Expiation. Don't forget, though, that *Resurrection* is a kind of *Crime and Punishment*, a story, like Dostoevsky's, of guilt and expiation, about conscience, or if you prefer, about neurosis. Raskolnikov's guilt, like Nekhludov's, has social and political implications, but Nekhludov's guilt springs not from an intellectual crime but from the social crime of Nekhludov's whole class. Tolstoy and Nekhludov, in *Resurrection*, turn against their class, their established place in society. In no other novel of Tolstoy—and in no other novel of the time in Russia—are the lower classes dealt with so extensively and so sympathetically.

Tolstoy's Views on the Fundamental Questions of Life. Though *Resurrection* cannot be considered a great work of art comparable to *War and Peace* and *Anna Karenina*, 1869 and 1877 respectively, it does contain the essence of Tolstoy's mature views on most of the fundamental questions of life. It contains Tolstoy's belief that:

- All judgment is not only useless but immoral; that judges and juries are not only not infallible but careless, ill-informed, and unworthy by their own shortcomings to pronounce sentences on their fellow men.

- Men in authority, from the public prosecutor to the lowest officer, are inevitably corrupted by the power they exercise and forget human considerations when acting in their official capacity.

- The organized Church has made a mockery of Christ's teachings and lent its authority to everything from the incantation over bread and wine to the practice of war, capital punishment, and all forms of legal restraint and violence.

- People are convicted and punished for being morally superior to their society.

- Taxation is robbery.

- Military service and the conditions of army life inevitably lead to depravity and the need to act against one's conscience.

- For the most part, educated society is selfish, corruptible (venal), mercenary, and hypocritical.

- Sexual relations are frequently degrading and offensive to human dignity.

- Only when evil men stop trying to reform evil men and all acknowledge their guilt before God, vowing not to kill, hate, swear, fornicate, or exact retribution (what TV's all about) but learning to respect as Christ (not the Church) commanded them, only then will there be any prospect of founding the kingdom of Heaven on earth.

All these beliefs are in *Resurrection,* expressed dogmatically, without compromise.

STRUCTURE

The novel's larger narrative plan in relation to theme (the evil consequences of government and the hypocrisy of the Church):

Part 1 is the offence (including Nekhludov's), the trial, the verdict, and the discrediting of the law. The satire of Part 1 is directed against legal institutions.

Part 2 is the attempt to use the law to right the law. The target of Part 2 is the bureaucracy.

Part 3 attempts to show that it is possible to change human beings. In Part 3 the strong satire against the oppressors gives way to an attempt to live with and understand the oppressed, the victims of state oppression. When we get to Solzhenitsyn, remember Tolstoy on state oppression and other abuses of state.

∅

Maxim Gorki, *Mother*

Although a poor novel by artistic standards, I am including Maxim Gorki's *Mother* (published about eight years after Tolstoy's *Resurrection* and about ten years before the revolution of 1917) because:

The Proletarian Hero. It heralds the advent of the proletarian hero, the later "positive hero" of Soviet literature, the leader of Russia's future in terms of socialist ideology.

Socialist Romanticism. It became (mistakenly, perhaps) the pattern for the rigid and doctrinaire "socialist (Soviet) realism" (more aptly "socialist romanticism"), with its idealized hero dramatizing an idealized (Utopian) future—a departure from nineteenth-century Russian Classical Realism and its radical (root) insistence of human truth.

Socialist Dilemma. It contains at least the seeds of the socialist dilemma of heart and mind, the sacrifice of human impulse to political (scientific, economic, historic, so-called rational) logic, as foreshadowed in Bazarov and Raskolnikov and treated later by Bulgakov, Pasternak, Sholokhov, Koestler, Solzhenitsyn, many others. In going through the text, I am going to emphasize the heart-mind conflict. Nilovna regards herself as a Mary-mother figure who must stifle her anguish for her son deep in her heart, subdue it to the higher cause of all her children, the world's children.

BIBLIOGRAPHY: Marc Slonim, *Modern Russian Literature*; Rufus J. W. Mathewson, Jr., *The Positive Hero in Russian Literature*

✄

Mikhail Sholokhov, *And Quiet Flows the Don*

INTRODUCTION - *THE QUIET DON*

And Quiet Flows the Don is half of a 2000-page, 4-volume novel titled *The Quiet Don* and published in Russia between 1928 and 1938 (Slonim says 1940). In English, *The Quiet Don* is usually published in two parts: the first, titled *And Quiet Flows the Don* (which you are reading), covers roughly Sholokhov's volumes I and II; the second, *The Don Flows Home to the Sea*, covers roughly Sholokhov's volumes III and IV. Sholokhov was born in 1905 and completed what you are reading by the age of 23 (not much older than most of you now), and the whole *Quiet Don* by age 33. *The Quiet Don* is definitely the most widely read and beloved work in Soviet literature, and probably the most widely read novel in the whole of contemporary literature. When the last volume was issued, crowds were standing in line in Moscow all through the night waiting for the bookshops to open. Sholokhov is the latest (1965) winner of the Nobel Prize for Literature.

The Quiet Don is basically the story of Gregor Melekhov (and the political story of the Don Cos-

sack region) from the time shortly before World War
I to the establishment of the Red (Bolshevik) government that is in the Don Cossack country. In
briefest summary:

Volume I. This volume concerns the pre-World War
I (Russo-German War) conditions of the Don Cossack country and Gregor Melekhov's involvement in
the war. Volume I includes the beginnings of the
Red Revolution and Gregor's emerging Red sympathies.

Volume II. Gregor takes up the Red cause, then becomes disillusioned.

Volume III. Gregor fights for the Whites against the
Reds in the Don Cossack region struggle. Gregor's
vacillations in sympathy are usually occasioned by
brutalities he sees on one side or the other.

Volume IV. Gregor deserts the Whites to fight for
the Reds, but they do not trust him and he becomes a fugitive, with Aksinia. The novel ends with
Gregor's capitulation to the new order. He is a
beaten man. Aksinia dies; Gregor buries her and
returns to the old family home on the Don, which is
not his, and to the son (by Natalie) who does not at
first recognize him.

Gregor as Tragic Hero. You should understand
from the beginning that although the character of
Gregor engages your sympathy and Sholokhov
seems to be neutral (Sholokhov is not discursive
like Tolstoy), Sholokhov intends his reader to see
Gregor Melekhov as a tragic hero, unstable in

character and tragic because of his individualistic Cossack spirit of independence. In his deep human sympathies and violent emotional reactions, he cannot see, because of brutalities on both sides, the course he should take: that is, the common socialist cause of the Russian people—the one that history and nature dictate as *the Don flows home to the sea.*

SHOLOKHOV AND TOLSTOY

The obvious comparison for *The Quiet Don* is of course Tolstoy's broad canvas in *War and Peace.* Both are huge portraits of life. But *Anna Karenina* will do for us, especially for making some contrast between the ideas of Tolstoy and Sholokhov.

Like *Anna Karenina, The Quiet Don* explores the meaning of human existence, the question of man's place in nature and society. Both novels balance the passionate emotional life lived for the individual self over against a more thoughtful (even reasoned) existence lived for purposes beyond the satisfaction of self and individual passions. I would like to put stress, as I did for *Anna Karenina,* on the balance in both novels of heart and head, of self and soviet, even though both authors ultimately tend away from justifying private satisfactions.

In the end, though Levin learns the importance of heart and feeling and the inadequacy of reason to know the purpose of life, the main thrust of *Anna Karenina* is toward man's communion with man in the divine plan and purpose. Likewise, though Sholokhov has sympathy with the fierce individualism of the Cossacks, in particular with Gregor Melekhov, he ultimately blames them for resisting the movement toward political community and Sovietization in their desire for individual freedom and separation. Sholokhov thinks Gregor is wrong for his inability to choose between his heart and his head, wrong in his vacillation, wrong for his inability to know the communion (communism) of man in the course of history. So Sholokhov is a Party man, and Tolstoy wants human community, love of Man.

But now note a big difference between Sholokhov and Tolstoy. Though there is a similarity in their zeal for brotherhood in the communion of man, Tolstoy, unlike Sholokhov, places man's destiny in the hands of God, even though man—each man, like Levin—finds God's purpose for man's relation to man within his own heart. Sholokhov belongs not to Christian Russia but to Soviet Russia, the new order. That which is beyond man is not the purpose of God moving inevitably towards man's destiny but the forces of nature, the course of history—also moving toward human communion in this world. For Sholokhov, the image of the illimitable steppes in *The Quiet Don* is the vast expanse of nature and history, and through it runs the course of the silent Don, flowing inevitably home to the sea, the source of all. Man's petty private feelings are drowned in the vast expanse of nature and history, impersonal and impassive.

Further, there is more thematic emphasis on the rational, on cold reason, in Sholokhov than there is in Tolstoy, as there is likely to be in Marxist thinking. This statement needs a lot of explanation and qualification. Tolstoy is filled with long discursive portions, rational speculations (the mind of Levin) that are largely absent in Sholokhov—yet in the end Levin abuses his reason. The whole point of Anna the woman is the importance of the private person, the individual heart, not the public person. Sholokhov works contrariwise: almost the total fabric of *The Quiet Don* is a presentation of immediate and passionate existence in the individual sensation of life, though quite objectively and dispassionately observed—yet Sholokhov's final emphasis almost brutally favors the subjection of private impulse to political necessity. In the end, Mishka Koshevoi, the calculating, almost cold-blooded man who sees the course history will take, displaces and is given precedence over the sympathetic, human Gregor Melekhov, the Gregor who vacillates and cannot stick to a course, the tragic hero who cannot adjust his individualistic qualities to the communal welfare.

It is almost as though Sholokhov's strong Cossack sympathies (Sholokhov was a Cossack) for the high-spirited, humane, individualistic Gregor are at war with his rigid Marxist doctrines. But then it could be said that Tolstoy quells the honest rational skepticism of Levin in a religious feeling that is an abdication of reason. From the viewpoint of a Marxist, *Anna Karenina* is a split novel; from the viewpoint of a Christian, Sholokhov is a split man. We ought to keep our focus in both novels on the human problems in them: today we speak of Christian humanists, and even Marxist humanists. With the contemporary emphasis on *this earth* and the possibility or impossibility of human love in the here and now, there have been more twentieth-century thinkers who have tied human development to the processes of nature than to divine Providence.

One point more: whatever their difference of emphasis at a particular time in human and national history, Tolstoy and Sholokhov share a common religious zeal for human community, for the communal welfare of men living on this earth. We should at least see their attempt to balance self and society. And it is easy to see why Soviet doctrine finds Tolstoy more compatible than Dostoevsky.

Boris Pasternak, *Dr. Zhivago*

Henry Gifford in *The Novel in Russia* states that the opening paragraph of Tolstoy's *Resurrection* sets the moral scale, the implicit values, for *Doctor Zhivago*. Let me read to you Tolstoy's first paragraph:

The sun warmed, the grass coming to life grew and showed green everywhere that it had not been scraped away, not only on the boulevard verges but also between flagstones—and birches, poplars, bird-cherry unfurled their sticky and scented leaves, the limes swelled their bursting buds: jackdaws, sparrows and doves with the joyfulness of spring were already preparing their nests, and flies buzzed by walls as the sun warmed them. Happy were plants and birds and insects and children. But men—fully grown men—did not cease to deceive and torment themselves and each other. Men took as holy and significant not this spring morning, not this beauty of God's world given for the welfare of all beings—a beauty disposing towards peace, harmony and love—but they took as holy and significant the things they themselves had plotted to dominate each other.

Says Gifford: "Pasternak's theme includes the self-deceit and the mutual tortures of men, but always behind and above stands the 'beauty of God's world' which Yuri celebrates in the midst of suffering, as does Lara." Gifford doesn't say so, but what Pasternak finds lacking in Russian Socialism (Communism, if you will) is what Razumikhin of Dostoevsky's *Crime and Punishment* finds lacking in the scientific determinism and socialistic community of François Fourier:

> They don't like the life process, because a living soul isn't called for in their system. A living soul demands life; a living soul doesn't obey mechanical laws. Nature wants life, the life process isn't over yet, it's too early for the graveyard. You can't vault over nature with logic alone.

A HUGE POEM

Doctor Zhivago is not simply a realistic novel; it is a huge poem dramatizing what the poems that conclude it express. It is a vast construction of symbolisms, a complicated allegory, or, best, a network of parables suggesting the situation of a living soul in time of Revolution. Obviously, I can't deal with every aspect of *Doctor Zhivago's* parabolic significances, but I can give you some idea of what is represented in the novel.

For example, and overriding, one part of the hero's name, the surname Zhivago, is the Church Slavonic genitive and accusative form of the adjective *zhivoi*, meaning alive-living, a one-word description of the doctor's basic loyalty. For Pasternak it combines and unifies life in nature and the life of the spirit, the pagan and the Christian, as suggested by two poems at the end, "Winter Night," and "Star of the Nativity." Doctor Zhivago (the character) represents life, that life which binds all together in nature and transcends nature in the individual soul. *Doctor Zhivago* (the novel) is a love poem celebrating life, the totality of human experience. The novel is not so much a rebuttal to Socialist doctrine as it is the assertion of something Pasternak feels is being lost in the new order.

In Chapter 3, Zhivago's dead foster mother, Anna Ivanovna Gromeko, represents what happened and is happening to Imperial Czarist and capitalistic Russia (her maiden name was Kruger); Zhivago's dead real mother, Marya Nikolayevna Zhivago, represents what happened and is happening to the Orthodox Church. (Compare Bulgakov's use of a dead mother and almost-dead brother.)

Also, in Chapter 1, the dialog between Yuri's uncle Nikolai Vedenyapin and Ivan Voskoboinikov is almost a debate on philosophical grounds between the opposing positions of Christianity and Socialism (Marxism) as Nicolas Berdyaev (White Christian existentialist philosopher) and Lenin would present them. The description of Ivan Voskoboinikov suggests things devilish; Yuri's uncle was once a priest in the Church, and Yura's teacher.

Of course, the very title of Chapter 1 is parabolic, the appearance of "the five-o'clock express." The late afternoon, the setting sun, the connotations of the word "express"—all are reminders of an era nearing death. The train, a mechanical dragon, symbolizes the Revolution rushing on towards its appointed hour. What happens to Yuri's father aboard the train (and off), in the hands of Komarovsky, has parabolic significance. Yura, Yuri, Yurii, other differences in names.

Through the novel Doctor Zhivago's successive loves, Antonina (Tonya) Gromeko, Larisa (Lara)

Guichard (Guishar in our text), and Marina Shchapova (Marinka) are all representative versions of successive Mother Russias, Lara being the most important for the life theme of the novel. Significantly, Marina, the last love of Zhivago, is a daughter of the Gromeko porter. As one critic observes,

In Pasternak's poetic novel, Yuri Zhivago not only writes love poems to Mother Russia but marries her three times—in the persons of Tonya Gromeko, Larisa Guichard, and Marina Shchapova, who typify distinct classes of Russian society.

Yuri never regards his country with loathing. He sees her as beautiful and compassionate but misguided, like Lara,/raped/seduced/betrayed by Komarovsky and Paul/Pasha Antipov-Strelnikov. Russia's heart, like Lara's, is naturally pure and loving, but it has been seduced by evil, bewitched by ruthless men, betrayed and driven to desperation and madness.

I suggested earlier that two poems of Yuri Zhivago at the end of the novel, "Winter Night" and "Star of the Nativity," suggest the fusion of the life in nature and the life of the spirit (pagan and Christian)—or they may represent two paths of revival for Russia: recreation from natural chaos by Revolution, or regeneration by Christian ideals, naturally, mythically, or both. Helen Muchnic in *From Gorky to Pasternak: Six Writers in Soviet Russia* says this about the poems: "The whole novel, indeed, all of Pasternak's work, may be said to follow the two lines of wonder represented by 'Winter Night' and 'Star of the Nativity.'"

☙

Aleksandr Solzhenitsyn, *One Day in the Life of Ivan Denisovich*
(1973)

LITERARY TRANSFORMATION OF AN UNEVENTFUL DAY

Georg Lukács (the most universally respected of all Marxist critics) believes that the point of *One Day* is not primarily the horrors of the Stalin era, the concentration camps, etc., but something more universal: the literary transformation of an uneventful day in a typical camp into a symbol of man's past, which has not yet been overcome, but will one day. And this past which has to be overcome, although it has nature-like features (inexorable, cruel, senseless, inhuman), is always and everywhere a social complex, exhibiting the consequences of human acts. Compare to Sholokhov.

Survival and failure to survive are seen by Solzhenitsyn, says Lukács, in social terms. Nature's essence is immutable, true, but can be subordinated to practical human knowledge—the kind of Ivan Denisovich Shukhov. The ultimate healthy attitude toward human existence in nature is a desire to change, improve, make human. Shukhov rescues human dignity.

Here is Solzhenitsyn's socialist optimism, according to Lukács, which you should compare with the optimism that Camus wrenches from his Absurd view of human existence. The failures, past and present, that contrast with Shukhov's modest triumph are preludes to a future normal mode of human relations, a real future life among men (cf. Tarrou).

Solzhenitsyn's attitude is basically very moral. Solzhenitsyn assumes a close relation between literature and morality, between art and life. He sees how bad men and their institutions can be, but he also sees man's basic virtues: comradeship and compassion, kindness and decency and loyalty, the capacity of men to endure and remain *men* under the inescapable and inevitable circumstances of fear, tyranny, and pain in prison, concentration camps, winter.

THE NOVEL

<u>Characters</u>. Ivan Denisovich Shukhov, a Russian peasant-carpenter, prisoner S 854, tells about the single day in the 8th year of his sentence, during January 1951, when the 104th squad of *zeks* (prisoners) builds a wall—and through him we are introduced to a cross-section of Soviet society: to the police, military, peasant, worker, intellectual, Russian, Estonian, Latvian, Ukrainian, gypsy, who inhabit the concentration camp world of Shukhov:

- Tiurin, squad leader of the 104th, a rich peasant's son, has been in the camp for 20 years.

- Buinovsky, a formal naval captain, is a confirmed Communist.

- Tsezar, a one-time film producer, represents the intellectuals.

- Alyosha is a Baptist convicted for religious beliefs.

- Volkovoi, a wolfish bastard, is the camp's security chief.

- Fetiukov, former government bureaucrat, has been reduced to a slobbering jackal.

The novel opens on a note of corruption that represents an infection of the Soviet society, and perhaps of man's nature: Tiurin, the squad leader of the 104th, has to bribe the senior official at the assignment center with salt pork to keep his squad from being assigned to building a settlement on the bare, icy steppe, where they would be terribly exposed. In the struggle of greed and corruption in the camp, the prisoners are even more cruel to one another than the guards. They fight viciously for the little food, rest, and warmth available to them in the camp, and sometimes find strength to survive in work or a faith: Alyosha in his Christian religion, Buinovsky in Communist idealism, Tsezar in his commitment to art. Shukhov takes pride in his workmanship, respects Alyosha, and seems to believe in God, but he does not find religion an adequate resource for hope.

<u>Tension between Materialism and Idealism</u>. The story of Ivan's day shows a tension between selfish materialism and altruistic idealism—an essential conflict that is in society and in men. Though Shukhov is a man with a survivalist ethic, it is not survival on any terms. He has standards of dignified conduct which he never abandons. These standards even help him survive. The shameless Fetiukov, who will do anything to live, is marked for death just because he does not have moral stamina. Shukhov's pride in his craft, the workmanship that goes into the wall, is Solzhenitsyn's pride in his craft of writing, his moral stamina in standing up against the corruption of the Stalin era.

Solzhenitsyn seems to be saying in *One Day in the Life of Ivan Denisovich* that men can achieve some measure of freedom in a concentration camp—or in the worst society. He seems to say that imprisonment of the body cannot ultimately imprison the spirit. Man can attain this measure of freedom if he is willing to sacrifice for morality and decency. Solzhenitsyn makes his point through the crude humor and ironic understatement of Ivan Denisovich who sticks to the facts of what was "almost a happy day." Some critics feel that restricting the point of view to an unsophisticated peasant increases the novel's realistic horror but limits its universality. I think quite the opposite.

        ঌঌঌ

ESSAYS AND REVIEWS

I cannot do all things, but I attempt to open minds
to everything.

—A. James Prins
"Teaching *Moby-Dick*," 1982

∂∂∂

Prins the Scholar

Kathleen Verduin

A. JAMES PRINS would not have considered himself a literary scholar. I remember visiting him one Thanksgiving vacation in the late 1960s and congratulating him on what was rumored to be his book in progress, a revision of his dissertation on Charles Dickens' *Bleak House*. "Oh, that's a lot of foolishness," he shrugged. The dissertation remains, of course, but the book was never written; even the four revised chapters, found among his papers and evidently intended for submission to an academic journal, were never mailed.

Yet Prins might have made a literary scholar, as he might have made a novelist: it was another road not taken, a path interrupted by his appointment to an institution where few professors published and quotidian obligations took precedence over research. Often, one observes, his lecture notes soar into the kind of interpretive sweep that makes a great critic. His admirably clear prose style, his faultless sense of composition, his workmanlike attention to academic documentation, and his respect for the scholarship of his generation—a period of prodigious de-

velopment in the discipline of literary study—
might have made him a real contender in the
field, had he chosen to contend.

Throughout the Sixties and Seventies, however, Prins produced—no doubt by pressing invitation—half a dozen literary essays and book reviews in local periodicals: *The Reformed Journal*
and *The Reformed Review* (now combined in the
journal *Perspectives*), *The Christian Scholar's Review*, *The Church Herald*, and Hope's student
newspaper, *The Anchor*. These pieces reflect, pre-
dictably, his passion for the novel—a genre, as he
insists in "Spiritual Frontiers," aimed at "the
heart of the matter." He engaged writers prominent in intellectual discourse of the time—
William Golding and Graham Greene, Kingsley
Amis and Muriel Spark—but always with an eye
trained on their ability to "probe the depths of
man's moral being." The moral and religious focus derived naturally from the imperatives of his
editorial venues, but it was in tune with the thematic *cantus firmus* of his own inner life, which
directed him by turns to the existentialism of Albert Camus, the Catholicism of Mauriac and Bernanos, and the numinous supernaturalism of
Charles Williams, among the most gifted of the
famous Inklings. Convinced of literature's importance on all levels of consumption, Prins even
took the time to address popular Christian narra-
tives, the volumes of Grace Irwin and Nicky Cruz
then turning up in the basement libraries of
churches all across West Michigan. Even here,
however, he holds such authors strictly account-
able, chiding one for evasion of personal culpabil-

ity but honoring another for her "genuine depth of self-discovery."

This section concludes with "Romance and Reality in *Bleak House*: The Death and Rebirth of Love in London," the revised final chapter of Prins' 1963 dissertation. I am gratified that this essay is at last to see the light of print, because it strikes me as a compendium of Prins' approach to literature. As in his lecture notes, the sustained attention to principles of form, aesthetic unity, and timelessness is strongly present: these were the literary articles of faith propounded by the New Critical and New Humanistic movements of his day. But we hear as well the undercurrent of Prins' relentless social conscience and profound compassion: his Calvinist insistence on human depravity, but simultaneously (and closest to the core) his truly Dickensian yearning that all the world's children might at last be gathered in by love.

☙

Spiritual Frontiers in the Contemporary Novel

The Reformed Journal, January 1960

THE SPACE AGE, the time in which we live, is the latest stage in the development of that world view which is the attitude of empirical science: the de-personalizing, dehumanizing habit of mind, inherited from the seventeenth century, which dominates twentieth-century thought and divorces sensibility from sense, imagination from intellect. This "scientific" approach to knowledge of our world is objective, quantitative, mechanical, technical. The Space Age extends this emphasis through the physical universe—out-ward.

I do not say that flight to the moon is not a subject for poetry. Nor do I say that Literature is uninterested in man's environment—natural or social or cosmic. But it is the distinguishing characteristic of poetry, drama, and fiction that they focus on what is peculiarly human about the way man experiences his environment, the way he reflectively feels it, enjoys it, is pained by it, morally evaluates it. It matters not a bit that Milton's cosmos in *Paradise Lost* is scientifically inaccurate, that he has the earth at the center of the universe: he has the human center right—man encountering God.

Literature is likely to move in a direction opposite to that of Space-Age Science. It probes the depths of man's moral being. It moves not toward the moon but inwardly to the heart and the soul and the spirit of man. These are the terms of poetry, not of Science; and it is significant that our time is characterized as the Space Age, a phase in the development of material progress, and not the age of poetry, a phase in the growth of the spirit.

The contemporary novel is no exception to the poetic impulse in Literature. Novelists today—those that count—are not concerned with the science-fiction of rocketry: they are not concerned with reaching the moon. They are concerned, as all great novelists, like Dostoevsky and Melville, have always been, with reaching, to use a poetic figure, the heart of the matter. A Christian critic of the contemporary novel, Mr. William R. Mueller, states in his introduction to *The Prophetic Voice in Modern Fiction*:

Wisdom remains, four hundred years after Calvin's definition, that knowledge of ourselves that convinces us of our sin and that knowledge of God which is our salvation. And it is frequently true that a man may come most directly to knowledge of himself when he sees himself anatomized in a contemporary setting and in an idiom, a language, which is of his own time. The voices of the past few decades which have pierced most decisively to the heart of the matter, penetrating most deeply into the anxieties of our generation and expressing most precisely our fears and hopes, have been those of the literary artists, and it is perhaps above all in the modern novel that we find the anatomy of our own age drawn with the greatest clarity. Contemporary novelists are concerned with the problems of the human soul and spirit. These are inner frontiers—not the frontiers of outer space. These are spiritual frontiers.

To exemplify spiritual frontiers in the contemporary novel, I will use Graham Greene's *The Heart of the Matter* and Albert Camus' *The Fall.* Both writers are significant contemporary novelists, and although neither novel is regarded as the author's greatest artistic achievement, each is typical of his thinking—and each is not only written in the theological terms of traditional Christianity, it cannot be understood except in a context of Christian doctrine. The two novels have complementary themes.

The Heart of the Matter

THE THEME OF Greene's *The Heart of the Matter* is Love; *apropos* the condition of modern man, it concerns what Mr. Nathan A. Scott, Jr., in *Modern Literature and the Religious Frontier* calls the "Myth of Sanctity." The central character of the novel is Major Henry Scobie, Deputy Commissioner of the police force of a British-governed town in West Africa during World War II. Though a sincere Catholic, Major Scobie makes what appears to be a mess of his life, because of a corrupting quality he has which Greene calls pity. Scobie is scrupulously just, in the compassionate sense. His immediate superior, the Commissioner, calls him, without irony, "Scobie the Just," a "terrible fellow." Scobie's flaw is an ex-

cess of pity: he cannot bear to watch disappoint-
ment and suffering in others. Scobie is, from the
standpoint of the law, too just—too prone to look
into the heart of the matter rather than to regula-
tions, too moved by compassion for human falli-
bility—to make a good policeman. So when the
Commissioner retires, Scobie is passed over for
the job. His socially sensitive wife Louise feels
humiliated; she begs him to send her away for a
holiday. Scobie cannot afford her passage, but,
feeling pity and responsibility for his wife, he bor-
rows the money from the only person who will
lend it to him, the Syrian Yusef, who is suspected
of working against the English cause in the war.
Thus Scobie compromises his official integrity,
but only in this way can he assume responsibility
and take up his wife's burden.

Soon after Mrs. Scobie leaves, Major Scobie
assists in rescue operations for the victims of a
German torpedo attack. Among the gravely ill is a
six-year-old child. As Scobie watches her dying
agonies and listens to her cry for her father's
presence, he remembers how his own young
daughter had died away from him, and he reflects that "one never really miss[es] a thing. To
be human one [has] to drink the cup." Pretending
a child's game, Scobie assumes the presence of
the father. Sweat breaks out on his brow as he
prays, "Father, give her peace. Take away my
peace forever, but give her peace." The little girl
dies in peace, but Scobie loses his own in deep-
ening pity.

God seems to answer Scobie further in another war victim—another object for pity—a
young woman, Helen Rote, who lies beside the

six-year-old girl, and lives. The young woman is terribly scarred, physically and mentally, by the horrors of forty days on the torrid sea in an open boat and by the loss of her husband. As Scobie views her ugliness and misery, he pities her—and is irresistibly drawn to her need. In offering the human communion that heals her, he later breaks the Seventh Commandment.

Mrs. Scobie returns early. She tries to persuade her husband to go to Mass with her. Scobie knows that she doubts his fidelity—is testing him. In the Roman Catholic faith a person must confess his sins through a mediating priest and receive absolution before he may partake of the Eucharist. Scobie can confess his sins to the priest, but he cannot repent and be absolved. He cannot promise God to grieve his mistress by denying her his company, nor can he grieve his wife by not partaking of the Communion, thus proving to her his infidelity. He chooses to eat at the Lord's Table with mortal sin on his soul; he desecrates the sacrament.

The paradox of Major Scobie's situation is that apparently every sin he commits is motivated by a tender heart. Finally, in guilty remorse for the death of a son-like servant who dies as a consequence of his compassionate dilemma, Scobie doubly damns himself in suicide, believing that by taking his own life he will cause the least pain to those he loves most. He carefully fakes a heart attack to spare his wife and mistress mental agony—and to give Mrs. Scobie financial security.

There are perhaps two corrupting aspects of Scobie's love, if it be truly love: he loves only that which is ugly or suffering, that which is in need of love, pity, compassion; and he has a kind of arrogant pride in carrying the whole responsibility for the world's suffering on his shoulders:

He had no responsibility toward the beautiful and the graceful and the intelligent [he thinks to himself]. They could find their own way. It was the face for which nobody would go out of his way . . . the face used to rebuffs and indifference, that demanded his allegiance.

Wherever there is a burden of pain, Scobie feels guilt—he must take up the burden like a cross. His thought at one point is that doing it is like the love of God, of Christ. Scobie is willing to die for love, to relieve the pain of another. He goes further, for in loving man he damns himself by breaking God's commandments, not loving God above all. As he takes the bread of the Communion, he echoes the wish of Paul in Romans 9:3. He prays, "O God, I offer up my damnation to you. Take it. Use it for them." His last words are, "Dear God, I love . . . ."

For Scobie, the heart of the matter is that one must give up his own peace for the peace of others. He believes he has forfeited eternal peace in taking the Communion in mortal sin, and in taking his life—or giving it. Has he? The heart of the matter is a complex spiritual problem. Greene gives the last word to God. At the close of the story, Mrs. Scobie rather self-righteously asserts to Father Rank the futility of hope for her husband's soul—to which judgment the priest furiously answers, "For goodness' sake, Mrs. Scobie, don't imagine you—or I—know a thing about God's mercy!" Mrs. Scobie protests that "the

Church says . . ."—and Father Rank replies, "I know what the Church says. The Church knows all the rules. But it does not know what goes on in a single human heart."

The Heart of the Matter explores a complex spiritual frontier, the paradoxical mysteries of love, pity, compassion in the human heart, the human limits of Christ-like love.

The Fall

THE THEME of Camus' *The Fall* is Guilt: *apropos* modern man's estate, it falls into Mr. Scott's category of "Myth of Hell." Guilt is related to love in that it is the inferno of the soul which is a consequence of not loving.

The Fall is a monologue delivered by a onetime Paris lawyer, Jean-Baptiste Clamence, who calls himself a "judge-penitent"—a monologue delivered to a silent drinking companion in the "Mexico City" bar, in Amsterdam. The novel strongly reminds one of the mariner and the wedding-guest of Coleridge's famous poem. The canal structure of Amsterdam is meant to suggest the concentric circles of Dante's Hell and symbolize the inferno of the soul to which the narrator has fallen. His recital is a confession of guilt.

Once, he tells his listener, he had lived blissfully in a kind of Eden of moral ignorance and complacency, one of the most respected lawyers in Paris, the protector of widows and orphans, in his own estimation. He had been at the height of his powers, successful, innocently happy, assured of his own righteousness and virtue—until one night he failed to risk his life to save the life of another; even more, he had failed to risk his life for the soul of another: he had failed to plunge into the icy waters of the Seine to save a desperate young girl from suicide. He had failed in a sacrificial encounter with human misery. Thereafter, he is plagued by an unidentifiable laugh that follows him everywhere, the ironic laughter of self-judgment. He confesses to his silent listener,

I have to admit it . . . I, I, I is the refrain of my whole life, which could be heard in everything I said. . . . When I was concerned with others, I was so out of pure condescension, in utter freedom, and all the credit went to me: my self-esteem would go up a degree.

Clamence's "fall" was a conviction of guilt, the discovery that his actions belied his motives, that the appearance of his outer-social self bore no relationship to the reality of his inner-spiritual self. "Modesty helped me to shine, humility to conquer, and virtue to oppress."

Clamence's further discoveries about himself are even more ironic and shattering to his pride. He rips off more layers of duplicity. He continues to his silent listener—who is also his own soul:

After what I have told you, what do you think developed? An aversion to myself? Come, it was especially with others that I was fed up. . . . The prosecution of others . . . went on constantly, in my heart.

The truth is that the whole purpose of Clamence's recital of confession is selfish—to gain from the listener a recognition of the listener's common involvement in human guilt, and thereby shift the burden of guilt from Clamence. Clamence tells the story so that he can accuse as well as confess. There takes place in his recitation a gradual shift from "I" am guilty to "we" are guilty. He says:

> This, alas, is what I am! . . . But at the same time the portrait I hold out to my contemporaries becomes a mirror. I stand before all humanity recapitulating my shames without losing sight of the effect I am producing, and saying, "I was the lowest of the low." Then imperceptibly I pass from the "I" to the "we." When I get to "this is what we are," the trick has been played and I can tell them off. I am like them, to be sure; we are in the soup together. . . . The more I accuse myself, the more I have the right to judge you. Even better, I provoke you into judging yourself, and that relieves me of that much of the burden.

With satisfaction, Clamence states: "I am for any theory that refuses to grant man innocence and for any practice that treats him as guilty."

Thus Clamence relentlessly pursues himself further and further into the pit—into the hell of self-knowledge; and therefore he ironically calls himself a "judge-penitent."

I have but skimmed over the surface of *The Fall.* The novel is rich in Christian allusions: the title, of course; and the narrator's name, Jean-Baptiste Clamence, which suggests, perhaps, a modern John the Baptist, crying (*clamans*) in the wilderness of his guilt for the mercy (*clemence*) of Christ, who must have felt, asserts the narrator, the guilt of complicity in the slaughter of the innocents by Herod. *The Fall* is so thoroughly dramatized in the ironic consciousness of Clamence that it is difficult to know the exact emphasis Camus meant. Does the novel mirror the hypocrisy of pious self-righteousness, or does it mirror the destructive effects of obsessive guilt feelings, the human limits of Christ-like assumption of guilt? Both, I think; but my aim here is to suggest, rather than to interpret or judge, particular novels. *The Fall* is another human dilemma of the soul. What is significant is that it probes the conscience of our time, a spiritual frontier.

LOVE AND GUILT, responsibility and the conscience of man: these are spiritual frontiers in the contemporary novel—if we accept Greene and Camus as representatives of the contemporary novel, and *The Heart of the Matter* and *The Fall* as representative of Greene and Camus. At least they are here to be read, with many more; and it seems to me that probing these spiritual frontiers is more urgent today than shooting the moon—or should I say, *especially* important at a time when the same rocket that probes the frontiers of space can, *and is intended to*, drive a hydrogen bomb to impersonal slaughter thousands of miles away. The mental and material resources of the nation expended on this "intention" would make good subject-matter for a sermon on the text of I John 3:14-16, a subtle problem of the Christian conscience more likely, ironically, to be explored in the pages of a contemporary novel than from the pulpit.

In *Pious and Secular America*, Dr. Reinhold Niebuhr says of the Christian faith that "it declares that God is love and that His love is the final source of harmony for men who know that they ought to love one another but who really love themselves." The Christian faith, Dr. Niebuhr continues, "is the answer to [man's] predicament and becomes meaningless if that predicament is not known." In probing the conscience of man, the contemporary novelist is making the predicament known. Mr. Mueller, with whom I much agree and to whom I am greatly indebted for certain ideas in this paper, puts the point well: "The novelist will not save us, but he may well bring us to the knowledge that we are in need of salvation." Mr. Stanley Hopper in *The Crisis of Faith* says it even more pertinently: "Poetry [and Greene and Camus are poets] will not save the world. But poetry can force the soul into the precincts of its last evasion."

Discovery in the spiritual frontiers is for the poet-novelist; decision, for the individual Christian.

☙

Golding Book Discusses Man's Fall

The Hope College *Anchor*, 2 October 1964

OVER A PERIOD of ten years, William Golding has written five novels: *Lord of the Flies* (1954), *The Inheritors* (1955), *Pincher Martin* (1955), *Free Fall* (1959), and *The Spire* (1964).

"I think of myself," Golding has said, "as a religious man." He likes to have his readers regard him as a maker of myths—of "something which comes out from the roots of things in the ancient sense of being the key to existence, the whole meaning of life and experience as a whole."

Free Fall is the myth of paradise lost, the Fall of Man. It is the story of Sammy Mountjoy, who rises from the slum of Rotten Row to become a successful artist and finds his Beatrice on Paradise Hill. Ironically, Sammy's mount of joy is a *Mons Veneris*; his rise to his Beatrice on Paradise Hill is a fall into the consciousness of guilt. Sammy tells his own story. He begins with a question:

When did I lose my freedom? For once I was free. I had power to choose. The mechanics of cause and effect is statistical probability, yet surely sometimes we operate below or beyond that threshold.

The novel is the retrospective search in Sammy's mind for the answer to that question: "When did I lose my freedom?" By loss of freedom Sammy means a purely private thing. He means to ask, at what point in his life did he make the choice to follow self at whatever cost?—the cost being the sense of guilt that now blocks the freedom of the self. That point is Sammy's free fall: his choice for freedom of the self that costs his freedom of the self because of the sense of guilt that checked his expanding ego.

The guilt-ridden Sammy goes back over the course of his life, looking for the point of fall. Tied to the retrospective technique of the novel is the idea that Sammy cannot know when he fell until *after* he has fallen: insight into the beginning can only come with insight into the end.

He quickly dismisses the poverty of his background, his illegitimate birth, his boyhood blasphemy against the Church. Sammy was essentially innocent then; his early sins were not the wickedness of self-will. He says,

There is no root of infection to be discovered in these pictures. The smell of today, the grey faces that look over my shoulder have nothing to do with the infant Samuel. I acquit him.

His attraction to the rational doctrine preached by an early science teacher and his youthful membership in the Communist Party also belong to this state of innocence.

Beyond the point of all are Sammy's seduction of the dependent Beatrice Ifor, his willingness to betray his comrades when a prisoner of war in

Germany, his dishonesties—but these were not causes; these were effects, the patterns established by a man already irrevocably fallen.

Where then did he lose his freedom? Where was the point of fall? Sammy finally localizes it in the deliberate decision to bend the will of the virginal Beatrice to his own sensual pleasure, to mount his own joy at the expense of another person, to stake everything on the satisfaction of his pride, his sensual ego. Beatrice Ifor, Beatrice for I; that is, for Sammy Mountjoy:

I said in the hot air what was important to me . . . her obedience, and for all time my protection of her; and for the pain she had caused me, her utter abjection this side death.

Here is the point of fall, where freedom was lost—not the seduction itself, but Sammy's decision to conquer another self for his own. And Beatrice's "utter abjection this side death" is exactly the consequence of Sammy's choice for self, plus the cost to Sammy, the sense of guilt that checks his pride, restricts his freedom.

Near the end of the novel, after the humiliation of Sammy's ego in a German prison camp, seven years after Sammy's desertion of Beatrice, Sammy visits her in a mental institution called Paradise Hill, a synonym for Sammy's surname, Mount of Joy.

Sammy learns that Beatrice has been there since his desertion of her. She does not, cannot speak to Sammy. When he tries to force her to recognize his existence, she urinates on the floor in fright.

Sammy tries to pin down just how guilty he is. Is he responsible for Beatrice's condition? The doctor's answer is equivocal:

"You probably tipped her over. But perhaps she would have tipped over anyway . . . . You may have given her an extra year of sanity. . . . You may have taken a lifetime of happiness away from her. Now you know what the chances are as accurately as a specialist."

The doctor's sensible comment questions the possibility of directly charging one person with the responsibility for another and tends to cut down Sammy's guilt. For even though the terrible effects of Sammy's sensual ego are horribly magnified in the deterioration of Beatrice's personality, making Sammy's guilt a medical issue, an exterior issue, softens Sammy's responsibility and hedges the question of the guilt of man.

This is the rational explanation that "drives back the mystery and reveals a reality usable, understandable, and detached." But it oversimplifies the nature of the man involved—the inner person of Sammy Mountjoy, where, he says, "all day long action is weighed in the balance and found not opportune nor fortunate nor ill-advised, but good or evil."

Sammy recognizes the interior issue: the doctor's approach to the essence of things in the world does not satisfy his personal experience of life; it does not bring to Sammy any grace of relief from the sense of guilt that exists in his private self:

At the moment I was deciding that right and wrong were nominal and relative, I felt, I saw the beauty of holiness and tasted evil in my mouth like the taste of vomit.

Sammy thinks of his private world, the world of his freedom and his guilt, as the world of the burning bush, where God is: "And so a sign to Moses that the Lord was present, the bush burned with fire but was not consumed." And he says, "To give up the burning bush, the water from the rock, the spittle on the eyes was to give up a portion of myself, a dark and fruitful and inward portion."

Sammy finds in that secret interior place at the center of himself a realizable essence, permanent and immutable, that judges between good and evil, between the "beauty of holiness" and "the taste of vomit"—in the face of which he is judged guilty.

Still, Sammy cannot join together his dual universe, inner and outer. The world of flesh is "real." The mind of Sammy is conscious of both but cannot make them fuse. "Both worlds are real. There is no bridge." This thought comes to Sammy on the last page of the novel. It is as far as Sammy's rational mind can take him toward a solution of the mystery he confronts in his search for the point at which he lost his freedom, but it is not quite the end of *Free Fall.*

It is significant for both the idea and the technique of the novel that Sammy's final insight comes, in a brief disconnected flash of memory that is a kind of revelation; his memory gives back to him a picture from his past, the last piece of the jigsaw puzzle of his experience, one over which we leave him pondering as though it were "the Sphinx's riddle."

Sammy is back in the German prison cell. There in utter darkness and aloneness he probes to the depths of his naked sensual self. On his knees, in an agony of self-knowledge, he cries to the black walls, "Help me!—and burst that door," the prison door of self.

"*Heraus!*" The cell door opens to admit a triangle of light. Before Sammy stands the camp commandant, not to judge, as he expects, but to pity, to tell Sammy he is free.

Sammy is absent-minded. The commandant asks, "You have heard?" "Have you heard?" The question occurs twice in relation to the incident, and its second form points the scriptural direction. "*Heraus!*" For Adam that meant "Get out! You are guilty." For Sammy it meant "Get up, off your knees! Have you heard you are free, forgiven?"

I give the last words on Sammy's insight to two lecturers in English at the University of Edinburgh who are writing a book on William Golding. This summer at the University of London, they contributed much to my understanding and appreciation of the contemporary British novel.

The cryptic ending is supremely tactful. Is it not a greater mystery than the "Sphinx's riddle'" of the nature of man, that the Sammy Mountjoy in man can be forgiven? He offers his tragic duality and receives an incredible gift. It is the miraculous operation of grace abounding that alone can fuse Sammy's split world and offer forgiveness, though he cannot see the fusion or accept the grace.

Yet the evidence is there, and the whole purpose of the book is, precisely, to point to it. (Ian Gregor and Mark Kinkead-Weekes in "The Strange Case of Mr. Golding and His Critics," *The Twentieth Century*, February 1960.)

Charles Williams

The Reformed Review, March 1967

The Theology of Romantic Love: A Study in the Writings of Charles Williams, by Mary McDermott Shideler, Pp. 243, $2.45; *Charles Williams: A Critical Essay*, by Mary McDermott Shideler, Pp. 48, 85 cents; five novels by Charles Williams, Grand Rapids: William B. Eerdmans Publ. Co., $1.95 each. All paperback, 1966.

THIS IS NOT so much a review as a long-overdue compliment to the William B. Eerdmans Publishing Company for reprinting five novels of the late Charles Williams, British poet, dramatist, novelist, literary critic, and religious thinker: *War in Heaven* (1930), *Many Dimensions* (1931), *Place of the Lion* (1931), *Shadows of Ecstasy* (1933), and *Descent into Hell* (1937). These novels have been called "holy thrillers"; they are adventures in the supernatural that dramatize theological concepts.

The novels of Charles Williams are for those who enjoy reading Dante and Dorothy Sayers, T. S. Eliot and W. H. Auden, C. S. Lewis and J. R. R. Tolkien. These names suggest the ingredients of Williams' fiction: Christian perspective, spiritual vision, and the fantasy of thrilling combat between the forces of good and evil. One may sometimes, even often, question Williams' technical merits as a novelist, and one may sometimes question, even be uneasy about, Williams' theology, but these remain open questions. For in every Williams novel the theological issue is a central one, and in each the forces of good and evil are powerfully dramatized in more than one character.

For example, the heroine of *Descent into Hell* (to my mind, the most successful expression of Williams' themes in the form of fiction) performs an act of atonement and redemption that dramatizes what is probably Williams' most important theme, the theme of "substituted love"—the doctrine of Exchange and Substitution. To Williams, the first law of the universe, a universe in which the natural and supernatural orders co-inhere, is that nobody can carry his own burden; he only can, and therefore must, carry someone else's. Pauline Anstruther's Christian name suggests from whom and through whom derives the doctrine she fulfills ("For continually, while still alive, we are being surrendered into the hands of death for Jesus' sake, so that the life of Jesus may also be revealed in this mortal body of ours. Thus death is at work in us and life in you"; "Help one another to carry these heavy loads, and in this way you will fulfill the law of Christ"). Pauline's redeeming and atoning act is Christlike in her willingness to carry for others that which in Nature is "terribly good"—a good which is "terrifying," "full of terror." This is Pauline's affirming "descent into hell"; it is balanced in the novel's narrative structure by the antithesis of negative descent, Lawrence Wentworth's fall into the darkness of self-absorption through worship of a succubus idol of lust made in the image of his selfish will. Pauline has her deepest insight when she thinks at the funeral of her aunt:

The central mystery of Christendom, the terrible fundamental substitution on which so much learning had been spent and about which so much blood had been shed, showed not as a miraculous exception, but as the root of a universal rule . . . "behold, I shew you a mystery," as Supernatural as that sacrifice, as natural as carrying a bag.

In the act of "substituted love" Pauline finds salvation for herself and others.

Pauline's burden, which is fearing to face herself (in the form of a *doppelgänger*), is carried for her by a poet friend and mentor (a *persona* of Williams); Pauline, in the exercise of Christian *caritas*, bridges centuries in carrying that fear—the fear of death by fire—of a martyred ancestor. In this chain of Exchange and Substitution, Pauline also points the ways to the City of Redemption for the soul of a suicide workman who has lost the way of love and is wandering in the eternity in which the temporal co-inheres. What Pauline learns is to love others not for themselves but for the divine qualities they and the universe exhibit, divine qualities that co-inhere in the natural world. Thus, her experience in the novel also dramatizes other concepts of Williams that are correlatives of "substituted love."

Such is the doctrine of co-inherence, the concept that nothing in the universe is isolated from the singleness of divine reality, from the eternal present of the Holy City. In *Descent into Hell*, as in all of Williams' novels, not only do the natural and supernatural worlds interpenetrate each other but past, present, and future are permutable, what has happened and what will happen are interdependent and interchangeable in the significance of what is. Co-inherence and substitution relate to another Williams doctrine, the way of Affirmation of Images: because the spiritual order co-inheres in the natural, the way of love is to affirm one's sense of the natural, one's sense of the world's body. This is the poet's way of love. It elucidates the Christlikeness of Pauline's act of charity as incarnation and atonement: the affirmation of images is the acceptance of the sense of the world's body, the natural order, as imaging the divine body of Christ, offered in charity, to close the gap between the eternal-spiritual and the temporal-material worlds.

In sum, since everything in the divine reality is single, co-inherent, Pauline can carry (substitute) the burden of anyone in any time by affirming (in an act of love) her sense of a "terribly good" Nature in which the spiritual co-inheres. Wentworth's direction is contrary to Pauline's; his selfishness splits apart the natural and spiritual orders, ruptures the singleness of divine reality. For Williams, Hell is in-coherence seeking to prevail over co-inherence, time and the natural seeking to prevail over the Holy City.

The preceding paragraphs indicate what happens when literary criticism tries to cope with the theological subtleties of a Williams novel and also, I think, what is likely to be the weakness of that novel: the dramatization of ordinary this-world human experience tends to get lost in the subtlety of concepts that link the ordinary and the extra-ordinary, concepts that underlie the action of the novel but which the reader only dimly comprehends. Those who seek guidance in the religious thinking of Charles Williams can turn to two other recent Eerdmans publications, *The Theology of Romantic Love: A Study in the Writings of Charles Williams* and *Charles Williams: A Critical Essay* (the first essay in Eerdmans' Contemporary Writers in Christian Perspective series), both by Mary McDermott Shideler. A student of the novel might wish that Mrs. Shideler had given more critical attention to the question of Williams' skill and effectiveness as a novelist, compared, let us say, with C. S. Lewis, but such is not her purpose in these books. Certainly, though, Mrs. Shideler knows more about the theology of Charles Williams than any other writer on Williams I have read. Certainly, too, she is right in saying that Williams' novels do succeed in creating a sense of the numinous.

∞

From Fiction to Fact

The Church Herald, 22 August 1969

CONTEND WITH HORSES, by Grace Irwin. Eerdmans Publishing Company. 284 pages. $4.95.

GRACE IRWIN, a Canadian novelist and teacher, introduced her preacher-hero as a young man in *Least of All Saints*, and continued his story in *Andrew Connington*. Now she concludes the Andrew Connington trilogy with *Contend with Horses*. The title is taken from Jeremiah 12:5: "If thou hast run with the footmen, and they have wearied thee, how canst thou then contend with horses?" The story is about running with the footmen; it concerns the ordinary, non-heroic ministry of a Toronto pastor in his middle years.

Central to the story are the personal problems that stem from the accidental death of Andrew's beloved wife Cecily six years before the time of the novel—a rebellious son who has become more and more estranged from Andrew since Cecily's death and a doting daughter who will feel hurt and cast off if Andrew marries a wealthy widow of the congregation. The situation is mildly Oedipal. After a slow start, because the reader must be filled in with the background of *Andrew Connington*, the pace of the novel picks up suspense, particularly in the wealthy widow's pursuit of the pastor, and the pastor's pursuit of an unscrupulous lady lawyer, to a stunning climax.

The whole novel has a natural and healthy flavor, and most readers will approve of the way Andrew resolves his problems—with good sense, grace, and presumably, humility. Still, I was a bit put off in sensing that the father and daughter, of whom, surely, the author greatly approves, are more pleased with themselves than they ought to be. Quite smugly pleased. This should not be, especially in a hero who is content to "run with the footmen."

RUN, BABY, RUN, by Nicky Cruz, with Jamie Buckingham. Logos International. 240 pages. $4.95.

In *Run, Baby, Run,* Nicky Cruz relates a horrifying tale of blood-letting violence that makes Andrew Connington's polite ministry seem irrelevant. Nicky Cruz tells his own story, from his arrival in New York City as a hate-filled youngster from Puerto Rico on the run, to his present position as director of Outreach for Youth in Fresno, California. In between are chapters that sometimes grip the reader with terror. Nicky records his bloody initiation into the Mau Mau gang; his participation in savage street wars, robberies, and beatings; his elevation to president of the Mau Maus. Nothing is sacred to Nicky except loyalty to the gang. There are seventeen killings during his period of leadership.

Then Nicky Cruz meets Pentecostal evangelist David Wilkerson, who converts him to the love of

Christ and sends him to the Bible Institute in La Puente, California, for study. There he receives his baptism in the Holy Spirit and meets Gloria, his wife-to-be. Together they return to New York and to Teen Challenge Center, where they minister in the ghettos to drug addicts, prostitutes, and alcoholics.

In his introduction, Billy Graham calls *Run, Baby, Run* "a thrilling story" and Nicky Cruz "a Christian legend in our time." Certainly, *Run, Baby, Run* contains sensational thrills aplenty and a grace so abounding that it covers the most bestial crimes with a minimum of self-analysis, soul-searching, or anguish over personal responsibility. Most of the blame for Nicky's crimes falls on Papa and Mama, Society and Satan.

EVERY WALL SHALL FALL, by Hellen Battle. Hewitt House. 318 pages. $5.95.

Hellen Battle's personal account of her ordeal in East German prisons reveals a greater depth of self-discovery than I found in the conversion of Nicky Cruz or in the ministry of Andrew Connington. This idealistic, impulsive young American girl, a teacher and student in West Berlin, was arrested on a visit to East Berlin, accused of helping an East German soldier escape to his fiancée in West Berlin, and sentenced to four years of hard labor in Bautzen penitentiary.

The reader shares the anguish of Hellen Battle's loneliness and despair as she struggles to break the barriers that separate her not only from the West but from her captors, her fellow prisoners, and her own true self. Hellen Battle is unjustly tried and sentenced. She endures more than a year of prison life. She is often harshly treated. Yet she finds her way from willfulness and self-pity to recognition of her own errors and to dialogue with those who persecute her.

I sensed a profound truth that went beyond East and West Germany, beyond the United States and the Soviet Union, beyond Communism and anti-Communism. It was the way of forgiveness, reconciliation, peace. It was the way of "love your enemy."

Hellen Battle's conclusion is that her first loyalty is not to her country but to the laws of God and to Christian love that break down the walls men build. She is right, but what she believes is not very popular among Christians.

❧

The Catholic Novel

The Christian Scholar's Review, Summer 1973

Gene Kellogg, *The Vital Tradition: The Catholic Novel in a Period of Convergence*. Chicago: Loyola University Press, 1970, 277 pp., $8.35. Melvin J. Friedman, ed., *The Vision Obscured: Perceptions of Some Twentieth-Century Catholic Novelists*. New York: Fordham University Press, 1970, 278 pp., $8.00.

PROFESSOR KELLOGG takes his interpretation of the "vital tradition" from Cardinal Newman's *An Essay on the Understanding of Christian Doctrine*, III, which states that the life of doctrines and views, like the life of organisms, depends upon the assimilation and interpenetration of external materials. He discovers such a growth and development in the history of Roman Catholic communities with their surrounding environments. To this vital tradition, this growth and development of Catholic doctrines and views through assimilation and interpenetration, the Catholic novel belongs as part and flower.

Kellogg strictly defines a "Catholic novel" as one whose mainspring of dramatic action depends upon Roman Catholic theology, or upon the history of thought within one of the world's largest Roman Catholic communities, or upon development of Roman Catholic ideas in Newman's sense. His method is clear and consistent throughout: first to describe the historical characteristics of a Catholic community, its internal dynamic and its relation to the surrounding environment, and to note the first stages of creative activity, then to examine thoroughly the fruits of convergence in close, perceptive studies of major Catholic novelists, François Mauriac and Georges Bernanos in "Revolutionary France," Evelyn Waugh and Graham Greene in "Protestant England," J. F. Powers and Flannery O'Connor in "Pragmatic America." Obviously, the conditions of conflict, inside and outside these Catholic communities, from separation to confluence with their surrounding environments, varied greatly.

Roman Catholic orthodoxy, according to Kellogg, possessed the attractions of a clearly defined faith, an eschatology that gave each person a sense of purpose and direction, and an insistence on the individual's free responsibility for his own fate. These, particularly the last, were in conflict with Jansenist beliefs within the Catholic community and with Protestant Calvinism and an increasing naturalism in the secular environment. Kellogg contends that the dynamics of cultural and religious growth, the assimilation and interpenetrations of external materials, attending abrasive convergence, "entered" into the thoughts of writers, who passed on their intellectual tensions as fiction in the Catholic novel. Catholic novelists, at their best, tend toward positions of opposition: opposition to the secular environment, or to the entire modern world, or to the corruptions within their own Catholic communities. Kellogg's most important conclusion is that a period of swift and intense convergence between Catholic communities and their surrounding environments (the mid-1920s to the mid-1950s, the period of the major Catholic novelists) "is highly stimulating to the dynamic of creative development." Bernanos, Greene, and O'Connor get highest marks and double space, especially when they successfully dramatize the tension between freedom and necessity in human action and preserve a central tenet in Roman Catholic orthodoxy: "the recipient of grace must be shown as free to cooperate or refuse."

Kellogg finds the vital tradition in decline by the 1960s, the creative spark waning with the loss of Catholic identity as Catholic communities (universally) approached confluence with their surrounding environments (forecasting the shape of Vatican II). Thus, "neither confluence nor isolation are productive of the flowering that produced the Catholic novels and the accompanying spiritual growth within the vital, centuries-old Catholic tradition"—a lesson also applicable, says Kellogg, to the "Jewish novel" and to the "Negro novel."

The collection of essays edited by Professor Friedman in memory of Frederick J. Hoffman covers the twentieth-century novelists designated by Kellogg as "major," and more. It could be said that these studies take up where Kellogg leaves off. Whereas Kellogg stresses the vitality of Catholic tradition and Catholic art produced by assimilation and interpenetration, they accent some more than others, the uncertainty and the loss of clear purpose attending convergence and confluence. Also, whereas Kellogg strictly defines a "Catholic novel," the contributors to Friedman's volume are less rigid in applying the classification "Catholic"; with the assimilation of not only secular but also Protestant elements, the question of identity is not so much a matter of Catholic outlook as of *Christian* outlook. What is "obscured," what is not easily perceived, is, variously put, a "metaphysical dimension" (Mauriac's term) of spirit, a transcendent reality, the grace of Divine presence, the Christian's traditional faith in union with God and the life everlasting.

Friedman introduces this theme by contrasting the moderated, sometimes uneasy, attitude of acceptance in Jacques Rivière and Alain-Fournier with the rejected Catholicism of James Joyce and the reluctant Catholicism of Anthony Burgess. He classifies the former, according to a distinction made by Martin Turnell in *Modern Literature and Christian Faith*, as "religious" in outlook, the latter as "theological" in outlook. George A. Panichas, in "A Metaphysics of Art," also introductory, does not differentiate Catholic art, or Christian art, but bears on these in asserting that any art to be great and genuine must be visionary in exploring the relationship of the seen to the unseen, the immediate to the eternal, and in revealing spiritual values that lie beyond temporal-material limits.

Being visionary in fiction is a difficult trade. In "J. F. Powers' *Morte D'Urban*: Secularity and Grace," John B. Vickery argues that "it is virtually impossible for a non-Christian age to yield

Christian and hence Catholic imaginative works" because an artistic economy firmly grounded in secularity provides no visible fictive means of aesthetically rendering the nature and experience of spiritual grace, of showing Divine presence in the world. There are no longer meaningful grounds on which to classify a writer as "Catholic" in any traditional sense: *Morte D'Urban,* says Vickery, ultimately makes clear the post-Christian nature of the twentieth century, ironically testifying to the dissolution of the Christian faith and the Christian Church.

Succeeding essays in *The Vision Obscured* take up, from different angles, this difficulty which the Catholic Christian imagination encounters when attempting to fictively represent the working of spiritual experience in a contemporary situation. Friedman's second piece detects "sacred objects" in the novels of Flannery O'Connor. There is in her fiction an "uneasy balance" between the sacred and profane, a reliance on "things" that manifest a supernatural reality, a cosmic hierophany, yet retain their ordinary physical identity. Barry Ulanov sums up the total work of Evelyn Waugh, from comic to serious, as a kind of spiritual "ordeal" for Waugh, the pursuit of grace in a graceless world. Waugh is a "furious partisan, fighting for ancient values" through an "allegory of irony." Irving Malin proposes that "the novels of Muriel Spark deal with religious themes in a deceptive manner." Mrs. Spark chooses the uncanny occurrence and the odd personality in a pattern of deliberate "deceptions" to signify that the ultimate meaning of the universe lies beyond normal perception, the eccentric design of a

Higher Power. Albert Sonnenfeld reminds us of Graham Greene's belief in sin, in mortal man's suspension between innocence and guilt from the moment of birth. In the lost innocence of "children's faces," Greene links the realities of saint and sinner, salvation and damnation, Heaven and Hell. Through the example of Georges Bernanos, Robert Champigny considers the problems that arise from the introduction of "spirits," supernatural entities, to the narration of fiction where logic is temporal. These problems are rationally insoluble, but the use of spirits in fiction is agreeable to us, humans, who still see ourselves as individual spirits, and aesthetically satisfying if authentically created in arranged tensions between physical and metaphysical elements.

Sacred objects, allegory of irony, deliberate deceptions, children's faces, authentic spirits—these fictive means attempt to reveal a transcendent reality.

There is much more in Friedman's volume: Germaine Brée on the novels of François Mauriac (she does not credit the "metaphysical dimension" claimed by Mauriac for his fictional universe); Jean Alter on Catholic imagination in the structural schemes of Julien Green's *Épaves*; R. K. Angress on the Christian surrealism of Elisabeth Langgässer; Pierre L. Ullman on moral structure in the development of Carmen Laforet's novels; William A. Sessions on transcendence in Giovanni Papini's Christian egoists of the spirit—plus an excellent checklist of criticism on the modern Catholic novel by Jackson R. Bryer and Nanneska N. Magee.

The two books reviewed here are valuable additions to Conor Cruise O'Brien's *Maria Cross: Imaginative Patterns in a Group of Modern Catholic Writers,* to be read with the studies concerning modern literature and Christian faith by Martin Turnell and Nathan A. Scott, Jr., not because of the uncomfortable title "Catholic novel" or "Catholic novelist" they help to define or clarify, but because they express a more significant catholicity for our times. They do what Turnell claimed for some of the novelists they treat: "remind us that human beings have immortal souls."

ℳ

A War on God

The Reformed Journal, October 1977

Kingsley Amis, *The Alteration*. New York: Viking, 1976, 210 pp., $7.95.

DURING A LATE May evening of the same day in 1976 that a Requiem Mass has been sung for England's King Stephen II in the Cathedral Basilica of St. George at Coverley, four boy choristers gather around a candle in the small dormitory of St. Cecilia, a choral school near Coverley, to read forbidden CW. CW (for "counterfeit world") is, in the words of Kingsley Amis' latest novel, "a class of tale set more or less at the present date, but portraying the results of some momentous change in historical fact."

What the boys are reading about is a world that corresponds to the world *we* live in, counterfeit to them because some of the "historical fact" which we know did not happen—neither Martin Luther's defiance of the Pope, nor Henry VIII's. Their world, one in which the secular authority of the Roman Catholic Church remains supreme, is, from our point of view, the Counterfeit World that Amis gives us in *The Alteration*. The novel is a kind of science fiction with theological implications. Amis imagines an alternative world, what the world of today might be if the crucial events of the early sixteenth century had been different.

In Amis' revision of English history, King Henry VII's eldest son, Prince Arthur, fathered a son, Stephen, on Catherine of Aragon. (In historical fact, Arthur died, without issue, a few months after his wedding to Catherine.) After Henry VII's death Stephen, the "true heir," with the support of the Holy See, led a "Holy Expedition" against "Henry the Abominable" in the "War of English Succession," resulting in a "Holy Victory" and the crowning of King Stephen II. There was no English Reformation, no Parliamentary Acts, between 1530 and 1535, that separated the English Church from Rome and put it under the control of Henry VIII. New England became "a place of exile and punishment for Schismatics and common criminals."

On the Continent, Martin Luther went to Rome and said, "If you make me Pope and promise the English it's their turn next and so on, all my followers will come around—and if I have to I'll declare a Holy War on Henry and restore Prince Stephen." Thus, Luther became the first Northern Pope, Germanian the First; Thomas More, rather than losing his head in the Tower, followed him as Hadrian the Seventh. In the world of *The Alteration,* papal authority and the spirit of medievalism continue to dominate England and Europe in the last quarter of the twentieth century. Amis creates the present as a direct extension of the medieval past. Temporal power in the hands of the Roman Church, fighting its enemies science (which seeks to disprove God) and the infidel Turk. Certain human beings have "absolute God-given rights" over others. Christians over Mahometans, clergy over laity, gentry over people of low condition, fathers over children, men over women. The status of women is trivial; they are little more than servants in their households. Sexual love is a sinful pleasure, hidden and coarsened by life-denying polity.

Particular developments from this medievalism are startling—sometimes amusing, often grim. Motorcars are powered by Diesel engines, started by clockwork. Streets and buildings are lighted by gaslamps. Electricity is officially regarded as witchcraft, experimented with only in the Republic of New England. The Eternal City Rail (a "railtrack train") runs non-stop from London, the seat of government (Coverley is the capital, being the seat of the Church) via "Channel Bridge, Sopwith's masterpiece," attaining a speed of 195 m.p.h. There are no airplanes, though dirigibles cross the Atlantic and, in New England, the Smith brothers have invented a flying machine.

Thomas Kyd's *Hamlet* is playing in Coverley. Shakespeare's plays are performed only in New England, where the playwright was transported after excommunication. A ten-year-old boy's reading includes *St. Lemuel's Travels*, *The Wind in the Cloisters*, *Lord of the Chalices*, and a collection of Father Bond stories. Monsignor Jean-Paul Sartre, a French Jesuit, has authored *De Existentiae Natura*. In the Republic of New England, where the national hero is Benedict Arnold and the capital Arnoldstown, several states and cities are named for dissenters: Cranmeria, Waldensia,

Latimeria, Wyclif City, Hussville. In Rome, the reigning Pope is John XXIV, a "broad, plumpish" Yorkshireman who refers to himself as "we." Among his cardinals are Henricus Himmler of Almaigne, Laurentius Beria of Muscovy, and Berlingauer, an Italian Communist. Though a policy of "detensione" has relaxed the strain between Christendom and the Turks, Pope John has decided for war "in the name of Christ" to relieve a population problem aggravated by the declaration of his predecessor (Innocent XVII) forbidding artificial birth control.

All this alteration of history makes possible the novel's central alteration, the alteration of Hubert Anvil, one of the St. Cecilia choristers who enjoys the secret reading of *Counterfeit World*. At the age of ten he is an unusually gifted soprano, "the best boy singer in living memory," and also a talented composer. Ironically, the novel opens with Hubert's solo performance in the *Agnus Dei* section of Mozart's "Second Requiem" at the service for the deceased King Stephen III. In the audience are papal emissaries who have come to judge the young soprano's capacities, and it will soon be clear that this lamb of God will be recommended for sacrifice *ad majorem Dei gloriam*, so that the "divine gift" may be preserved.

Their recommendation generates several conflicts. The Lord Abbot of St. Cecilia and his Chapelmaster want Hubert for the Cathedral of St. George, the mother church of all England at Coverley; Pope John wants him for St. Peter's, Rome. St. Cecilia's Prefect of Music, Hubert's teacher, objects to the operation on the grounds that Hubert's career as a singer will prevent his development as a composer. Tobias Anvil, Hubert's father, a pious merchant, consents to his son's emasculation, viewing it as a duty to God and His Holy Church, but is opposed by the family chaplain, Father Lyall, whose signature to the document authorizing surgery is necessary. Dame Anvil, the boy's mother, by way of an affair with the chaplain, seeks that priest's aid in saving Hubert from the knife that will cost him the kind of joy she has found. Hubert himself is at first not recalcitrant to what the Church calls God's will for him; then, as he gropes toward some adolescent understanding of the manhood he will miss, he has his doubts: "I know it's glorious to have God's favour, and I'm as grateful for it as I can be, but I can't prevent myself from wishing it had taken another form." His resistance grows. Nobody, of course, has any power to resist what has been decided by the Pope. "We can indeed do as we please throughout Christendom. We are the Holy Father."

So Hubert runs. First, with the assistance of his dormitory mates, he flees to the house of the Ambassador from New England in Coverley. His Excellency, a liberal-minded Schismatic with the Netherlander name van den Haag, is not in Coverley, but his servants help Hubert to London, where his brother succeeds in getting him into the New Englander Embassy, "the soil of the only nation in Christendom into which the Pope's servants could not enter at will and of right." From the Embassy, disguised as an Indian page (though the New Englander Schismatics are less repressive in their social distinctions than the Roman Church, they do force *apartheid* on the Indian, whose "brain is smaller"), Hubert is smuggled to the coast of England and safely aboard a dirigible bound for New England.

Hubert has escaped the tyranny of the Church, but not, it seems, God's. Soon after he flees from St. Cecilia, the Lord Abbot prays for him: "Enter into his heart and mind, O Lord, and send him the desire to return here among those who care for him. Or, if that is not Thy purpose, bring it about in Thine own way that he forsake the path of rebellion and outlawry and be brought at last to serve Thy will." That latter is apparently what happens—by an arbitrary act of God that destroys life.

It is not easy to determine what Amis is up to in *The Alteration,* the exact point he wants to make. He is not totally for the progress of science; there are plusses for medieval tyranny. After all, Coverley (pronounced Cowley, to suggest both cowl and a suburb of Oxford), has a better sound in this spelling that the Cowley we know stands in its place. The unspoiled countryside, the gardens, the flowers of Coverley are more charming than the congestion, the giant automobile factories, the gasoline fumes of Cowley. In all of altered England there is less urban blight and more green grass than there is in the 1970s England of historical fact. Because motor cars are fewer and tobacco-smoking is not socially approved, the air is purer everywhere, and in New England passenger pigeons cover the sky like clouds. A world in which Thomas Sopwith built bridges rather than fighter planes is more stable than ours; there is even a kind of satisfying harmony in stories, paintings, pieces of music, all consistently expressing sanctified devotional themes (like Soviet art bound to an ideology).

Nevertheless, the price of this stability and harmony, the cost to human freedom, is too great. Amis is four-square against Christian totalitarianism. *The Alteration*'s puzzling resolution seems to be an attack on God, or, more precisely, on what Amis thinks is the traditional Christian conception of God: a loveless, life-hating God for whom "Thine own way" is brutally crushing human feelings and desires to a monolithic order, the sort of God Dostoevsky's Ivan Karamazov and Camus' Dr. Rieux indict for the suffering of children. Ivan and Dr. Rieux are, of course, nihilists; for them (and perhaps for Amis) a God whose purpose justifies such suffering is a rational absurdity. In *The Alteration* this God's victim is life at its source of sexual pleasure, in the mutilations of Hubert and Father Lyall, in the aborted loves of Dame Anvil for the chaplain and Hilda (the New England ambassador's daughter) for Hubert. Father Lyall admits to Hubert's mother, when she asks whether he believes in God, "The Church holds without the slightest equivocation that everything you and I do together is a sin. I know that to be false. Therefore . . . ."

That is also probably the logic of Amis. In an essay "On Christ's Nature" he states, "What troubles me [about Christ] is the association of a man who has many claims on my respect and sympathy with a God who has none on either. 'Son of God' I can accept; 'son of *God*' I cannot. I am one of that company (large and rapidly growing, I hope) which says: 'I think the traditional God of Christianity very wicked'."

The Alteration is not a jolly book, not like the extremely funny *Lucky Jim* (1954) and Amis' other social satires of the next ten years. True, there are many amusing surprises in its fabricated world, but the consequences of tyranny are nothing to laugh about: ultimately, "thirty million Christians dead, men, women, and children" to reduce population and save the Church's authority. *The Alteration* continues Amis' angry mood that began with *The Anti-Death League* (1966). The League makes war on God, a sadistic brute who delights in playing nasty jokes, like leukemia and breast cancer.

The same kind of grotesque jest is at the center of the theological problem. In *The Alteration*, how (and why) is Hubert, the lamb of God, fortuitously mutilated, just when his freedom and fulfillment seem assured? Fundamentally, *The Alteration* goes beyond an assault on the Church and the Church's God to a kind of comic nihilism. Surely, Amis intended the vehicle of *Counterfeit World* to suggest a false dominion, a world "founded on one great lie," says a friend of Father Lyall—"at first a lie nobody had the slightest use for, since become the sole necessity." At bottom, the anger of Amis is directed at the tyranny of life itself, with death inherent. The perfect art of Hubert's voice can be preserved only by the mutilation of life; even before Hubert receives it from Hilda, the blue cross, token of her love, is annulled by the silver crucifix he wears around his neck in flight. Be it Providence or the nature of things, Hubert Anvil never had a chance.

In *Ending Up* (1974), Amis sums up life as "bloody horrible," a monstrous farce. In this geriatric horror five characters struggle through the miseries of old age on their way to the "scrap heap." One of the five, Bernard, faced with terminal cancer, finds his only relief in playing malicious pranks on the other four. But even spite fails him. *The Alteration* is that sort of gesture.

♉

Romance and Reality in *Bleak House*: The Death and Rebirth of Love in London

A revision of the final chapter of Dr. Prins' 1963 Ph.D. dissertation, "The Fabulous Art: Myth, Metaphor, and Moral Vision in Dickens' *Bleak House*." Although the essay was prepared for a scholarly journal, there is no evidence that Dr. Prins ever submitted it. Neverthelss, it stands as the best and most heartfelt of his scholarship.

> I told her that my heart overflowed with love for her; that it was natural love, which nothing in the past changed, or could change.[1]

DICKENS' *BLEAK HOUSE*, romance or realism? What is the relation of romance to reality? Austin Warren states that "the two chief modes of narrative fiction have, in English, been called the 'romance' and the 'novel'. . . . The novel is realistic; the romance is poetic or epic: we should now call it 'mythic.'"[2] No one would seriously challenge that there is a large portion of social realism, of social criticism, in the story of *Bleak House*: the evil of Chancery delay, the desolation of the slum Tom-all-Alone's, the corruption of the pauper's graveyard. Such studies as those of Humphrey House and John Butt on the topicality of Dickens' novels and their relation to the particular world of Victorian society have demonstrated that social realism clearly.[3] Just as clearly, too, the social realism is permeated with and colored by romance, with the poetic and mythic. Dickens' stated intention for *Bleak House* was to dwell upon "the romantic side of familiar things" (p. xxxii).

Should a novelist so mix the modes of narrative fiction? The question of literal or figurative significance in *Bleak House* is well stated by Murray Krieger in a footnote to his discussion of Kafka's *The Trial*. In regard to Kafka's "failure to relate in any workable way" the actual and symbolic levels of meaning in that novel, Krieger praises, by contrast, Dickens' *Bleak House*:

How much more promising, for example, is the arrangement with which Dickens begins in *Bleak House*, where the legal court and the absurd court merge in the impossible actuality of Chancery. The world of social-economic reality and of nightmarish fantasy, the political and metaphysical levels, have a single narrative source full enough to sustain both at once. We feel the symbol of Chancery as Dickens creates it supports an equal sense of cogency on either level.

But, says Krieger, "this rooting of the symbolic level in the bedrock of a detailed social reality comes at a cost." He believes that there is an unresolved conflict in *Bleak House*: the detailed social reality, demanding its own resolution, threatens the symbolic level; the symbolic level threatens the credibility of the actuality from which it springs.[4]

The novel from its beginning held romance and realism in tension. In a perceptive essay on the "equívoco" of *Don Quixote*, where discussion of the novel as a distinct genre should probably begin, Ángel del Río notes that

> the new literary genre in *Don Quixote* (later to be called 'the modern novel') arose out of a changed situation of man in history, one in which incongruities between individual intentions and individual capacity for realizing them became apparent, and in which truth became a problem—not in the abstract nor in relation to transcendental forces but relative to man's own existence.[5]

Georg Lukács once defined the modern novel as "the search for the expression of the irrational, the soul, in and through an alien and hostile reality; the principle of its form is derived from the consciousness that 'inwardness' has its own independent value."[6] Putting aside for the moment the question of what is "really real," we can say that the prerequisite to defining the novel is understanding in its structure and meaning a culturally generated split between what have become opposing poles of human experience: romance-realism, fantasy-reality; though the novel recognizes the dominant empirical idea of reality, and is greatly bound to that idea, polarity is the definitive element in it. The contention for *Bleak House* here is that Dickens uses the forms and figures of myth and poetry to shape his topical matter to an inner and universal meaning. The unity of *Bleak House* is effected by its mythic and poetic qualities; its most significant meaning is discovered in the organizing patterns of fable and folklore, and in the radical identifications of metaphor and symbol.

Dorothy Van Ghent has argued persuasively that

> two kinds of crime form Dickens' two chief themes, the crime of parent against child and the calculated social crime. They are formally analogous, their form being the treatment of persons as things; but they are also inherent in each other, whether the private will of the parent is to be considered as depraved by the operation of a public institution, or the social institution is to be considered as a bold concert of the depravities of individual "fathers."[7]

Bleak House can be read as a fable of deserted children, the recurrent motif being that of young dependents who are forsaken by father or mother or parent society, like the lost children in the nursery rhyme about "The Babes in the Wood" and in the ballad of "The Children in the Wood." Looked at in this way, the story of *Bleak House* is a complex of characters and incidents, all related to deserted children, that supports a double plot, the Chancery Story and the Dedlock Mystery, two distinct but interrelated lines of action which dramatize the two aspects of child abandonment by parents: the public crime and the private crime.

These social and personal failures (guilts) in *Bleak House* inhere in each other and are inseparable. They are reciprocal and spring from the same root: the "parent" society corrupts (infects like a disease) individual parents, and the individual parents corrupt the "parent" society; the guilt of the parent society (Chancery) for the "wards in Jarndyce" (Richard Carstone and Ada Clare) and the guilt of Lady Dedlock for her lost child (Esther Summerson) both spring from a denial of parental affection, or, more broadly, a denial of humane compassion—what Esther Summerson calls the "natural love" she has in her heart for her mother. Thus with the mythic suggestions of a fable Dickens relates and unites two worlds: the private inner reality of human lostness and need for love with the public reality of social delinquency and need for social conscience.

These mythic suggestions in Dickens' fable of deserted children fit Alan Watts' description of myth as a "complex of stories—some no doubt fact, and some fantasy—which, for various reasons, human beings regard as demonstrations of the inner meaning of the universe and of human life."[8] *Bleak House* contains "story in time," story of the kind that Edwin Muir regrets the passing of in poetry: "[story in time] reminds us of the pattern of our lives; and within that pattern it brings our loves, our passions, their effects, and unavoidable chance"—because it moves in time, and because we live in time. This "story in time" is "the most pure image we have of temporal life, tracing the journey which we shall take." The contemporary novel, says Muir, that is "concerned mostly with relations that space imposes on us," that "deals, at its most typical, with society . . . gives us a description or a report, not a clear image of life"—and thereby destroys the poetic "story in time," the fable, the myth of human experience.[9]

Images of sunlight and shadow, patterns of light and darkness, evoke persons and places in *Bleak House* and progressively reinforce the Chancery Story, the Dedlock Mystery, and the enveloping story of Esther Summerson, to give moral meaning to the plot. The central image of *Bleak House* is the sun, in its presence or absence, an archetypal symbol that has universal significance, representing vision or blindness, good or evil, fertility or sterility, and ultimately, for Dickens, a concept of love, or its antithesis, humane compassion, secular responsibility, as opposed to the cruel, coldhearted desertion of "children," public and private.

Like the fable of deserted children, the mythic-poetic sun metaphor, from which spring the images of sunlight and shadow, relates and unifies the two worlds of *Bleak House*, the public reality and the private reality: the archetypal images of light and darkness link the particularity of person and place and plot to common human experience, giving a deeper psychological significance to Lady Dedlock and Tulkinghorn, Richard and Vholes, Esther and John Jarndyce, the Court of Chancery and Chesney Wold, Hertfordshire Bleak House and Yorkshire Bleak House, the lives of Lady Dedlock and Richard and Esther.

The sixty-seven chapters of *Bleak House* are almost equally divided between two alternating and complementing points of view: that of a third-person narrator who speaks in the present tense, and that of Esther Summerson who reports retrospectively. Though the third-person narrator stays close to the story of the private

crime, the Dedlock Mystery, and Esther Summerson tells most of the story of the public crime,
the Chancery Story, both points of view contribute significantly to both stories: together they
share the searching for two secrets, the telling of
two tales that are concurrent in time, concen-
trated in place, related through characters and
events, and common in theme. Esther Summerson is the central character in *Bleak House*, the
integrating voice. She turns out to be Lady Dedlock's daughter, and she tells the story of the
wards in Jarndyce, to whom she has a motherly
relation; the tragic resolutions of the Dedlock
Mystery and the Chancery Story are climaxes in a
larger story, the story of Esther's life. It is the
point of view of Esther, the naive simplicity of innocence, that envelops the public and the private
stories, and they are finally resolved and blended
in the mythic timelessness of her fairy tale: "I was
brought up from my earliest remembrance—like
some of the princesses in the fairy stories—by my
god-mother" (p. 11). Once upon a time, in the fable of the deserted child, means always.

The two points of view also complement each
other in tone and attitude. The third-person narrator speaks with the urgency of the present
tense, with angry indignation denouncing the
immediate evils that he sees close about him. He
speaks to the conscience of man, and not without
hope that the darkness in the heart of man and
in human society will be lightened, though that
hope be but "a distant ray of light" (pp. 116 and
167), like the light that shines from a small act of
kindness upon the crossing-sweeper Jo. Esther
shares the third-person narrator's attitude to-

ward coldness of heart and cruelty to children, sees the evil, public and private, but her voice does not have his tone of angry indignation: the third-person narrator's stress is on the cruelty to children, the evils of the Chancery world; Esther's stress is on the cure, on kindness of heart. She complements the present urgency of the third-person narrator, his rational clarity, with the optimism and good cheer of a retrospective look—with the simple faith of fairyland's deserted child that the crimes against children, public and private, are redeemed by kindness of heart.

Esther's point of view, in complementing the third-person narrator's, fulfills the compensating role which C. G. Jung ascribes to the archetypal child motif in psychology:

> The child motif represents not only something that existed in the distant past but also something that exists *now*; that is to say, it is not just a vestige but a system functioning in the present whose purpose is to compensate or correct, in a meaningful manner, the inevitable one-sidedness and extravagances of the conscious mind. It is the nature of the conscious mind to concentrate on a relatively few contents and to raise them to the highest pitch of clarity. A necessary result and precondition is the exclusion of other potential contents of consciousness. The exclusion is bound to bring about a certain one-sidedness of the conscious contents. Since the differentiated consciousness of civilized men has been an effective instrument for the practical realization of its contents through the dynamics of his will, there is all the more danger, the more he trains his will, of his getting lost in one-sidedness and deviating further and further from the laws and roots of his being. This means, on the one hand, the possibility of human freedom, but on the other is a source of endless transgressions against one's

instincts. . . . Our differentiated consciousness is in continual danger of being uprooted; hence it needs compen-
sation through the still-existing state of childhood.[10]

Esther's progress toward maturity of self in *Bleak
House*, from darkness to light, achieves a synthesis, a balance, between the state of childhood and
the differentiated consciousness.

So again, in using the double point of view to
interrelate two stories that are together a fable of
public and private crimes, Dickens integrates the
worlds of public and private reality. The sophisticated intelligence of the third-person narrator,
speaking prophetic tones of denunciation and
damnation about particular Chancery abuses
and Lady Dedlock's personal failure of heart, creates an image of Hell that is complemented by an
image of Heaven in the simpler consciousness of
Esther Summerson who looks beyond her shadowed childhood and the tragedy of Richard Carstone to "the world that sets this right" (p. 659).
In the complementary points of view, the public
reality of Chancery becomes a mythic Hell; the
mythic Heaven of Esther's private vision becomes
the hope of social salvation—becomes the distant
ray of light.

Mark Schorer, in writing on Blake, with whom
Dickens has some affinity, stresses the unifying
function of myth in literature:

Great literature is impossible without a previous image—
imaginative consent to a ruling mythology that makes
intelligible and unitive the whole of that experience from
which particular fables spring and from which they, in
turn, take their meaning.[11]

To Schorer,

myths are instruments by which we continually struggle
to make experience intelligible to ourselves. A myth is a
large controlling image that gives philosophical meaning
to the facts of ordinary life; that is, it has organizing
value for experience.[12]

In this sense of myth as a comprehensive primary
impression that orders human experience, a
metaphoric identification of public and private,
outer and inner, reality, Dickens goes deep into
the human consciousness for his large controlling images, his related unitive myths: to the inner experience of lostness and foundness, the
myth of quest and fulfillment in the fable of deserted children; to the inner experience of life and
death, the myth of good and evil in the sun symbol and the images of light and darkness; to the
inner experience of innocence, guilt, and redemption, the myth of Paradise, Hell, and Heaven in
the two voices, the complementary tones and attitudes in the double point of view.

There is an even larger, more subtly unitive
"controlling image" in *Bleak House* which relates
its two worlds of public and private reality: that is
the impression of tension between the public and
the private stories, between the patterns of
sunlight and the patterns of shadow, between the
two voices. It is the image implicit in such terms
as balance and counterpoint, polarity and antithesis, ambivalence and ambiguity. The weights
suggested by these terms may be differently opposed, differently counterpoised; they may tend
toward emotion or attitude or idea, toward the

sensory or the abstract, but always they are tensively related and complementary, symmetrical, in that they are mutually completing parts of a whole. Balance, for example, can be described as a complementary tension that maintains an equilibrium, a synthesis, between two polar forces. This image of tension is central to the art of *Bleak House*: the counterpoint, the complementary contrast and interplay of elements in Dickens' handling of the story, the images, the point of view.

In the story, the corollary aspects of child desertion are counterpointed: the private crime, the personal guilt in Lady Dedlock's denial of her maternal instinct, is counterpointed by the public crime, Chancery society's abandonment of its child Richard Carstone (and its child Jo). These complementary failures, inherent in each other and inseparable, are reinforced by numerous other bad fathers and bad mothers, public and private desertions of children. The counterpointed public and private failures are themselves counterpointed by *good* fathers and mothers, public and private kindness and responsibility, notably in the sentiments and actions of John Jarndyce and Esther Summerson.

Counterpointed images of darkness and light impress their affective qualities on the public and the private stories. Patterns of sunlight and shadow lighten or darken places and persons and plot development with suggestions of counterpointed good and evil, benevolence and malevolence, life and death.

In the double point of view, the subjectivity of Esther Summerson who speaks in the first person counterpoints the objectivity of a narrator who speaks in the third person; the slow tempo of Esther's past-tense reminiscence (which counterpoints her first-person subjectivity) counterpoints the immediate urgency of the third-person narrator's present-tense observation (which counterpoints his third-person objectivity); Esther's simple heart counterpoints the third-person narrator's rational intelligence; Esther's mood of sentimental cheer counterpoints the third-person narrator's tone of ironic anger. The counterpointed voices of Esther Summerson and the third-person narrator, speaking alternately to move the public and private stories forward, create a highly complex image of tension in the narrative structure of *Bleak House*: the third-person narrator, personally detached from both stories, moves only the action of the private story, the mysterious inner drama of Lady Dedlock, commenting meanwhile on both public and private matters in a tone of lofty ironic indignation; Esther Summerson, personally involved in both stories, concentrates on the public story, Chancery's abandonment of the wards in Jarndyce, but finally draws together both stories, accommodating them to the slow tempo and cheerful optimism of her retrospective look.

This artistic counterpoint, the complementary contrast and interplay of elements, pervades the whole of *Bleak House* with an impression of tension that pulls together the aspects of private and public reality: self and society, personal confession and social history, the mystery of inner experience and the moral of outer existence:

every noise is merged this moonlight night,
into a distant ringing hum, as if
the city were a vast glass vibrating. (p. 503)

In the rhythm of blank verse, this image of London the night of Tulkinghorn's murder suggests the full tensive reality of *Bleak House.*

Philip Wheelwright says that reality—What Is—"as envisaged through the medium of poetry and the poetic consciousness," has three characteristics. It is presential and tensive; that is, it contains an inner sense of something unseen within, amidst, or behind—and in mysterious contrast to—the familiar things of the outer world. It is also coalescent and interpenetrative; that is, the inner world and the outer world, the private and the public, grow together and qualify each other to blur the boundaries between them. And it is perspectival and latent; that is, it reveals itself only partially in the prospect of a certain point of view, and is therefore constantly to be created in shifting angles of vision.[13] The fable of deserted children, the images of light and darkness, the double vision create such a reality in *Bleak House,* a reality that is more profound and universal in human experience than the public reality of Chancery. In *Bleak House* Dickens draws the public world of Chancery in such a way that it is transformed into an image of the spiritual world, the private reality.

The public and the private dimensions of *Bleak House* are reciprocal and coextensive: the suggested tension between the Angelic and the Demonic on the private level of mythic experience polarizes good and evil in the public world of

Chancery; in turn, the tension between good and evil in the Chancery world polarizes the Angelic and the Demonic in a modified myth—a myth of Chancery. In this identification of the inner and the outer worlds of human experience, the private reality and the public reality, Dickens' art is mythopoetic, making out of the legal incubus of Chancery and residual mythic patterns a "story in time," to use the phrase of Edwin Muir once more—that is, a sort of modern myth of being "in Chancery." *Bleak House*, at its deepest and most profound, is a dark journey of the human soul, from the death of love in the lost innocence of childhood to redemption and the resurrection of love in maturity. It is the death and rebirth of love in London. And London is London, but London is also the whole world of human experience.

The death and rebirth of love: this is the fullest meaning of *Bleak House*—meaning as revealed by the fable, the images, the inner and the outer perspectives. Readers of Dickens have always seen in all of his novels the theme of Christian charity, the injunction to love one's neighbor. More recently, critics have found in them a deeper and darker Christian meaning: the need for man's redemption. Two examples of such interpretation point to the first and to the last of Dickens' novels. W. H. Auden, in a critical testament, reflects that "the appeal of mythical characters transcends all highbrow-lowbrow frontiers of taste" and that "every such character is symbolic of some perpetual and human concern." Auden then says:

The conclusion I have come to is that the real theme of the *Pickwick Papers*—I am not saying Dickens was consciously aware of it and, indeed, I am pretty certain he was not—is the Fall of Man.[14]

John Gross, introducing a collection of essays on Dickens' significance for the twentieth century, remarks that

[Dickens'] Christianity is more relevant than one tends to think nowadays. . . . Dickens may have thought of Christianity primarily in terms of a diffuse loving kindness . . . but he was also profoundly attracted to the ideas of redemption and resurrection. John Jasper betrays more in Cloisterham than respectability.[15]

I have stressed the dramatization, in *Bleak House*, of two evils: the public crime and the private crime, the public guilt and the private guilt, reciprocal and inherent in each other. When Lady Dedlock seeks out Jo in Tom-all-Alone's to question him about the recently deceased law-writer Nemo, Dickens asks:

What connexion can there be, between the place in Lincolnshire, the house in town . . . and the whereabout of Jo the outlaw with the broom, who had that distant ray of light upon him when he swept the churchyard-step? What connexion can there have been between many people in the innumerable histories of this world, who, from opposite sides of great gulfs, have, nevertheless, been very curiously brought together! (p. 167)

Dorothy Van Ghent answers that what brings Lady Dedlock and Jo together is "the bond between the public guilt for Jo and the private guilt of Lady Dedlock for her daughter, these two offering for each other—as usual in Dickens—the model of parental irresponsibility. . . ."[16] To balance the private guilt of Lady Dedlock, there is also the public guilt for the wards in Jarndyce. This bonded guilt, like "original sin," in the corrupted child-parent situation of the Dickens world "requires an act of redemption," a symbolic act of love by the child, who must assume the guilt for what has been done, that would redeem the living dead (in heart), that would "redeem not only the individual fathers, but society at large"— a redemptive act "adequate to and structural for both bodies of thematic material, the sins of the individual and the sins of society."[17]

Mrs. Van Ghent believes that *Great Expectations* is the only novel of Dickens that succeeds in an adequate redemptive act. *Bleak House* also succeeds: Esther bears the inescapable effects of both the private and the public crimes, the stigma of her mother's shame ("Your mother, Esther, is your disgrace, and you were hers") and the disfiguring marks of fever ("I was very much changed—O very, very much"), carried to her by Jo from the public slum (pp. 13 and 382). Esther's acts of kindness seek to relieve the effects of parental delinquency, public and private. A close analysis of Dickens' art in *Bleak House*, Dickens' handling of story, images, and point of view, shows the redemptive act of love to be adequate to and structural for both bodies of thematic material—the sins of the individual and the sins of society. Dickens' meaning in *Bleak House* goes beyond the public and the private crimes. If we keep clearly in mind that Dickens is pointing toward the triumph of kindness of heart and social conscience in *this* world, the secular world, we can say with truth that the fullest meaning dramatized in *Bleak House* is the basic Christian doctrine that love is the beginning of redemption. To his hopes for the human heart and human society, Dickens gives the force of the Christian myth of redeeming love and the reward of Heaven. Dickens clearly sees that a redemption is required, clearly sees the darkness from which the human heart and human society must be redeemed.

So, despite the pervasiveness of evil and darkness and death in *Bleak House*, its meaning tends toward goodness and light, the rebirth of life and love. In the fable of deserted children, the public and the private crimes are redeemed by the deserted child and the benevolent father, Esther Summerson and John Jarndyce. "Lord Chancellor" Krook, through whom Dickens parodies that gloomy Hell the High Court of Chancery, symbolizing the public crime, dies "the death of all Lord Chancellors in all Courts, and of all authorities in all places under all names soever, where false pretenses are made, and where injustice is done," a death "engendered in the corrupted humours of the vicious body itself"—death by "Spontaneous Combustion" (p. 346). Black Tulkinghorn, the torturer of Lady Dedlock's private heart, finally lies "face downward on the floor" of his murky room, significantly "shot through the heart" and turned forever from the light he never reflected (p. 504). Images of darkness are at the end dispelled by images of light, and the corrosive irony of the third-person narrator yields to the simple faith of Esther Summerson, who looks always to "the bright and sunny landscape beyond" (p. 504), to a "radiant" prospect that is "like a glimpse of a better land" (p. 193).

All three stories begin with images of death. We follow the story of Richard and Ada from the day Miss Flite greets the wards in Jarndyce and ominously links the Great Seal of Chancery with "the sixth seal mentioned in the Revelations" (p. 25)[18] to Richard's death when the Chancery suit dissolves. But the evil spell of Chancery that saps the will of Richard is lifted before he dies "to begin the world" (p. 659). His redemption is symbolized in the smile that "irradiates" his face when he departs for "that pleasant country where the old times are" (p. 659), and his strength is reborn in the strength of a new Richard, a son born to Ada after the death of her husband—in the "strength of the weak little hand" whose "touch could heal [Ada's] heart, and raise up hope within her" (p. 663). We follow Lady Dedlock from her prefiguring swoon that is "like the faintness of death" (p. 11), when Tulkinghorn surprises her with a document in the handwriting of her one-time lover, to the moment when she lies "cold and dead" (p. 615) at the graveyard gate. But Lady Dedlock, too, is redeemed in her ordeal of the heart, and reborn in her identification with Esther, the deserted child. We follow the enveloping story of Esther from a childhood that is loveless, and therefore lost; images of cold and death mark the start of Esther's "progress" to maturity: "an old hearthrug with roses on it . . . hanging outside in the frost and snow" and "dear old doll" buried "in the garden-earth" (p. 17). But Esther recovers her lost love in the exercise of her own maternal affections, in the discovery of her mother and her own identity. She goes through a transfiguring illness that symbolizes a rebirth, a transformation of character. The dark shadow of her childhood is dissipated and the agonies of death and loss are healed by the warmth of John Jarndyce's paternal benevolence, that is "like the sunshine," "like the brightness of the Angels" (p. 649).

By story's end, the dead November sun, the London sun of Chapter 1, is eclipsed by the name that Esther is destined to fulfill, by the summer sun of Yorkshire, by the sunshine of Esther's wedding day. Still, the tension between good and evil, light and darkness, life and death, remains, as it remains in the reality of human experience. Call it a rhythmic tension that remains, to the end and past the end of *Bleak House*. The reality of *Bleak House*, its truth, is the mythic reality of seasonal rhythm; its tension is the experience of spring's rejuvenation and summer's fullness of life held in the consciousness of autumn's dying and winter's death: the experience of autumn's dying and winter's death held in the consciousness of spring's rejuvenation and summer's fullness of life. "Both the world of fashion and the Court of Chancery," says the third-person narrator (Dickens), "are things of precedent and usage . . . sleeping beauties, whom the Knight will wake one day, when all the stopped spits in the kitchen shall begin to turn prodigiously!" (p. 6).

The story of the Sleeping Beauty[19] is pertinent to the rhythmic tension in *Bleak House*.

The story of the Sleeping Beauty, like the story of the Children in the Wood, is a universally popular tale with mythic roots. On the mythic level it symbolizes the long sleep of winter and the awakening of spring, the rejuvenation of the earth by the sun. The Princess, symbolizing the Earth goddess, is pricked by the distaff spindle, winter's seasonal death, and falls into a deep sleep from which she (now the Sleeping Beauty, or Briar Rose) is awakened after one hundred years by the Prince (the Knight), symbolizing the Sun god, who has searched far for her. When the Prince awakens the Princess, the hedge of briar thorns that encloses the castle where she sleeps bursts into a bloom of roses. In Romance, the Prince's awakening kiss is the redemption of love from evil, from death.

Chapter one of *Bleak House* introduces the Chancery Story, the story of public guilt, and the sterile world of the High Court of Chancery with the image of a dead sun: "flakes of soot . . . as big as full-grown snowflakes—gone into mourning, one might imagine, for the death of the sun" (p. 1). Chapter two, where we find the allusion to the story of the Sleeping Beauty, introduces the Dedlock Mystery, the story of private guilt, with a similar image for the closely associated world of fashion: "it is a deadened world, and its growth is something unhealthy for want of air" (p. 6). Images of sunlight and shadow lighten and darken the whole of *Bleak House,* the world of Chancery and the world of fashion, places and persons and plot patterns. Clearly, the public and the private worlds of Chancery and of fashion, of the Court and Lady Dedlock, are cold and sunless worlds, and clearly, too, their lack of warmth and light is a lack of love—a lack of social conscience and kindness of heart. And these "sleeping beauties . . . the Knight will wake one day" (p. 6).

Both John Jarndyce, whose beneficent kindness is "like the sunshine," and Esther Summerson, the summer sun, are closely associated with the revitalizing power of the sun that symbolizes redeeming love. Esther—"like some of the princesses in the fairy stories" (p. 11)—can be seen, too, as the Sleeping Beauty, the deserted child pricked by the sunless-loveless chill of shadowed childhood and warmed to life by the genial sun-love of John Jarndyce. But close correspondences are not to the point here. *Bleak House* has the mythic rhythmic tension of sunlight, "the ripening weather" (p. 649), and shadow, "chilling the seed in the ground" (p. 468): moving regularly from winter solstice to summer solstice to winter solstice to summer solstice over two and a half years, it has the rhythm of death and rebirth that is symbolized in the story of the Sleeping Beauty. The Sleeping Beauty will wake one day, and the spits in the kitchen shall begin to turn prodigiously. Dickens means to say that the world of fashion and the Court of Chancery, the dead past, will be redeemed by the sun of love, by a rebirth of social conscience and kindness of heart.

NOTES

1. Charles Dickens, *Bleak House*, Riverside Edition (Boston: Houghton-Mifflin, 1956), p. 386. Numbers in parentheses after quotations in my text refer to page numbers in this edition.

2. Austin Warren, *Theory of Literature* (New York: Harcourt, Brace and Company, 1949), p. 223.

3. Humphrey House, *The Dickens World* (London: Oxford University Press, 1941); John Butt, "*Bleak House* in the Context of 1851," *Nineteenth-Century Fiction*, X (June 1955), 1-21.

4. Murray Krieger, *The Tragic Vision: Variations on a Theme in Literary Interpretation* (New York: Holt, Rinehart and Winston, 1960), pp. 138-40.

5. Ángel del Río, "The Equívoco of *Don Quixote*," *Varieties of Literary Experience*, ed. Stanley Burnshaw (New York: New York University Press, 1962), p. 215.

6. Quoted from *The Theory of the Novel* (*Die Theorie des Romans*; Berlin, 1920) by Roy Pascal in his "Foreword" to Georg Lukács, *Studies in European Realism*, trans. Edith Bone (London: Hillway Publishing Company, 1950), p. v.

7. Dorothy Van Ghent, *The English Novel: Form and Function* (New York: Rinehart & Co., 1953), p. 134.

8. Alan Watts, *Myth and Ritual in Christianity* (London: Thames and Hudson, 1954), p. 7.

9. Edwin Muir, *The Estate of Poetry* (Cambridge, Mass.: Harvard University Press, 1962), p. 29.

10. C. G. Jung and C. Kerényi, *Introduction to the Science of Mythology: The Myth of the Divine Child and the Mysteries of Eleusis*, trans. R. F. C. Hull (London: Routledge and Kegan Paul, Ltd., 1951), pp. 112-113.

11. Mark Schorer, *William Blake: The Politics of Vision* (New York: Henry Holt and Company, 1946), p. 29.

12. *Ibid*, p. 27.

13. Philip Wheelwright, *Metaphor and Reality* (Bloomington: Indiana University Press, 1968), pp. 153-73.

14. W. H. Auden, *The Dyer's Hand and Other Essays* (New York: Random House, 1962), p. 408.

15. John Gross, "Dickens: Some Recent Approaches," in *Dickens and the Twentieth Century*, ed. John Gross and Gabriel Pearson (Toronto: University of Toronto Press, 1962), p. xii.

16. Dorothy Van Ghent, "The Dickens World: A View from Todgers's," in *The Dickens Critics*, ed. George H. Ford and Lauriat Lane, Jr. (Ithaca: Cornell University Press, 1961), pp. 223 and 226.

17. *Ibid.*, pp. 435-36. See also *The English Novel: Form and Function*, pp. 136-37.

18. In Revelation 6:12, at the opening of the sixth seal, "the sun became as black as sackcloth of hair."

19. Varying versions of the story are found in the fifty folk tales of Giovanni Battista Basile's *Il Pentamerone* (1637), "The Sleeping Beauty in the Wood" in Charles Perrault's *Contes de ma Mère l'Oye (1697)*, and "Briar Rose" in *Kinder- und Hausmärchen* (1812-1814) of Jacob and Wilhelm Grimm.

ℒℒℒ

REMEMBERING PRINS

Jim Prins was something of an enigma, an enigma in a positive sense. It took some considerable effort to penetrate his shyness, his reserve, and to grasp the brilliance of his mind. Walking down the street, reading a book, he was an Ethan Frome, of whom one of his favorites, Edith Wharton, wrote: "He seemed a part of the mute melancholy landscape, an incarnation of its frozen woe, with all that was warm and sentient in him fast below the surface; but there was nothing unfriendly in his silence."

—Bruce Van Voorst, Class of 1954

ΦΦΦ

Coming to Terms: Jim Prins as I Knew Him

Kathleen Verduin, Class of 1965

THE FIRST TIME I saw him, he was standing outside his office, looking down from the second-floor balcony in old Van Raalte Hall. Just looking: not looking for anyone or anything, just gazing thoughtfully at the students, myself among them, ascending the creaking stairs. *Who's that*, I remember thinking, *he looks like Lincoln*—not just the height and the gaunt, angular frame, but something in the expression, a sense of dignity and self-communion.

That was in the fall of my sophomore year, when Prins's name was invoked so often around the *Anchor* and *Opus* offices that it seemed to hang in the air with all the smoke. "Well, *Prins* thinks," somebody would begin, or "*Prins* was saying this morning," another would add, and the respect in their tone was unmistakable: this "Prins" loomed almost as an archetype, a totem, who stood in some important way for intangibles held in common.

When I enrolled in his American Novels course the following year I began to understand this for myself. It was first of all, of course, a matter of presence: as I had known from the brief glimpse on the stairs, Prins was naturally a man you noticed, watched, wanted to listen to (when he lectured on *Moby-Dick*, I was reminded of Rockwell Kent's austere engraving of Captain Ahab). It was certainly his command of literature: he had read widely, appeared to know the novels almost by heart, and spoke easily of scholarship on the subject. But it was most an unspoken but profoundly evident conviction that what we were doing, this shared activity of reading, was worthy and honorable, the work of adults in the real world we students were only beginning to know. In a letter recommending him for a fellowship, Dr. Clarence De Graaf, then Chair of Hope's English Department and a legend in his own right, once credited Jim with "the spark that is needed to challenge and galvanize the students," and he was certainly right.

"Coming to terms with the novel" was a phrase Jim Prins repeated often: the novel as an opaque but numinous object, yielding great treasure to patient and attentive contemplation. In his classes he would speak for the whole hour—occasionally a student would make a comment, to which Prins would listen politely, but for the most it was just Prins and the book in front of him. Never did I find this tedious, and if any of my classmates had ventured the word "boring" I would have held them in disdain as hopeless Philistines. I was rapt in Prins's classes: there was always something of the vatic about them, so that the vaulted ceiling of Winants, with Sargent's frieze of the prophets hanging on the wall, seemed entirely fitting. One wanted to lose oneself in that voice, in the literary worlds it brought to life: I remember more than once even shedding a few secret tears. Never did I feel "lectured to," dominated, in any sense oppressed: what went on was somehow not about Prins himself, but about the high privilege of reading literature.

And yet of course it was about Prins. As another student of my vintage said, "it wasn't so much what Prins taught: it was what he was" (another told me he had gone to graduate school expecting all his teachers to be like Prins, "but nobody was, so I left"). Prins had the air of speaking from a perspective of wisdom; his illuminations of passages seemed drawn from deep experience, profound knowledge of humanity as by turns noble and fallen. I remember his comment on the ending of Balzac's *Père Goriot*, where Rastignac shakes his fist at the venal and mendacious Faubourg Saint-Germain and vows, "Now there is war between us!"—only to turn around immediately and accept a dinner invitation from one of Goriot's odious daughters. "Well, what else could he do," Prins shrugged, "except get up on a cross somewhere." We understood, of course, that Prins meant getting up on a cross was exactly what Rastignac should have done, but that the likelihood of his doing it, people being what they are, was next to nil. It was, among many other things, that kind of moral realism—that seasoned awareness of The Way Things Are—that impressed us about Prins. We knew he had been "in the war"—I remember him remarking once that he had lost a friend at Omaha Beach—and supposed that that had had something to do with it. And yet his lectures could not be described as sombre—I remember unexpected moments of humor, as when he noticed the rain as class was ending and offered protection of his raincoat—on the condition, he said (flashing us that rare but wonderful grin), that he could screen the applicants. Or the time he wound up his remarks on one of his favorites, Camus's *The Stranger*, and then said that what the novel proved after all was (in reference to the eternal debate of Dutch Reformed Sunday Schools) that no, you shouldn't go to the beach on Sunday.

In his relations with his students, he was neither judgmental nor solicitous of our approval: but we knew, consciously or unconsciously, that he took us seriously, even when we fell short. I remember the first time Jim and I ever spoke face to face: he stopped me in the Pine Grove to ask why I hadn't managed more than a paragraph on James's *The Ambassadors* on his last essay test, ready to hear an explanation even when it was perfectly obvious I simply hadn't finished reading the novel. He listened gravely as I stammered a confession, then told me what I had written about Hemingway's *Farewell to Arms* was "rather marvelous." In fact it had not been marvelous at all, but I had commented on the novel's title from a sonnet by George Peele, invoking clumsily but I hope sincerely something I thought I knew about the Elizabethan awareness of love and death: youth always giving way to mortality, an awareness more poignant in wartime. Perhaps it struck some chords of memory for Prins. Looking back, and in this year of the sixtieth anniversary of D-

Day, it seems to me that "the war" still held us all; Jim had brought back an English wife from "the war," and when he and Iris and the children, charmingly named Christopher and Robin, agreed to share a meal at Voorhees Hall with my roommate Susan Spring and me, it seemed only right that Robin should take home with her one of my Christmas angels, sent as a gift from Germany because my father had befriended a prisoner of war. The moral questions urgent after the Holocaust, the intellectual dismissal of facile optimism that simultaneously prompted, in theology, a resurgence of attention to the "problem of evil," formed a context for contemplation of literature as a human record.

Following graduation I saw Prins now and then when I came back to Holland to visit my sister Eileen, who like me had responded deeply to Prins's classes; in the 1970s, as an editor for Hope's alumni magazine, she wrote what I think remains the classic appreciation of Jim's gifts. It still amazes me, though, that in the fall of 1978 I, when others were so much better suited, should have enjoyed the privilege of returning to Hope as Prins's colleague. It can be imagined how I shied from the prospect of working with my two most beloved professors, Jim and Henry ten Hoor, but they were kindness itself, pretending, at least, to have forgotten my former delinquencies. I liked hearing Jim and Henry talking together in Henry's office across the hall from mine, Jim settled back in the big chair. Now and then I would stop outside Jim's classroom and listen, and as Hemingway's Nick Adams put it in "Big Two-

Hearted River," I felt all the old feeling. The passion was still there, the pace and cadence of the sentences. There were still students who loved him: I remember one beautiful dark-haired girl who lived for her independent study with Prins. But I realized almost from the first that he was also wearing down: the sense of human tragedy that so informed his lectures was cracking him, the Lincoln was becoming a Lear. I resolved then that I would not permit this grand ungodly godlike man (Melville's appellation for Ahab, the way I liked to think of Prins) to go out in obscurity, and I began plotting a surprise retirement celebration. I wrote first to alumni of my own generation and carefully kept a list of every former student Jim ever mentioned—a growing list, because he always spoke warmly of his students, remembered them with interest and care. Jim, meanwhile, raged against retirement and was clearly in profound dread of the end of his career, mandated for May of 1981. In a summary gesture of resistance, he declined to attend the English Department's farewell party. As his former student, I had been designated to give the valediction, some of which I reproduce here:

I guess he's always had a morose side, an itch to point out just how bad things were. But in these times of the happy face and have a nice day, when we're consoled that "inch by inch life's a cinch," I'm glad to have known a man who's respected and honored the tragedy of life, and its ironies, and therefore felt compassion and charity for its victims. He was never exactly a pious man, especially in these last few years. But what a fine old Protestant he was, in the truest sense of the word—a man in an eternal posture of protest, and a man who stood forth his own inexorable self and never let anybody come between him and his conscience.

Well, Prins wouldn't come to our party. He goes down not gracefully, but like the old Ahab he is, still nursing his animus, still getting his jabs in the whale. But those of us who know him know that even this absence is a gift and a legacy: it's Prins making his last stand against the perfunctory and inauthentic, things he's been against all his life. And the gesture is so true to what he is that it seems a kind of benediction.

However, the "real" retirement party did indeed take place, on a perfect afternoon in June at the Castle on Lake Michigan, the week of Jim's sixty-fifth birthday: more than seventy of Jim's former students attended, spanning the whole range of his teaching career, and one by one they testified to Jim's importance in their lives. Jim, a little dazed at first (thanks to Iris, he had had no idea where she was taking him), and manifestly nonplussed when a few of the women kissed him, listened with the same thoughtful silence I remembered, then after a few minutes rose with that impeccable dignity of which he was capable and, as though with words prepared, thanked all of us for what we, astonishingly, had given him.

That was the same year I met my future husband at the International Congress on Medieval Studies at Kalamazoo; Leslie Workman and I married two years later (I a blushing bride of forty, he a confirmed bachelor I must have caught in a weak moment). My attention was absorbed by my teaching and by the scholarly journal my husband had founded, *Studies in Medievalism*, and in time by its accompanying annual conference. My resolve to stay in touch with Jim and Iris lapsed. But I ran into the Prinses around town—they were great walkers—and it was always wonderful to see them and hear about their joy in their grandchildren. Larry Helder, an English major who wanted to study the Russian novel, pulled Jim briefly out of retirement, an interval Larry still talks about. Jim and Iris still took trips to England some summers, and Sundays they often spent with Jim's old friend John Pershing Luidens, one of the most naturally courtly men I ever met, and John's wife Marcelle, like Iris a war bride. When I gave a course called "War Stories" in 2000 Iris came one afternoon and spoke beautifully and evocatively of those years.

My husband's death in the spring of 2001, after a long and wearing illness, coincided almost exactly with the beginning of Jim's terminal decline: for some time unsteady on his feet, Jim had fallen at home and pulled a grandfather clock on top of him as he reached for support. The resulting back injury put him in Rest Haven for a few weeks, where I visited him: I remember the strangeness of those long limbs stretched out on a bed, but also the grace and composure of his expression. But his increasing frailty, both physical and mental, soon decreed that he could no longer stay at his home on Paw Paw Drive, and his family reluctantly moved him to Oak Crest Manor.

I didn't want to visit him there—I had had enough of hospitals and nursing homes by that time, and I had never really gotten over feeling shy around Jim. What would I say? How would I end the visit without offending him? But I forced myself, one afternoon in the early fall, and followed the carpeted corridor to his room. Not a bad room, as such places go: it was large and quiet, and he had it all to himself. An intricately inlaid chest of drawers stood near his bed, made by his father, a skilled carpenter; there were photographs of his parents and his grandchildren, and Iris had brought a finch in a cage. And as it turned out, Jim made it easy for me to talk with him; the body on the bed was wasted, almost motionless, but the voice and the smile were the same. I asked him some things about his life: I felt presumptuous doing it, the whole thing had a kind of self-indulgent Tuesdays with Morrie dimension, and I realized guiltily that I was already thinking about some kind of memoir. But it was also fun: Jim talked about his early years, and I learned a lot. His days as a student, when he was so poor that he lived on ice cream sodas—so many that a doctor thought he was diabetic. His affection for his University of Michigan professor Joe Lee Davis, a sardonic Louisianian who introduced him to Zola. His eagerness to enlist after Pearl Harbor, frustrated by a 4-F classification because his weight was too low; he surmounted this, he told me, by drinking gallons of water before the next medical exam (only later did I learn that a childhood illness had also left him nearly blind in one eye). Commissioned as a military policeman, he was stationed near the docks in Southhampton, England, guarding a public building (this of course was where Iris first met him; he and his future brother-in-law Hubert, like many G.I.s, attempted to ingratiate themselves with American Hershey bars). Like many World War II vets, he deprecated the dangers of war, joking about the buzz bombs that fell around his barracks in France.

On another occasion—and they were far too few—it occurred to me that I could bring Lambert and Joan Ponstein to visit; Bert had taught in Hope's Religion Department for many years, and I remembered his telling us, in one of his classes on the Old Testament, of a long and apparently mutually gratifying conversation with Jim about Jean-Paul Sartre. In the car Bert warmed, reminiscing about the circumstances of Jim's marriage—his agonized indecision about whether, after years of correspondence ("so literate," I remembered Jim calling her letters), he should propose to Iris. "Let's take a walk," Bert had said, and I worked hard to suppress a smile at the picture of Bert, fully a foot shorter than Jim, trotting along trying to counsel him. "Do you love her?" Bert had demanded. "Yeah, I love her," confessed Jim. "Then tell her you want to see her!" Bert was still thinking about this when we reached Jim's room. "You have a nice wife," he pronounced as an opener. Then they commenced a long memory-lane session that all of us thoroughly enjoyed.

The last time I saw Jim, he was lying alone in his quiet room, and I asked him if he was bored. "No," he said complacently. "I think, and somehow the time passes." "What are you thinking about today?" I asked. "Dogs," he said. This was of course the last thing I had expected to hear. But the dog was his boyhood pet Cherry, a reddish-brown cocker spaniel whose death he had never forgotten: as the family approached their house walking back from church, she had bounded joyfully to meet them, never seeing the truck. She was killed before their eyes. It was a quintessential Prins moment: the ecstasy of love, natural to all of life, tragically cut short by the indifference of the cosmos.

A few months later he was found dead in his room. Iris and Robin came and sat with the body until it was cold.

I'm in my seventh decade now, and find myself looking back a lot—and the impetus behind this essay, as perhaps behind this volume, is transparently a desire to come to terms with Jim Prins, and what he meant to me and to generations of Hope students. What was the man about, anyway? What was it that made so many of us revere him, sometimes almost worship him?

The sheaf of lecture notes salvaged by his son Christopher helps bring it all back: Jim's true voice, thankfully, is there, and I realize how ignorant we were to think he ever lectured off the cuff—"in stream of consciousness," as one student quipped—even though it always looked so spontaneous. Reading over his book reviews, and, for the first time, his dissertation, I see that he was indeed highly intelligent, well abreast of contemporary criticism, and a very fine writer to boot. But at this distance, of course, I notice other things too. As a literature teacher myself, I see Jim imbued with the principles of the New Criticism, the methodology pioneered by Cleanth Brooks and Robert Penn Warren in the 1940s and 50s: close dissection of the work of art, the "verbal icon," in order to reveal its artistic whole-ness. Jim's dissertation on Dickens, finally com-pleted in 1963 between the distractions of teach-ing and child-rearing, in fact defines itself in the introduction as "a 'close reading' of an individual novel, *Bleak House*," and his class notes show his own approach as fundamentally formalist, organ-ized by reference to structure, symbolism, point of view, and all the other "elements" of literature. His course on literary criticism was titled "Practi-cal Criticism" after the book by I. A. Richards, a precursor of the New Critical principles.

His teaching was shaped, in other words, ac-cording to prevailing directions in the profession. Yet Prins also transcended his training: for one thing, he chose as his *métier* the novel, a genre usually too irregular for the New Critics but onc better suited to his interrogation of society and human nature. Like other professors of his gen-eration, he chafed at the onset of the culture wars, as documented by this letter sent me by the late Bryce Butler at the time of Jim's retire-ment:

On my latest (last?) visit to Hope, he was the only one who received me at all cordially, for which I was grateful. It was 1970 or thereabouts—all the sensibilities of the late sixties were in full flower. Prins had asked his class what they thought of the novels, and a black girl had complained that there were none she could relate to; nothing about her experience. Prins had not liked the answer. [Prins believed, Butler goes on, that even a novel like Ellison's *Invisible Man* was universal.] And in any case, the reader could transcend his particular experi-ence when reading a great novel.

Apparently Jim waxed fairly eloquent on this, but it is significant that shortly thereafter he incorporated Richard Wright's *Native Son* into his course, and his Last Chance Talk of 1966 reveals his outspoken anger at the Vietnam war. Literary universality aside, Prins despised bigotry and injustice in all forms: I remember his contempt for a Holland congregation's evident discomfiture when a brown-skinned man walked in wearing what Prins sympathetically described as "his pickle shirt." "I'm a Democrat," he told me once. "The Democrats have always cared about the poor." For the record, he never looked down on his female students either, and he quoted no critic more often than Dorothy Van Ghent.

Prins startled us by invoking Freud sometimes too—he knew about phallic symbols and deltas of Venus, obviously, and called on these tropes as ways of affirming an important underlayer of human life too often still repressed, especially at the Hope College of those days. (There's the story, probably apocryphal, that during a lecture on *Moby-Dick* he swooped down on the front row and demanded, "You DO know what SPERM is, don't you?") He had grown up Christian Reformed, after all, and among his most painful memories was the discovery that his mother had been pregnant before marriage—the child had died—and in the custom of the day had to stand before the whole congregation to confess. Her son could vicariously feel the shame: "And she was a be-YOO-ty-ful woman," he said, pronouncing "be-YOO-ty-ful" in the way I had heard the word from the old Dutch people of my childhood. Something of that memory, surely, informed his teaching of

The Scarlet Letter and *Tess of the D'Urbervilles*—as his powerful appreciation of *The Grapes of Wrath* must have derived from seeing his father, during the Great Depression, bent over the kitchen table, face hidden in hands, weeping because he could not feed his children.

Like all of us, this man came from somewhere, had parents, a social matrix—though one he clearly defined himself against. When I taught a course called "The Dutch and American Literature" in 1982 to mark the bicentennial of Dutch-American diplomatic relations, I invited Jim, along with Henry ten Hoor and some others, to talk about the western novelist Frederick Manfred, who as Feike Feikema had attended Calvin a few years before Jim matriculated there in 1934. Prins duly considered the invitation, but (in a note starting "*Ja*, but") finally begged off in favor of others he thought better qualified: "All these people have known F/M at Calvin, have memories and recollections of him there, have no resistance to professional Dutchism and Dutchists (particularly Frisian and Calvin-oriented). I don't (have recollections and memories), and do." Rebel and *isolato* though Jim was, did he take anything from the Dutch culture? I think he did: he shed the narrow prejudice and fear of the larger world, but he retained what I like to think was best in the tradition, a strong moral sense, a prodigious independence and contempt for all who curried favor, a dogged and residually Calvinist insistence on the darkness in human nature. It was an insistence he could in fact transfer almost whole to the world of literature and literary criticism: if the New Critics stressed structure, postwar literary criticism was also energized by the high moral seriousness and specifically Christian consciousness exemplified by Auden, Eliot, and C. S. Lewis, and one of the most prominent novels of the era, Golding's *Lord of the Flies*, radiated an Augustinian severity. This was a world view Jim had learned early and proved by experience. Representative are these words from the final chapter of his dissertation:

Bleak House, at its deepest and most profound, is a dark journey of the human soul, from the death of love in the lost innocence of childhood to redemption and the resurrection of love in maturity. It is the death and rebirth of love in London. And London is London, but London is also the whole world of human experience.

The death and rebirth of love: this is the fullest meaning of *Bleak House*—meaning as revealed by the fable, the images, the inner and the outer perspectives. Readers of Dickens have always seen in all of his novels the theme of Christian charity, the injunction to love one's neighbor. More recently, critics have found in them a deeper and darker Christian meaning: the need for man's redemption.

Jim was likely able to take the Christian vision imparted to him in youth, winnow out the cultural contingencies, and find that freshened vision reflected back to him in works of literature, where his lifelong quest for truth could operate within the freedom of doubt. "God will be kind to Camus," he said once. I think too that the kind of passionate faith in literature that inspired writers of the 1920s and 30s, the writers revered by his own generation, was transmitted to him as a young man, even in the relative cultural isolation of Calvin College, where he spent his freshman year: something was in the air there that led even young Dutch-Americans like Manfred, Peter De Vries, and David Cornel De Jong to venture with confidence into the literary world. These men were only a few years older than Jim; I remember too his telling me to read Wessel Smitter's 1910 novel *F.O.B. Detroit.* Coincidentally, the 1930s was a period of prodigious activity in American literary studies, and colored to some extent by the backwash of H. L. Mencken's sardonic anti-Puritanism. Mencken's famous definition of a Puritan as one tormented by "the haunting, haunting fear that somewhere, someone may be happy" certainly paralleled the anti-Calvinism driving the generation of De Vries, and it is interesting that Jim wrote his master's thesis on the Edwards-Chauncey controversy of the Great Awakening, the revival that spelled the end of Puritan dominance in colonial America. In a sense, then, Jim's cultural context helps explain him: but of course it goes only so far.

So, finally, how does one "come to terms" with Jim Prins? At the time of his retirement I came across a quotation from the novelist Thomas Wolfe, his notion that

the deepest search in life, the thing that in one way or another was central to all living, was a man's search to find a father, not merely the father of his flesh, not merely the lost father of his youth, but the image of a strength and wisdom external to his need and superior to his hunger, to which the belief and power of his own life could be united.

Perhaps it was something like that: Jim, unperturbed by inhibitions we attributed to the surrounding culture, paternally guided and approved the path of intellectual inquiry on which we were hesitantly embarking. But the word that best defines him for me is "sorrow." Melville writes in *Moby-Dick*,

> that mortal man who hath more of joy than sorrow in him, that mortal man cannot be true . . . . The truest of all men was the Man of Sorrows, and the truest of all books is Solomon's, and Ecclesiastes is the fine hammered steel of woe.

Jim's woe, to tell the truth, could range from the sublimity of the Man of Sorrows to the lugubriousness of Eeyore, and even he knew that: I remember him saying with some satisfaction that he "wasn't affable," and he was therefore always a haven for students a little disaffected. Witness another passage from Bryce Butler's letter:

> During my Junior year, or Love's Young Nightmare period, I came up to see Mr. Prins one time. I was depressed, of course, I was always depressed that year. I knocked, and he came to the door and said, "What can I do for you," conveying with his whole manner that, with the best will in the world, no one could do anything for anyone. "I'm depressed," I said, "and I'm looking for someone more depressed than I am, and I knew I could count on you." "Come in," he said, and we both felt better. As a teacher, I think, he lived in part for such moments . . . . In a way his teaching was aimed at such meetings, and they were what made him tolerant of people like me, although he did get tired of my habit of not turning up at class and then coming around to his office to meet him one on one.

Sherwood Anderson writes in his introduction to *Winesburg, Ohio* that embracing one truth of life to the exclusion of others makes us, in his word, "grotesques," and I guess something like that was taking place in Prins as he aged. But in this time when sorrow is pathologized as a treatable syndrome, when the endurance of Oedipus and Lear is discredited as a socially irresponsible mystification of pain, it comforts me to think of Prins, his stubborn affirmation of the dignity of human suffering, his unbounded charity to sinners. That was his vision, he made no apologies for it, he considered it a truth worth passing on; and every time I adapt to the latest upbeat, de-centered-classroom pedagogical trend I think of Prins, stationed tall and upright and alone before his students, and fight the nagging sense that I'm betraying him. Through his reverence for the medium of literature, he showed us the complexity and richness of life: he opened our eyes. I don't now remember when I heard Jim quote this passage from Joseph Conrad's preface to *The Nigger of the Narcissus*, but I know he loved it, and it may stand as his epitaph:

My task which I am trying to achieve is, by the power of the written word, to make you hear, to make you feel—that is, before all, to make you see. That—and no more, and it is everything. If I succeed, you shall find there according to your deserts: encouragement, consolation, fear, charm—all you demand—and, perhaps, also that glimpse of truth for which you have forgotten to ask.

℘

Recollections of Jim Prins as a Boy

Jay R. Vander Meulen

JIM'S MOTHER AND MINE were sisters, and we lived near each other in Holland—his family at 116 East 20th Street and mine at 103 East 24th. Jim was the oldest grandchild of Grandpa and Grandma Dogger, and I played with him in the 1930s when he was in high school and I was in grade school. He had his own gang of friends from Christian High—Roscoe De Vries (who later was the Ottawa County drain commissioner), Ralph Brouwer, and Vern Rose—but for a while I was like a puppy dog, with him all the time, and he welcomed me as the brother he never had.

The Prins house was also near to Jim's grandparents. Every Friday night Jim and his parents (my Uncle Albert ["Appie"] and Aunt Coba ["Cobie"]) and his sister Julia ("Juke") would visit the Doggers in their big white house at 750 Lincoln. On Christmas day all of Grandpa and Grandma's nine children and their grandchildren would be there. We would open presents around the Christmas tree and then at 8 or 9 p.m. have a big lunch that always ended with Grandma's chocolate cake with marshmallow frosting.

Jim's dad refinished damaged furniture at West Michigan Furniture, and the family wasn't well to do. Uncle Appie never had a car, and I remember him taking his bicycle with a basket in front to get groceries from the A & P at 10th and River. Jim walked to Central Christian School, about half a mile from his house, and on Sundays the family would walk to Maple Avenue Christian Reformed Church. Jim and his sister both had bicycles, and I learned to ride on hers (a girl's bike was easier to ride). During college Jim lived at home and he walked to Hope. (He had a scholarship to Calvin and started out there but didn't like it.) When he was in graduate school he hitchhiked back and forth to Ann Arbor for a while and then bought a car, a Ford—before he knew how to drive. I had been driving a milk truck since I was fourteen, so I taught him, on 20th Street, in front of his house. He was very excitable and not a good student.

The neighborhood had a number of good places to play. Uncle Appie put up a backboard for basketball on the neighbor's property, and just beyond that, at the southwest corner of 20th and Columbia, was Van Voorst's sand pit. They would dump the sand off the bank on the northeast corner down to a factory below, where they made cement blocks on the site where Hope now has a maintenance garage. (There's a house made from those blocks on 16th Street just east of the foot of Hazel Avenue.) After the city paved Columbia Avenue between 22nd and 24th between Prospect Park and the old Bush and Lane piano company, they closed it for roller skating. I went there with Jim, who had skates that clamped on over his shoes. One day he came home from there with a dog. His mother wouldn't let him keep it, but a neighbor lady took it in; he named it Poochie. Across the street from his house he used to hit golf balls on the ball diamond. One day when I was with him he sliced a ball through a porch window. No one was home there, and Jim hid his clubs. When the owner came back he found the window broken and a golf ball on the porch. Jim was going to try to get out of it but then confessed, and I think he ended up paying for the window.

During the Depression the city set up an area for people to have gardens in the swamp north of 6th Street. Uncle Appie had one—up College Avenue, beyond the dump, toward the river, next to the hot water crick that came from the turbines from the power plant. He raised potatoes, and getting them home was always a bone of contention between Jim and his dad. I would help Jim pull a wagon of them to his house on 20th Street, where his mother stored them in a cold cellar. Jim had his own uses for them. He would sneak them out of the bin, and we would hike up 20th Street, across the fairgrounds (now the back of Pilgrim Home Cemetery) and through Van Dragt's apple orchard to what we called "Spreechie's Pond" on the north side of 24th Street near Waverly Road. We would make a bonfire, wrap the potatoes in clay, and roast them in the coals. The place is now a Menards parking lot.

Jim and I didn't stay in touch after he went off to war and met his wife in England. I would occasionally bump into him when Vander Meulens were doing carpentry work around Hope, but I didn't see him much. When we did talk, though, he would always bring up memories of when we were young.

᷐

War Years

Iris Prins

WORLD WAR II BEGAN September 3, 1939, a few weeks before my fourteenth birthday. The early months were eerily quiet; we waited apprehensively for the unknown. People busied themselves digging air raid shelters in back gardens. Housewives put up blackout material over windows, and wondered how they'd manage with food and clothing ration books. Gas masks were issued and fitted, and carried on our shoulders until war's end. And when it seemed that nothing would happen, the first air-raid siren shattered the quiet, and the bombing began.

Before the first year of war ended, France surrendered to the superior strength of the German Army. Thousands of troops from the British Expeditionary Force were stranded on the beaches of Normandy, there to hold out until the Royal Navy, and hundreds of small boats, crossed the Channel to rescue them.

Morale was low. An invasion was feared. Prime Minister Winston Churchill's speech rallied us:

"We shall defend our Island, whatever the cost may be. We shall fight on the beaches, we shall fight on the landing grounds. We shall fight in the fields and in the streets; we shall fight in the hills. We shall never surrender."

Port cities, Southampton's extensive docks, were prime targets of the stepped-up bombing, and, farther inland, the industrial cities suffered in turn. The Blitz of Southampton lasted forty-eight hours, beginning as the fires from incendiary bombs lit the path for the heavily-laden bombers. Those who survived the ordeal looked out on a wasteland of craters and smoking ruins.

In what may have been a prelude to invasion, the Germans sent waves of Fokker Fighters over the coast of Southern England. On a beautiful summer morning, the dogfighters raged overhead. Over the countryside, planes and parachutes fell in flames. At the end of the day, the R. A. F. were victorious, and of the airmen, Churchill said:

"Never in the field of human conflict was so much owed by so many to so few."

The Allied Forces began the invasion of Normandy June 6, 1944. As the armies pressed into France, air raids over England became less frequent. But in their place, V Rockets visited new terror on London.

I was on transfer to a London office when the war in Europe ended. That night I joined the delirious throng on its way to Trafalgar Square. We cheered and the lights turned on again in England.

Time does not erase the horror of war. Long after—and sometimes now—a low-flying plane can cause my heart to jump. In the street where I lived in Southampton, every other house was damaged or destroyed. Friends lost homes, lost family members, with little time given to grieve. Our family was spared that pain, but my brother became one of the many tuberculosis victims. He spent his last years in a miserable, makeshift building on the grounds of Southampton's crowded Chest Hospital.

I remember his courage, his cheerfulness, his appreciation for a banana I'd scrounged from a Dock warehouse. I remember the water-logged shelter, the nights of terror, my sister's nails digging into my hand as we huddled in fear. I remember meager rations, the walks to a dimly-lit bus stop amid invisible, jostling crowds. I remember the joy of a shared chocolate bar, the anticipation of ice cream at war's end. And I remember the young faces of German prisoners, behind barbed-wire fences in Southampton's parks.

In April 1944, P.F.C. A. James Prins, 36191895, with Company C, 796th M.P. Battalion, disembarked in Scotland from the converted luxury liner *Queen Elizabeth*, and left by train for Southampton. For the next four months, P.F.C. Prins did guard duty on the No. 2 Gate entrance into Southampton Docks. From the second-floor window of the bomb-damaged Docks Branch Post Office where I worked, I first saw the tanned, long-legged, khaki-clad soldier. My window vantage allowed me a spot to see him often. He looked, I thought, like Gregory Peck. But my shyness and reserve would not allow for more than a greeting when I walked by. I gave him my address the day I heard he was soon to leave for France.

Letters came infrequently from France and Belgium over the next two years. In 1946, Jim was discharged from the army. Later that same year, he began his teaching career at Hope College. Our correspondence continued until 1949, when I came to Holland to visit Jim and his family. I think I knew I would not use my return ticket home to England. In Thanksgiving break of 1949, Jim's uncle Arnold Dykhuizen married us in his church in Marion, New York.

☙

Jim Prins: A Memoir

Victor Nuovo, Class of 1954

MY RECOLLECTION of Jim Prins goes back a half century, when he was young and I was barely out of adolescence. I took two of his courses, one on the American novel and the other on literary criticism. I recall them well, better than other courses that I took as an undergraduate or graduate.

Why is this so? First and foremost, because of Jim himself. I have said that he was young, but it was a youthfulness interrupted by the experience of war that came too soon in his life. His voice, indeed his whole manner, was melancholic. I contrast this with the ebullience of John Hollenbach, the gravity of Clarence De Graaf, and the irony of D. Ivan Dykstra, all teachers whom I recall with affection and respect. That mood fit the themes that he reflected upon, human frailty, the sources of tragedy and comedy, compassion and acceptance. His melancholy and his uncompromising honesty were the sources of the spell he cast over us students and made him such an effective teacher. They suited the presentation of themes from American novels, although, I'm sure, they would have applied as well in a course on the Russian novel. After I had graduated and entered seminary, Jim wrote to me that I should read the great Russian novels, especially Dostoevsky. I did.

Jim's course on literary criticism, which he offered in the Spring semester, 1954, was a new and, I suspect, daring venture for him and for Hope College. Looking back, it seems that this was the first time in my experience as a student that I came to see my role as one not of a mere student but as an intellectual called not just to receive what was given, but to join in an uncertain project of enquiry, interpretation, and, perhaps, new understanding. I don't think I realized what a poem was until then. The experience was philosophical in the profoundest way.

I took another course that spring with D. Ivan Dykstra that had a similar effect, a seminar on the philosophy of history. But because the style of both men was so different, the effect happened differently. D. Ivan displayed his learning and in a wonderful way; it flowed over us and moved us forward. I guess I could say that D. Ivan made me a lover of learning.

But Jim never claimed to be learned, indeed he denied it. He was a pure enquirer; and his attitude was so unmistakably genuine and so searching that one could not resist adopting it. Jim's authority in the classroom was real but not imposing. He never condescended or presumed to speak from a superior vantage point. But he was always the teacher. I think that his authority derived from the truth that he sought, and that he knew could only be discovered if one remained intellectually honest and open.

My deep regret is that I lost touch with him as the years went on. I hope we will meet again. If so, since by then he will have become a seasoned explorer of eternity, I will gladly submit to him again as a teacher and guide. I say this not idly, nor sentimentally. In eternity we shall see God face to face, and also each other, free of the protective camouflage with which we surround ourselves in this life. Then our enquiries will be as pure as pure light, and the prospects that open to us satisfying beyond imagination.

☙

Jim Prins

Jane Gouwens Bach, Class of 1958

Delivered at the memorial service for Dr. Prins, August 17, 2003.

IN THE NINETEEN-FIFTIES I took several courses from Jim Prins. My first class with him was World Literature, and my first strong memory of him consists of a moment in his lecture on Homer's *Iliad*. Jim invited us to look closely at the scene in which the hero Hector—about to go into battle—bids farewell to his wife and their little son. Jim pointed out the tenderness with which the child was described, the dignity and heartbreak of the hero's speeches, the way his shining plumed helmet both fascinated and frightened the little boy. Such a moment, in a literary work thousands of years old! The emotion in Jim's voice and the rapt attention he gave the text created an epiphany for me. For the first time, I realized the power of literature to strike deep into the heart—to show that throughout the ages human beings experience the same emotions. Grief. Love. Courage.

Jim Prins educated our hearts, whether the
subject matter was an ancient Greek epic or a recent British novel.

In the novels courses, Jim's approach was
very disciplined, carefully organized, and
thoughtfully responsive to selected critical resources. He systematically demonstrated that the
fictional work of art, in all its components, evokes
not only a thematic idea but also an atmosphere
and attitude unique in itself. Throughout each
analysis, however, pulsed the force of Jim's passion for literature. We students could see, as he
explored a novel with us, that his own feelings
and those in the book went deep, and out of such
depths came the power that had created the
work, that perceived it, and that enabled us to
share it. Thus every class session was balanced
between feeling and reason, passion and thought.

Jim welcomed discussion. He treated student
comments with the intense attention that was his
trademark. When three or four of the more articulate students raised questions, he welcomed
their challenges, and became even more involved
and animated than before. He would stand with
one foot on the floor, the other foot planted firmly
on the desk. The novel was open in one hand.
With his free hand he gestured, with the mobile
expressions of his face he revealed whole se-
quences of feeling, and with his sudden laugh he
caught us off guard—a good reminder of the ambiguities of a passionate devotion to literature.

Once during Jim's time as an advisor to the
student literary magazine, he and Iris invited the
Opus staff into their home for a meeting with a
student author whose work the staff liked but

had reservations about. I can't remember the reasons. What I do remember was that there—in that serene and welcoming environment—I first experienced the difficulties of making judgments, trying to be fair, trying to articulate a critical response without denying the strength of a fellow student's writing. That particular student went on to become a college president. Perhaps he too remembers that evening, and the tension, and the effort on all sides, fostered by Jim, that one needed to be fair, honest, and involved at every turn. Not just in the classroom, but everywhere that students and literature came together.

As I remember all these things and reflect on them, I realize once again how lucky I am to have had Jim Prins as a teacher. I sense that my own life, including my experience as a teacher, would have been far more meager, had I not been one of his students. Throughout our lives we have benefited from witnessing his profound devotion to literature and especially to the way it incarnated deep thought and deep feeling, conjoined. Every session in his classroom took us a little closer to those two cherished ideals: a passionate mind, an educated heart. We are grateful to have been the students of Jim Prins.

∽

And When My Students Thank Me

Gardner Kissack, Class of 1959

Delivered at the retirement celebration for Dr. Prins, June 6, 1981.

WHO IS Dr. A. James Prins and what's he doing here in a nice place like this on such a beautiful afternoon? Wouldn't you rather be home dandelioning or weeding?

(Monica ad-libs: "That's my grandfather!" Audience erupts in appreciative laughter. AJP grins proudly at the tot's perfect timing. Speaker: "That's right . . .")

Teddy Roosevelt, raising his sons late last century, told 'em, "Boys, in matters of right and wrong, never be neutral!"

Ring Lardner, late in his short, tragic life, fought against *risqué* lyrics in the popular songs of the late Twenties and early Thirties . . . without much success, you may conclude if you've listened hard recently.

J. P. Marquand, in his 1941 novel *H. M. Pulham, Esquire*, has Harry Pulham tell his friend, "You and I, Bill, we have our rules."

Gordon Liddy, when he visited Northwestern University in Evanston several months ago, told his audience that the world was not Evanston on a nice day, or Beverly Hills, California, or Chicago—or, he might have added, Holland, Michigan, on a sunny Sunday afternoon. "The world," he said, "is a bad neighborhood at three-thirty in the morning."

Joshua Loth Liebman, in his 1946 bestseller, *Peace of Mind*, has that key paragraph in the last chapter:

Out of this hero worship instinctive in all of us, a sobering truth emerges. If we are influenced by powerful personalities around us, may not we, in turn, influence others? Yes, for better or for worse, we do. Constantly, without our knowing it, we are sources of infection for good or evil. We are carriers of health and disease—either the divine health of courage and nobility or the demonic diseases of hatred and anxiety. As we live, we make the world freer or more enslaved, nobler or more degraded.

Cut to 1957, Boone's City Kitchen *(audience laughter)* on 8th Street, just around the corner from Vogelzang's Hardware . . . a long, narrow room with close tables crowded near the front *(additional slight laughter as audience remembers)* and the long formica counter in the middle. Hot beef sandwiches—with lots of potatoes and gravy—35 cents! Hot chicken sandwiches, 40 cents. And once a week, club steak: $1.25! *(Audience silent, either in pity for the speaker or sorrow for his lost youth/$1.25 club steak.)* Of course, milk or coffee was ten cents extra. But you can still get a cup of coffee for a dime at Russ' drive-in on 8th. Ah, the nineteen-fifties!

Do you know what one of our big worries was then? Whether Professor Prins' two-tone, two-door `47 Chevy fastback would get safely across the dangerous intersection of 8th and Chicago Drive. *(Mild laughter. AJP nods, fondly remembering good old car?)*

My Zoology professor encouraged me to attend summer school, and so I enrolled in the summer of 1957 in Dr. James Dyke Van Putten's Modern American Diplomacy and Professor A. James Prins' Modern European Novel. Nine novels in six weeks . . . Tolstoy, Dostoevsky, Turgenev, Balzac, Flaubert . . . . *(AJP: "And a lot more too!" Audience laughter. Speaker upstaged again. Who next? Beautiful Robin? Magnificent Iris? Time for bag of tricks.)*

I have here three novels I bought on June 17, 1957—and as is my custom, I dated them when completed: June 18, June 20, and June 29—must have hit a weekend. So wherever I went, a novel went with me. It was read, read, read.

One late-June evening, after supper at Boone's, I walked or biked to Kollen Park where I usually read from six until eight or so, depending on the mosquitoes. I was just settled, starting to read, when very suddenly I was struck by the realization that I had walked out of Boone's without paying for my supper! Walked right past the cash register, novel in hand! Embarrassment. Shock. Surprise. A little shame. And amusement. How could such a thing happen? What had happened?

I know now and I suppose I began to realize then—as some of you know—it was the P. E.

To make a book, a novel, a fictional character—Madame Bovary, Bazarov, Anna K., Pierre—

real, alive . . . live . . . and more important than, well, than food—or at least paying for it. Well, that was something. That was a first for me.

Call it what you will. Describe it somewhat differently . . . most of you know about the P. E.— the Prins Effect? *(Audience acknowledges: nodding, knowing glances; slight, brief buzzing.)*

It was that summer that my education truly began—oh, not merely terms: "ethics," "amorality," "hedonism," "existentialism," "egalitarianism," and "omniscient." But having a professor who was able to make—to allow—an author's thoughts to be mine. That was new.

The next summer, the English Novel. Encore. My senior year, the American Novel. Encore. And more new friends: Moll and Jane and Pip and Ishmael and Tess and Nana and George and Lenny and many more. I went over my novel notes last week in preparation for today and found that I have more notes on *Great Expectations* and its author than any of the others. Just imagine if *Bleak House* had been in paperback that summer.

To make, to allow the author's meaning clear and real—and vital. It still impresses and amazes me.

In a small way, I have attempted to share that appreciation and understanding and enjoyment of the novel in the novel classes that I have taught since 1967—not so expertly of course, not so technically to be sure . . . but I have shared Melville and Twain and Crane and Wharton and F. Scott Fitzgerald and J. P. Marquand and even Hemingway and Steinbeck . . . and recently, Jack Finney.

And when my students thank me, they thank you. *(Speaker nods to AJP.)*

Thornton Wilder, in the last act of *Our Town,* has Emily ask, "Live people don't understand very much, do they?"

And the Stage Manager replies, "No . . . the saints and the poets—they do some . . . ."

Which are you? Perhaps a little bit of both? *(AJP, having removed glasses, shakes head, denying both—thereby acknowledging at least one.)*

And maybe a little bit of George Bailey in "It's a Wonderful Life"—you remember Jimmy Stewart in Frank Capra's film? *(Audience murmurs approval and appreciation for Stewart/Bailey-Prins comparison.)*

". . . for you have spread the infection of the divine health of courage and *the world is nobler because of you.*"

And when my students thank me, they thank you, Dr. Albert James Prins . . . and so do I.

♫

Remembering A. James Prins

Jim Michmerhuizen, Class of 1963

JIM AND IRIS PRINS—and Robin and Christopher, when they were still little—lived in Holland Heights, less than a mile from the house on East 8th Street where we moved in 1945. I knew him from my senior year at Holland Christian High—when a friend who had been translated to collegiate status a year or so earlier arranged an invitation and a visit—through the early Eighties, when I visited several times with Rosemarie and my daughter Kate.

Through that entire time, Jim Prins stood for something unique in my life. He did something, every day, that I couldn't do, and wouldn't learn to do until many years later: he lived, as one person, in two worlds. He breathed, and spoke, and moved, in the world of my Dutch Calvinist upbringing, and equally in the world of learning, of literature, of careful thought and pleasurable speech. Without ever, so far as I am aware, setting out to do so, he became an example to me.

Early in my life I abhorred examples. "Exemplary lives" bored me; and when my elders, attempting to correct my misbehaviors, reminded me of the example I was supposed to set for others, I wanted to run away.

I've done a complete about-face on this issue. Everything important in human culture is transmitted, not by discursive thought or by the written word, but by personal example. I don't mean that thought and word are not significant; they are, but only individual persons can bring them to our attention, and, by their own example, give them meaning. Every well-lived life is an ostensive definition of the ideas on which it is founded.

Jim Prins was from the same background as myself. In fact, Clarence De Graaf, Henry ten Hoor, and A. James Prins were all from that background, they were all graduates of Holland Christian High School; my father knew them; he and De Graaf had been classmates.

I, at Hope, knew only that I was Dutch and Christian Reformed; but what else I might be, I had no idea, and I got dizzy in my head when I tried to imagine that. I was living in two worlds—at least two—and was only just beginning to realize that they existed on two different foundations.

One of those worlds had Sunday School and catechism, and church twice on Sunday, farm bullies at Van Raalte public school, interminable sermons, prayer before meals and a Bible passage afterwards. The other world—had Bach and Messaien, Kafka and Faulkner and Henry James, Wittgenstein and Russell and Gabriel Marcel.

Jim Prins had found his integrity, I think, early on. His conversation—both in class and in my visits to his home—always came directly from his center—a center that I could only obscurely sense, not yet having one of my own. His conversation was never oblique; it was never shaped by other concerns. In particular, he paid no homage to the idols of academia—the idols whose worship consists of opposing these two worlds to each other, and imagining that we must—or even can—choose only one as our spirit's home.

In conversation with him, there were never prohibited topics, nor prohibited perspectives. He loved argument; he had no use for mere debate.

I honor him now for that integrity. During the time that I knew him, it fed me; my two worlds came into contact, became permeable to each other, and merged. That took a long time; without Jim Prins' example, it would have taken longer.

I think that he must have played that exemplary role, or one very similar, for many Hope students and friends during his tenure there. But this little testimony will have to do: Jim Prins has come to stand, in my experience of him, for the principle that all learning is personal, and that the goal of all such learning is personal integrity—to be one person, no matter the number of worlds there are to live and act in. It was the only sort of learning that he recognized.

It occurred to me once that there are more kinds of people in the world than there are people. If this is so, then A. James Prins, all by himself, was a cloud of witnesses, as numerous as the number of his students; one of whom I was forty-five years ago, and respectfully and gratefully remain to this day.

%

The Soul of the Matter

Linda Patterson Miller, Class of 1968

UNTIL I ENTERED Hope College in the fall of 1964, I read voraciously and indiscriminately from the books I gathered weekly from my local Park Ridge library. Only when I took (in compelling succession) Dr. Prins's three novels classes did I learn to read for my very life.

I can still see Prins striding into Graves Hall. I don't know why I remember this entrance so vividly, since invariably he stood on that staged podium anticipating our arrival. It speaks to the unrelenting power of his intellect that we never dared to sneak in late. We knew he noticed everything, and we also did not want to miss a word. But in my mind I watch him now, not so much striding as loping, his body leaning forward (tilting at windmills, I would think later). His arms seemed too long for his body, and everything about him seemed angular and skewed toward truth-telling.

We knew that class was ready to begin when he would drape himself over that podium, seeming to embrace it, and then look up. I never felt that he looked at us, though. His gaze often seemed distant and detached, and I never knew where his mind would take us. I found this both mesmerizing and terrifying. I remember one time when he stepped off the podium stage to walk over to his right, where the windows of Graves fronted the Pine Grove. The afternoon sun slanted sideways through the windows, and as he looked out, he continued to talk (was it about Nick Carraway's noncommittal stance, or Gatsby's impossible dream, or that green breast of the world that recedes daily before us?). All the while, as Prins stood in silhouette against the light outside, and we sat beside him in the contained space of that classroom, the world beyond us lurched and shifted faster than any of us could hold it.

When I try to analyze now what made Prins so memorable a teacher, no one quality predominates. He took the best from the New Criticism techniques of his day, homing in on textual analysis by isolating and reading to us aloud passages that illuminated key structural and thematic patterns. In the overall patterning of his courses, themes emerged that illustrated the care with which he had initially organized his courses wherein nothing, save life's own unpredictability and its daily losses, seemed left to chance. I still have my notebooks from all the courses I took with Prins, and I am struck to this day by the pristine orderliness of the notes I kept of his lectures: clear summaries of the literary and cultural contexts for these works followed by a representative selection of scholarly voices weighing in on the texts. But it was Prins's own voice (at once wry, bemused, irreverent, melancholic, telling) that made the day. We heard that voice most as he read, with some occasional asides, the passages from each work that he chose to highlight. I have these passages underlined in my original texts (most of the bindings now shot), and in the accompanying marginalia to these selected passages, I hear yet again Prins speaking. He seemed most impassioned when he read from Hawthorne's *Scarlet Letter*, metaphorically offering up to us, his students, a flower plucked from the rosebush that, "by a strange chance, has been kept alive in history." "It may serve, let us hope," Prins reiterated, "to symbolize some sweet moral blossom that may be found along the track, or relieve the darkening close of a tale of human frailty and sorrow."

I believe that Dr. Prins was attuned to life's underlying darkness, and that he knew things he did not always want to say. This comprised, for me, a large part of his mystery and power. If I seldom knew where he was looking, I came to realize soon enough that it was usually inward. This was the gift he gave to all of us who over the years experienced the transformative power of his teaching. I include Prins among the professorial triumvirate that ruled Hope during the 1960s. D. Ivan Dykstra gave us the life of the mind and Arthur Jentz gave us the will to believe in the life of the mind; but James Prins gave us our souls.

꙳

The Coat on the Platform

Bruce Ronda, Class of 1969

For Bryce Butler (1944-2001), Hope College Class of 1966

AMONG OURSELVES we always called him
Prins. For some other English Department professors we had nicknames, none of which I will
repeat here. Perhaps in face-to-face conversation
we called him "Dr. Prins," but always in private
he was simply Prins, and nothing else. A few
other Hope faculty merited such naming: Arthur
Jentz was always "Jentz," Jim Malcolm just "Malcolm." This was not disrespect, you understand,
but quite the opposite. Last names (one could not
then imagine calling professors by their first
names!) suggested seriousness, intensity, devotion to one's subject matter or art. You would not
call Herman Melville "Herman" or Ludwig Wittgenstein "Ludwig." Jim Prins was always just
Prins.

The "we" in the preceding paragraph needs
some explanation. For three of my four years at
Hope College (1965 to 1969) I lived in Crispell
Cottage with ten or twelve other young men. Although the group's make-up changed yearly, the

identity of Crispell during those years came from the handful of us who were English or Philosophy or Foreign Language majors, worked on the *Anchor* and *Opus*, listened to classical music, and took ourselves very, very seriously. Well, mostly. There was also a zany, Beatles-like quality about Crispell—whimsical, absurd, indebted to "Beyond the Fringe" and Mike Nichols and Elaine May.

Ours was also a straight male world. It wasn't as if there weren't women in our lives. Most of us had "girlfriends," some were involved in very serious relationships, and like other testosterone-laden late adolescents we fantasized and talked about women constantly. One or two had boyfriends, although homosexuality was simply beyond conversation, even for us talky types, in those pre-Stonewall years. A few of our English professors—notably Joan Mueller, Jean Protheroe, and later Betsy Reedy—were women, and some of the most brilliant English majors in the mid-1960s were women—Sue Spring, Carole Osterink, Mary Hesselink. But the humanities were still a very male and officially heterosexual world in the mid-1960s: we read a male-dominated canon, we competed with each other for the austerity and brilliance of our seminar contributions, we relied on the old-boy network to get us into good graduate schools and first jobs.

It sounds almost monastic, the way I describe it: a handful of undergraduates devoted to those close readings of literary and philosophical texts, encouraged by professors themselves devoted to reading and teaching, though not often writing about, classic texts and works of art. For all its limitations, the world of the humanities at Hope in the mid-1960s was a haven from religious conservatism and social conformity. For me, and I suspect for others as well, Prins was very near the core of that humanities experience.

Thinking back on those years, I realize how little I knew of Prins's life, his family, his background. Perhaps others did, but I never went to his home, surprising when I think of it, since I was a visitor in the homes of other professors—John Hollenbach, Joan Mueller, Jim Malcolm—and lived for a year with the family of the historian David Clark. This now seems even more surprising since at one time Prins was my advisor, counseling me, I suppose, on course selection and perhaps even on my future.

No, my knowledge of Prins derived from the triangle of teacher-text-student. Clearly there were other students in those novels classes for the requirement or the ride, but for us readers, it was all about intensity. We burrowed into the American and English and European novels he assigned, came up gasping for air to absorb his lectures, and then plunged back into the reading. The whole experience had a terrific concentration about it. You were, in a sense, the only person in the room with him, despite the fact that there were maybe fifty or sixty others in Winants Auditorium along with you.

Each class session was an encounter with Prins the teacher. I recall that he engaged in no small talk, though sometimes offered a disarming smile and a grimace about something, but no idle chat with students as we teachers often do today, seeking, alas, to be our students' friend as well their mentor. Prins would stride into Graves moments before class was to begin, shucking off his trench coat and flinging it, while still some distance away, toward the raised platform. There was something so intense, so focused, so unworldly about that gesture, it always took my breath away. That memory links in my mind with a passage from Alfred Kazin's 1951 memoir *A Walker in the City* (a book I often teach), in which he recalls his friend David, whose Brooklyn tenement dining room was adorned with photos of political leaders and racial violence from the 1930s, and little else: "Yet far more than the poverty of that orphaned and rotting house; more, even, than the sense of impending death, it was some deep, brave, and awful earnestness before life itself that I always felt there."

Gaunt, Lincolnesque, perpetually in anguish, Prins towered above the podium, meant for people of ordinary stature. He was in anguish over the moral dilemmas in the novels, anguish about the aesthetic decisions writers were forced to make, anguish over his fragile ability to convey all this to complacent young people just awakening from the sleep of the Fifties. Perhaps some of it was an act, dramatization like good pulpit oratory, meant to awaken the dozers in the back row. Some undoubtedly derived from his own Calvinism, transfixed by the soul's dilemma of choice and election, free will and fate. I like to think, though I have no real evidence, that Prins's lectern manner—the self-deprecation, the grip on the podium, the outstretched hands, palms forward, brow furrowed as he sought the right words, the emotional reading of the most fraught passages—came from his own existential struggles, his own desire to make sense out of life.

I still have my notebooks from those courses. In fact, I consult them periodically, especially the spiral-edged one from American Novels (fall semester, 1966, almost forty years ago), since I regularly teach some of those novels myself in various courses. If the notes are any indication, Prins focused, as did virtually the entire literary profession, on form and structure, and to the extent that there were larger themes to be drawn out, they were about "man" and "consciousness" and "the west," those huge generalizations soon to be exploded by a new generation of readers, ours, it turns out. Our American novels were all by men; the scholarship recommended to us nearly all by men. Teachers today draw from a larger and more diverse range of works to teach, and often try to avoid the kind of sweeping statements favored in an earlier era of teaching and scholarship.

In one way, then, Prins was among the last of the old school, dramatic, anguished, an eccentric who would surely now be out of place in our era of witty and ironic postmodernism. In another way, however, he shaped the next generation of teachers and readers who passed through his classes. Although Holland, Michigan, seemed a quiet corner of the world in the mid-Sixties, it was beginning to be troubled by the civil rights movement, anti-Vietnam War protest, and the women's movement, all of which gained momentum on Hope's campus throughout the late sixties and early seventies. In the midst of that turmoil, Prins infused what he taught with a kind of moral urgency, a sense that these books were hot to the touch and aroused, through the alchemy of reading, the same conflicts and dilemmas and drives that provoked their writers and their earlier readers. These books encouraged great imaginative leaps into the worlds of seventeenth-century New England, nineteenth-century Russia, or twentieth-century Ireland. Through these novels, Prins had opened the world to us; it was now our turn to inherit and transform it.

ℒ

Two Dreams

Kenneth Kulhawy, Class of 1971

I FIRST MET JIM in the autumn of 1969, when I took his American Novels class. We talked often during and after class, and became friends. I left Hope at the end of that semester, but we wrote to each other semi-regularly for many years. I was thrilled to be able to attend, and participate in, his surprise retirement party in 1981. In the summer and autumn of 1993 I returned again to Hope to complete my degree (yes, those dates are correct) and I was a frequent guest at the home of Jim and Iris, to watch Saturday football and drink beer. I say all this to explain that I knew Jim for a long time, and in varied contexts.

He was a brilliant lecturer. We all knew this. Literature was alive to him, and through him it became so to us. One afternoon, twenty-four years after I took his course, we were chatting in his den and an idea came up, and I said, yes, you used to trace that, and I listed back to him the entire order of his American Novels syllabus: *Scarlet Letter, Moby-Dick, Rise of Silas Lapham, Huck, The Ambassadors, Sister Carrie, Gatsby, Farewell to Arms, Grapes of Wrath, Sound and the*

Fury. He was very surprised at my memory, but said, well, you actors, you remember everything. But no, I argued. I remember that because the content was fired into my brain, like the wedding of glaze and clay in a kiln at 2300 F. I remember because what you taught was so memorable. That embarrassed him, so he deflected the subject and we drank another beer.

But I'm sure he knew what I said was true, as I really could swiftly list those novels still after twenty-four years AND trace the thought through them—Jim's theme throughout the course, that the American Dream was somehow squandered, that we were Gatsbys chasing after empty Daisys, our ideas emotionally arrested at the moment we saw Caddy's dirty pants in that tree. A deeply sad theme, but there it is. And I still knew it because I had been properly taught it. *Educo, educare*—to lead out. With a solid foundation. That's what Jim did. And I was proof back to him that what he did had worked. I'm very grateful I was able to show him that, that afternoon.

He passed to me, and I passed back to him. And yes, the Dream is squandered. But the Dream is also one generation teaching another to live, and Jim knew that, too, of course, and when he read aloud to all of us the last pages of *Grapes of Wrath*, we understood that we could, if we tried, turn that squandering around, reverse that fall, and make a new world. Jim read that to us, and I still hear it oh so clearly today:

Rose of Sharon loosened one side of the blanket and bared her breast. "You got to," she said. She squirmed closer and pulled his head close. "There!" she said.

"There." Her hand moved behind his head and supported it. Her fingers moved gently in his hair. She looked up and across the barn, and her lips came together and smiled mysteriously.

And all of Hope College wept.

All for a Good Book

Larry Helder, Class of 1982

DEAR JIM,

I remember when I was a little boy, seeing you and Iris diligently gathering sticks around your yard, and neatly stacking them in a column between two trees. To a little boy it seemed odd. My house was two blocks away. You knew my parents. Many years later, when I was a student at Hope, you asked me about them. After my father's death in '82, you wondered aloud how my mother was getting on. Thank you for asking.

Before I took your class in American Novels, a friend, an English major, warned me not to take a class from you. I don't recall the context of that warning, but I ignored it, in retrospect, happily. I hope you haven't forgotten I pulled you from retirement for two novel tutorials: Russian and European. We found common ground: love for a great story, a need to question Calvinism and the Church, and a passionate belief that literature could address the pain and hope of the soul.

I remember, in particular, we read and reveled in Russian novels, because individual souls were at stake in those books. And because Russian authors attempted nothing less than the salvation of Russia itself. I still, sometimes, carry this feeling with me when I pull a book from the shelf: "Will this book save me, 'open my eyes,' change me?" You may have been the last teacher on earth to believe that a man's soul could be redeemed by reading a novel. Did Literature save you? Why didn't you become a great writer, instead of a great reader?

I like to think of myself as your last student. You were my Ancient Mariner, clutching at my arm with your passion, your sudden booming laugh, the shared intimacy of your own disappointments, offered as asides, but strangely relevant to the material at hand. You made people uncomfortable. You were not pleasant or nice—these characteristics being lukewarm. I remember some years after your retirement, while in a conversation with Dirk Jellema, that he, Dirk, wished he could visit you to talk about novels, but was unsure if you'd open the door. If you could put off Dirk Jellema, what did you do to many of your students? I don't mean your disciples, but rather all those filling their Humanities requirements. Like Captain Ahab, you "have your humanities," but did you need be that intense?

The last time I saw you and Iris was at the old Herrick Library during a winter blizzard. Apparently, you'd walked all the way from your home in the Heights, a five-mile round trip. You were covered in snow, a stocking cap pulled over your ears. You did not recognize me; you had come for the books.

✺✺✺

Four Decades of Reminiscence

JIM WAS ON A PANEL whose charge was to discuss the values of literature and history. A history professor claimed that a primary value of history was that "it deals with the facts, and that is one of the things that separates history from literature, something that makes it more worthwhile, of more value." Jim let the panel member finish, then offered this acknowledgment. "Yes, you are correct. You deal with the facts; whereas, I deal with the truth."

—Jack Ridl, Professor of English

ℒ

I REMEMBER with grateful heart the blessing of shared moments with Jim Prins, a professor with notable literary savvy and a keen humanity.

Jim was and continues to be a gift and challenge for me. He modeled an intellectual curiosity, a world view, a morality, and an example of life-long learning as important as any particular consideration of Hawthorne's *Scarlet Letter* or any of the other works he illuminated.

What can I say about his love of literature, especially Dickens, and his loyalty to his students? His Socratic approach with questions, questions, and more questions got his students to thinking and thinking hard.

Jim became for me and for others, too, I'm sure, a kind of benchmark against which to measure one's growth in understanding important truths found in literature, indeed in life. Jim whetted one's appetite for a lifetime of learning.

How well I recall his rational kindness. Jim and I were in his department office, there at my request, to discuss a grade less than I had expected. After some reasoned discussion I said something which put an improved grade at his mercy. "The quality of Jim's mercy was not strained." Jim changed the grade.

It seems fitting that of all the British ladies finding our GIs attractive during America's friendly occupation of England during World War II, it was Iris who caught Jim's fancy and Jim whom Iris fancied in return. His special lady saw in Jim a lanky Yank of rugged handsome features whose MP facade hid a gentleness which matched her sensitive, caring nature.

Iris, I discovered Jim's and your caring natures when on the occasion of having our second child and in need of a babysitter, you and Jim met our need.

Your kindness warmed me. Your friendship engendered optimism about a world in which such friends abide.

Thank you, Jim, for your patient teaching and for bringing Iris back from England.

—*Harold Saunders, Class of 1952*

DR. PRINS WAS ONE of my English profs when I was a Hope student. I respected him as a person and as an instructor. He was dedicated to his profession at a time when monetary rewards were much less at Hope than what they were elsewhere, but he chose to stay at Hope and I, along with many other students, am grateful for that decision and dedication.

He was kind to those of us who were science majors and took his classes as electives. We weren't treated differently from the English majors.

One thing I remember is his respect for his wife. He often said that she had given up much to marry him. He said that if there were an emergency in her family, they would not be able to afford a trip for her to return home.

He had to cross the bypass every day between his home and Hope. He often said that the odds were against him and that he knew one day he wouldn't make it across safely. Thankfully, that prediction never came true. However, I often think of that comment when I cross the bypass on my way into Holland.

I took a summer literature course from Jim Prins the summer between my junior and senior years at Hope, and had to read one hundred pages every day in order to complete the required nine books. I enjoyed the course and liked living in an apartment for a summer. However, I swore off reading for many months after my Hope graduation (I had read twenty-seven books for three consecutive lit classes) but rescinded that decision a few years later.

I appreciate this opportunity to express my gratitude and appreciation for a man who played a part in my Hope education. I will remember him with gratitude for many years to come.

It is surely a tribute that his students from almost fifty years ago still remember him with fondness and will travel to Holland to pay tribute to him.

—Loraine M. Pschigoda, Class of 1959

℘

DEAR JIM,

Kathleen Verduin, of the Hope College English Department, contacted me about your memorial of August 17th. Wish I could have been present.

I always thought much of you. You guided me through American and English Novel, introduced me to Charles Dickens. For most of my pastoral life, and leadership in Native American Affairs, has been devoted to making change, for the futures of the boy "ignorance" and the girl "want" as presented by the ghost of Christmas Present.

My own humble efforts at getting published have resulted in a book of poetry, a book of short stories. Now, I have a work in progress, on the subject of motivation.

You and Henry ten Hoor were the men I looked up to. Ms. Protheroe was also an inspiration to me. As I never knew my own father, you, along with Eugene Osterhaven at Western Seminary, hold a special place in my spirit. I wanted to be like you fellows.

Over the years, we have spoken a few times, exchanged notes. You applauded and encouraged me in my writing. Thank you.

I can still see that turtle of John Steinbeck, crawling across the road. The first driver, at peril, avoided hitting the turtle with the "old humorous eyes." The truck that came down the road next struck the edge of the turtle's shell, landing it wounded, and on its back. Recovering, the turtle went on, planting three wild oats for a future harvest. My own shell wounded, my toes have "slipped a fraction in the dust." Still, I continue to look forward to the harvest, and sitting under the shade of a big oak tree on a breezy day with you, and the Brontë sisters.

As you greet my friends and relatives, up there, tell them I still greet the Omahas, and say: "Washkonga Ho Cuga." That means, Good health and may God bless you, my friend. Until we meet again.

—*Frank V. Love, Class of 1961*

&

MR. PRINS WAS ABLE to communicate with his expressions and tone of voice better than any other instructor I've ever had. I particularly remember Mr. Prins talking about how his son, who must have been three or four years old at the time, would object when he would put on a dress shirt, a sign of imminent departure. He said that Christopher would point to a casual shirt and ask his daddy to "put that one on." Many years later what he said and what he must have felt came back to me when my own son was about that age and could not understand why I couldn't take him with me on a trip to the Mideast.

—John Draper, Class of 1962

☙

HE COULD make me sit up in class and read the assignments the night before so that I could contribute: he made me want to think, to care, yet even then he didn't know it. In short, he gave me the best, the only gift a teacher can give a student.

—Tom Vandenberg, Class of 1964
(quoted from the Hope College Magazine, *1969)*

☙

WHAT I REMEMBER vividly was his face. He had a beautiful face, all long and sallow planes with incredible warmth in the eyes and smile. He would perch his Ichabod Crane body on the desk. One long leg folded, knee up, sock falling, and the other in perilous equilibrium on the floor. Book in hand, he surveyed us from this incredible position. Dr. Prins danced before us, he danced around us, and is still always dancing beside us . . . inviting us to his celebration.

Now a funny story. Maybe curious would be a better way to describe it. We were talking about predestination in class. I do not remember how this came up, but what a heavy subject for the young students that we were. Suddenly I said, "What makes you think that I'll come walking in through the door next time we have class? I may be sick or something else may happen."

We all agreed that whatever happened it would have been predestined anyway. Well, next time we had class I went early, made sure that the window latch was not locked, and went to wait outside. When class had started, I climbed up the fire escape and burst into the classroom through the window.

The surprise was great and Dr. Prins frowned . . . this was the first time I had ever seen him frown. I turned to him and, raising my arms halfway up my body, palms open, shrugged my question to him.

Dr. Prins gave me an affectionate but stern look and said, "De Velder, you are an ass." And I was one. I had disturbed the class and proved nothing. Thank you for the lesson, teacher.

Once, on another occasion, he did say however that I had a fertile mind. I was so proud. Of course, he did not say if I was using it properly or not.

Dr. Prins used his whole mind . . . the right and the left brain. He even got us in touch with our "reptile" brain for some of the more somber literature we studied with him. He never taught by monologue, but dialogued with us. He pushed and cajoled us to think, to experience, to put into practice the fine lessons to be learned from the written word. In his lessons he let us put things into place ourselves. Lessons of honor, lessons of humility, lessons of humanity, lessons of love. Love of man. Love of God. Always the love of literature.

I will never forget his smile. It started small
and tentative, then went wide and generous.
Then into the eyes, so kind and expressive. Then
into laughter, the like of which I have never heard
before nor since. A building and building into an
explosion, both infectious and communicative.
He sounded like a bell, pealing deep and harmo-
nious, and it was oh so fulfilling to laugh with
him.

—Dirck de Velder, Class of 1965

❧

THE QUINTESSENTIAL revelatory Prins happened one spring day when he walked into class
and commenced, without so much as a hello, to
wail on the college administration for plastering
the image of a particularly attractive co-ed on all
of its promo material. Exploitation and cruelty,
he called it, and hardly befitting the posture of a
Christian college that cared about *who* its students were. There was probably more that he
loosed upon us that day, but I don't remember it,
so enthralled was I with the white-hot purity of
his indignation and compassion—and all of this
long before feminism and its protests about the
objectification of women.

For me at least, that was a confirmation of
sorts, an emphatic indication that all Prins did
and said in behalf of the stories he taught really
did have real and immediate consequence for the
living of one's own very real life. You suspected
all along that the reason he was in the teaching
business was that literature harbored some
pressing connection to how we spent our days.

With Prins, all those many, and sometimes very long, novels—about one a week, regardless of length—laid bare the complex tangles that invariably engulf the mysterious creatures that we are. And such riddles were not only interesting but of urgent importance for how one understood and, because of that, chose to live. The cascade of words he daily bestowed upon us all, his own and from the critics, struggled toward putting a verbal fence around that mysterious and finally inscrutable thicket of wonder—what he himself likely suspected could not be said and made clear, no matter what the effort, but golly, he came close, ever so close. And, remarkably, he got others to join up.

That day he fumed about the college was as personal as A. James ever got, for class time was given over entirely, for him and for us, to the utter submission to the subject matter at hand, the teasing out of puzzles of meaning in literary texts, the longer and more daunting the better. For his self-appointed crusade, Prins seemed like he was sent straight from Central Casting, and he probably was. All ascetic leanness, he sometimes came into class looking for all the world like some crazed monk who had wandered in from the desert. Or, in his supreme cragginess and a thatch of hair, a bent-over 6'4" or so, and, what, maybe 160 pounds, heavily tweeded so to keep the meager flesh warm, he most resembled a character from the stories he taught: Ichabod Crane or maybe Don Quixote, and, for sure, Isaiah. Or maybe simply a milder, sweeter version of Ahab, an earlier existential Quaker-Calvinist caught in the fierce scramble to know what God knows. If one was going to bother with being alive, one ought then to find out a few things about it.

All of this sounds larger than ordinary life, and it was. For that only two words will do, though repeated over and over: thank you, thank you.

—Roy M. Anker, Class of 1966

☎

WHILE REFLECTING upon the legacy of Dr. James Prins, I came across an address given by Professor Henry Zylstra at a teachers' conference in October of 1948. Zylstra taught English at Calvin College from 1941-1956. In his address, entitled "The Role of Literature in Our Times" (later published in his *Testament of Vision*), Professor Zylstra argues that literature should be considered as part of humane letters rather than one of the fine arts. Teachers of English, he goes on to say, should teach it as an "exacting discipline"; they should teach it "intensively rather than in historical surveys"; teachers should make their students achieve "the personal experience of literature"; and they should give it more time in the schools than currently done. In an age of pragmatism, Zylstra warned against literary study "sneaked edgewise" into curricula overburdened with grammar, rhetoric, and composition. And during the heyday of formalist criticism, he argued for the notion that literature is about "seeing life steadily and seeing it whole."

These points summarize rather well James Prins's teaching of literature. In his courses on the American novel and the European novel, Dr.

Prins taught the great works of the canon in their entirety, no matter what their length. In the course on the European novel, I recall thirteen novels, including *Anna Karenina, Madame Bovary, The Plague*, and *And Quiet Flows the Don*. With erudition and great finesse, he would discuss the historical, social, and political contexts of the works examined. Then, after dwelling on the style of the novel, its plot lines, characters, themes, world view, he would muse on its human significance. "Mme Bovary, c'est moi," he quoted, identifying with Flaubert's anguish at the writing of his tale. For too-brief moments, he enabled us to imagine worlds apart, he gave us space and freedom to feel, to dream, to love literature.

—Anne M. Larsen, Class of 1970

ॐ

I STILL HAVE, marginally marked, my copies of many of the novels we read with Jim Prins. I recall the large lecture hall in Graves where he stood on the platform looking haggard even at what must have been, from my current perspective on aging, his fairly tender years in the late `60s. I recall reading *Anna Karenina* and *Crime and Punishment* in a weekend (I was younger then) so I could take a test on Monday morning. I remember that I wanted to take his courses, as everyone else did, and I remember some years ago my father's remembering him from the days of his instructorship in the late `40s as being already the man I came to know twenty years later. Beyond that, little except a sense of constant low-level torment and struggle in the cadence of the voice or the gaze out the window or the pause in a lecture, of a life that advertised itself as having seen more than it wanted to of life, and of the seriousness with which he seemed to take everything even while laughing—how important and ultimate everything seemed to be whether in the world outside the lecture hall or in the texts we were reading. That's all well and good, and a *persona* like that is perhaps particularly appealing to the college-aged. As in all pedagogical scenes, I guess, the professorial performance mediating the texts is more important and longer remembered than is the substance of the course.

My most vivid memory of Prins, however, is from long after the fact. A couple years ago I read the then new Richard Pevear and Larissa Volokhonsky translation of *Anna Karenina*, a book that I can hear myself claiming long ago had changed my life in college. As I grinned and chuckled my way through its pages I marveled that Prins, perhaps abetted by Constance Garnett, hadn't told me this novel is a comedy of manners. *Anna* is one of the few novels I have ever reread, but the shadow over thirty years later of that Prinsly, as I recall it, anguished or, on tamer days, weltschmerzy experience of *Anna* testifies to something at once clichéd and profound about how books read the reader, how life stages or context or, if you portentously will, history and texts interact. No longer cowed and inspired by what I must have taken in college as the "adultness" of his experience of the texts we read, this tension in memory is enough to remember now and write, and enough to be grateful for.

—*Robert Kieft, Class of 1970*

ℒ

I REMEMBER WELL taking every novels course offered by Jim Prins, using them to fulfill electives for my political science major. I was absolutely captivated by his lectures. He made the characters come alive. He prodded me to look for meaning deep beneath the words of the story. I most vividly remember his lectures on *The Scarlet Letter*. He became so animated, and in the process challenged me to think more deeply about moral issues.

—Glenn G. Lowe, Class of 1970

ℒ

AS A TRIBUTE to his unpretentious character and humility, Dr. Prins left a lasting impression on me when he once told this little story in English class.

He and his young son were traveling in their older (already somewhat dilapidated) car down the streets of Holland, Michigan.

The son asked his father, "Dad, why are the people staring at us?"

Dr. Prins answered, "Because they think we're migrant workers, son."

—Adelheid Holthuis Fuith, Class of 1971

ℒ

I JUST READ in today's *News from Hope College* about the death of Dr. Prins. Another Hope legend gone. I remember his Modern Novel lectures in Graves Hall, the way he stood up there looking like Abraham Lincoln, his long expressive fingers curling around as he talked, pointing, jabbing the air. We were all so young and naive, and he introduced us to dark worlds—the worlds of Madame Bovary and Raskolnikov and Kafka—the world of Europe, which was so different from the cheery "Hi-ya" Midwest. He helped us understand the sexual symbolism of Faulkner, and we couldn't believe he actually said those things right there in front of us. He helped us learn that the things we were beginning to fear ourselves, the late night anxieties, were nothing new—this was the stuff of literature. It made us want to be English majors!

God bless him. I will certainly pray for him. He was a wonderful teacher, a good man.

—Nancy Forest-Flier, Class of 1971

⅘

I HAD JIM PRINS for several classes and they were my favorites. In one he yelled at my friend and me—well, he didn't really yell AT us, but he suggested that those not paying attention should get the hell out of his class. We had been joking a bit in the back and making wind noises to each other in response to the picture of the title character on the front of the book, while Prins was taking *Tess of the D'Urbervilles* quite to heart. But that, of course, is what he was all about. Taking the books to heart.

There was not a lot of technical English talk in his classes. Metaphors and motifs were not the coins of the realm in a Jim Prins class. Instead we discussed the characters and their motivations, their decisions and the repercussions, as if they were real. And in that classroom they were.

I've been teaching English and literature for twenty-four years, and the characters in the books I teach are like old friends. I can't wait to revisit them every year. I suspect my classroom manner owes more to those hours spent with Jim Prins than I've ever acknowledged. But I want to thank Mr. Prins for showing me that books are foremost stories about people and lessons in life.

—*Bill Weller, Class of 1976*

$\mathscr{Q}$

WHEN I STARTED at Hope College, an advanced placement score allowed me to start taking 300-level classes as a freshman. This first one of these classes I took was Russian Novels with Dr. Prins.

I will never forget the thrill of sitting there in an assembly hall filled with upperclassmen, listening to Dr. Prins go over the syllabus. Over the course of my years at Hope, I had several classes with Dr. Prins, all of them surveys of literature, and I remember not only the great themes he taught, but also his unfailing courtesy and kindness. He always started the semester by apologizing for the small type in the paperbacks he ordered through the bookstore. Then he would invariably explain each time that he had looked for the least expensive version of the book that he could find, so as not to burden us with extra costs in his courses, which required numerous books. He addressed students with respect and listened to questions patiently and attentively. I always felt comfortable in his classes.

One time, Dr. Prins questioned a student who had been absent for a number of classes. The student told Dr. Prins that his grandfather had died. Dr. Prins said how sorry he was, even while some of the students, disbelieving the story, chuckled in the background. Dr. Prins gently chided them, saying that they had no reason to doubt the student. Then he said something I'll never forget. He said, "Even if you don't believe him, I do. And that's because I'm a teacher. It's my *job* to trust you and believe you."

Since that day in Graves Hall, I've tutored students, worked in elementary classrooms, and taught as an adjunct instructor at Grand Valley State University. Any time I privately doubted a student's excuses, I hope that I never let it show, always remembering the words of this dignified and compassionate man I had been privileged to have had as a model.

—*Kathryn Solms Wheeler, Class of 1976*

⌀

I NEVER KNEW a better reader than Professor Prins. At the start of one of our novels classes, he confessed he was a swift reader when younger but now could not manage more than twenty pages an hour. His progress through a book was exhaustive: he noticed everything. As I get older myself, my reading, too, increasingly has grown deliberate, but no matter how I race to match him, I always see Prins outdistancing me.

That lean, lank body was an apt illustration of Prins' reader's soul. He was folded and creased almost to an abstraction, the better to insert himself between the meanings of words. I seldom saw him after his retirement. For all I know, he lived long enough to read the entire world in a single word. Perhaps, at the end, even the silence spoke for him, his mind finally spinning out original interpretations in a resonant, cosmic thrum.

—Christopher Wiers, Class of 1981

$\wp$

MY RELATIONSHIP with Dr. Prins began the day we discussed *The Great Gatsby*. He kept saying that Gatsby was under the assumption that "everything was possible" if you did what was necessary. Gatsby, he said, personified the American Dream. I was thoroughly engaged in his lecture. At the end of the class I approached him, near tears, and cried, *"Isn't* everything possible?"

He understood. He understood that I mourned for Gatsby in a very personal way, because I lived the novels I read. He understood because he did, too. We were kindred spirits.

I loved his classes. I loved the books. I loved the way Dr. Prins communicated his love of literature. I loved the fact that simply reading the books was enough; he didn't assign a lot of papers. He could tell instantly whether or not a student had read the book. I have to admit, I found his classes easy. Reading was play. His lectures were a joy. His courses were a break from French verbs and diminished seventh chords. I don't know how I would have survived Hope without them.

I was a very confused kid. I didn't know what I wanted to do with my talents. My mother and grandfather were journalists, and I loved to read and write. Unfortunately, journalism left me cold. I wasn't interested in current events. I wanted to write poetry. After graduating from Hope, I used to joke that I minored in music so I would have something to fall back on.

Now I am a musician. I teach voice, so I still get to indulge my love of poetry and foreign languages, in the form of song literature. I perform early music (pre-eighteenth century), so I get to indulge my love of history. I still read for pleasure. I used to try to write, but my two children and my students take up too much of my time.

I am a very good voice teacher. I am passionate about my subject matter. I love my students. I love helping them succeed. I try to communicate my love of music in all its variety. My philosophy is to teach them as many songs as possible before they go off to college (in addition to working on technique, of course). It occurs to me that Dr. Prins very much lives on in my work. It occurs to me as I write that I was deeply influenced by the man.

—*Nancy MacArthur Smith, Class of 1982*

ℒ

WORKING FOR the Hope College English Department during the 2004-2005 school year, I had the privilege of viewing and transcribing some of James's class notes. Unfortunately I never had James as a professor, but I feel that through these notes I was privy to a slice of who this man was as a professor and as a human being. His questions on literature were not exclusive to the passages he quoted, but included questions on life in general. They were questions we ourselves might often think of but never really form into words. I learned a great deal from James Prins. He didn't give me too many answers, but he certainly made me ask questions.

—*Meaghan E. L. Elliott, Class of 2005*

ﾂﾂﾂ

Ultimate Freedom:
Remembering A. James Prins

Jacob E. Nyenhuis, Provost Emeritus

He came in a vision last night.
They were all there, the giants of the past—
Henry ten Hoor, Bert Ponstein, D. Ivan Dykstra,
John Hollenbach—
But it was A. James Prins
Who demanded center stage.
He strode, no, loped again
Down the corridors of
Third-floor Lubbers.
Battling his demons in the guise of
The Brothers Karamazov and others
In the rogues' gallery of
Tolstoy and Dostoevski,
He railed against injustice,
Assailed mandatory retirement.
Abandoning friends of a lifetime,
He followed Kazantzakis's Odysseus
To ultimate freedom—death.

✍

A Poem for (A) James Prins

Edward S. Small, Class of 1963

Read at the retirement celebration, June 6, 1981.

My Michigan Mentor—
I am told that we may
Bring thee gifts; let
This poem stand for mine.

Alliteration fails to
serve my thanks
to thee,
Who set me
On my course;
Yet I come in
confusion
Not knowing whether
To kiss thy cheeks
In gesture of
Gratitude profound,
Or to punch the
forebones of thy
calves around,
With deft
little kicks:

(to shin.)
For this mess
That I am in
Results from thy
illusion.

There was a time
When you and I were young
(Younger than we dare now dream
we could be):
You were then
My age now;
And I? Too young to
Remember: transformed by
Thee since, scheming on
To other things (yet)
Still emulating
Your ideals.

When I knew you
(When you were my age)
You were legend,
Emblem for academe
(ech) excellence.
Now (that I am
Your age, then)
I know I'll never
be as good as Thee
As:
Teacher
Mentor
Humanitarian Philosopher
Existentialist
Actor Saint . . . whatever.
But (all) academe

Ain't what
it seemed
to be, then—
Some twenty years ago
This day
When play of mind
Was on my mind
(Mirrored by your own
designs)
And profound expectations,
Great expectations
(See?) Can allusion
Serve poor me
Better (than alliteration, see?)
To assure you
That I, after all,
I learned something.
And that Edward Small
Learned well
Those thoughts,
Ideas so
Well expressed
With such singular methodology

So what was illusionary?
Your grace: you made it
Look so easy
And so much fun. (Yet)
Today's academe
(the mess I'm in)
Suffers broadcast bureaucracy:
Which ain't much fun
And ain't easy,
Worse—the intellect
(I suspect)

Ain't no gate to
God. Does
That pilgrim's quest
(what you taught best) say
art may still provide
a way?

Recall Keats' (structuralist)
equation: "Truth is Beauty
                Beauty, Truth—
                That's all ye
                Know (and)
                All ye need
                to know"
Upon this Earth which gives
Us birth (to)
Christ's beyond.

Beyond for you (now)
Will be beyond for me
(then, when you are old
or returned heavenfold).
For the interim
Let your mentorship
Remain.
Again give me call
And guidance,
Lest I fall,
Go down this drain
Of drainèd intellect,
Or the lesser limbo of
Cathartic Art,
Or just fart
Around expanding resumes.
Tender thy advice

Tell me what is meet
And nice
About these years that remain
Before I reach your (`81) Age then;
And then
Maybe
You can tell me
What to do
After,

After Eliot's
cups
Marmalade and Tea
Eliot's talk:
(You and Me):
When Eliot's
Balled-up universe
Is in reverse,
From us
and our
Angelic machinery.

Maybe you can (still)
Tell me what-to-do
To get me through
This interim,
My present and
Your past.
Can you mentor
My present passage
(and perhaps my last)?

On Attending the Memorial Service of A. James Prins

Judith Tanis Parr, Class of 1967

The August ceremony in Mulder Chapel gathered
the family,
the former students, the former colleagues,
friends from near and far—
rememberers all—and an unexpected guest.

Whether through open window or open door,
whether allured by the sensual music of Chopin
and Debussy
or by the peaceful shade,
there it was, the thing with feathers, Emily's
"Hope," a sparrow.

What does one do with a sparrow in a memorial
service?
Cover one's head? Try to ignore it?

Yes, try to ignore it.
Focus on the reflections:
      . . . learned heart and passionate mind . . .
Focus on the poetry reading:

. . . guardian butterflies . . . children building
sand castles . . .
. . . and the waves wash them all away . . .

And there was that bird again, flitting on high
from ledge to ledge.
Focus on the scripture reading:
"then came Jesus, the doors being shut, and
stood in the midst, and said, Peace be unto
you."

That bird, now sailing in the nave, circling,
wheeling, reeling,
Turning and turning in the widening gyre . . .
Yeats?

Yes, of course.
Literary criticism, Van Raalte Hall, 1967,
explicating poems:
"Among School Children"?
"Sailing to Byzantium"?
"The Second Coming"?
And T. S. Eliot:
"Journey of the Magi,"
"Love Song of J. Alfred Prufrock":
Let us go then, you and I . . .
There will be time, there will be time . . .
Do I dare? Do I dare disturb the universe?
I grow old . . . I grow old . . .
"I am Lazarus, come back from the dead,
Come back to tell you all, I shall tell you
all."
Somewhere in time . . . aloof . . . that bird . . .
observing:
Surely some revelation is at hand.

Was it the late professor sneaking in to attend his
own funeral?
Giving one last chance speech? Giving us the
bird? One final protest?

My eyes are on the sparrow, the vulnerable bird,
the Venerable Bede:
   Our life is as the bird flying in from the winter
darkness
      through one door, into the warmth of the
mead-hall,
         then out the other.

And Pascal:
   When I consider the short duration of my life,
      swallowed up in the eternity of before and af-
ter . . .
      the eternal silence of these infinite spaces
frightens me.

And Milton: "When I consider how my light is
spent . . ."

When I consider . . .
Focus on the text, . . . the words, . . . the Word:
   "because thou hast seen me, thou hast believed:
      blessed are they who have not seen and yet
believed."

ℒ

Jim

Delwyn Sneller, Class of 1967

I

From Graves you spoke
Forever in that brown suit.
You laughed and wept with words.
Felicité's stuffed parrot
Haunted the Pine Grove
And the tiny beetle
From Anna Karenina's haystack
Ran across our hands.
You mocked reason's sand hinges
And welcomed our dreams
To parades of drummers and clowns.

You always carried the college
In your tattered briefcase.
With a father's love
You fretted over wickedness
And often you were afraid.

II

You liked
My old sonnet about sand castles—
How beachcombers topple them
And waves wash them away,
The way even poems
Are leveled and lost.
But other children find the lake,
The sand, the haze of midsummer noon—
Playthings more durable than minds.

All that matters is our children—
The jaws of forgetful landscapes
Around their ankles.
Turgenev, Hawthorne, Hardy—
These mean nothing
Until we see our children
Playing in the sand;
Their castles and walls
Built to last.

III

I remember a golf game with you
Mostly in swamp and woods.
You saw no worth in it,
And claimed it struck
The flammable part of your soul.
The poison ivy was interesting, you thought;
Something Whitman could make into
"LITRITURE."
We shared golf clubs, my ten dollar set,
And laughed
At the impossible bridge

And huge hot lawn.

IV

Let me tell you something:
I love you
Because you counted
The trees in your yard
And valued
The common agate, the ordinary day.
You named
The angry red butterfly
That guarded your porch
May through October.
You kept the locusts' willow,
The map burning in the chimney
A wife, children, grandchildren—
All more precious
Than anything written.
The only way to travel home
Is on foot
Together.
You said this, my teacher;
You did not lie.

V

You stood in the middle of the weather
Knowing taproots guessed your heart.
Along hushed hills
Ghosts shook water
From glass faces. Slow
Autumn huntings followed
A grey pirouette through windless woods;
She chilled sunlight and pulled

Stars into chains.

She asked why you tried to be
What you already were.
You escaped (or said you did)
Remarkably intact—ghosts back
Under cracked basement floors
And you to bones and books.

Everything we do returns,
For time, like wind, hurls
Our dust ahead of us.

You were a simple pilgrim
With stones in your shoes.
You loved the sky,
The sky,
Stronger than almost
Every birth.

VI

The night that holds you now
Allows no wave goodbye, no kiss,
For death despises courtesy.
But we believe a broken hand
Has passed above your soul
And light has gathered time
Into another world
Where we will once again embrace.
And you will find a scarlet butterfly
Upon a porch and shores
Where castles made of sand
Are swept away.

❧❧❧❧❧

ACKNOWLEDGMENTS

Articles from *The Hope College Magazine* and *The Anchor* are reprinted by permission of the Office of Public Relations, Hope College.

"Charles Williams" is reprinted from *The Reformed Review*, March 1967, and appears by permission.

"From Fact to Fiction" is reprinted from *The Church Herald*, August 22, 1969. Copyright © by *The Church Herald*. Used with permission.

"The Catholic Novel" is reprinted from *The Christian Scholar's Review* II:4 (1973). Copyright © 1973 by *The Christian Scholar's Review*. Reprinted by permission.

"Spiritual Frontiers in the Contemporary Novel" and "A War on God: Kingsley Amis" are reprinted from *The Reformed Journal*, January 1960 and October 1977. Reprinted by permission.

The editors gratefully acknowledge help and encouragement from Iris Prins, Robin and Philip Bakker, Yvette Hopkins, and David Vander Meulen, and, at Hope College, from David Klooster, Peter Schakel, Stephen Hemenway, and William Pannapacker of the Department of English; Mark Cook, Director of the Hope-Geneva Bookstore; Elton Bruins, Van Raalte Institute; Geoffrey Reynolds, Joint Archives of Holland; and Tom Renner and Greg Olgers, Office of Public Relations. Brian Cook designed the dust jacket and cover. Kate Maybury, Chris Gould, and Andrew Bredow, Office of Computing and Information Technology, gave invaluable technical assistance, as did Sally Smith, Office Manager for the Departments of Philosophy and Political Science. Myra Kohsel, Office Manager of the Department of English, worked tirelessly and with skill at all stages of production. Meaghan E. L. Elliott, Stephanie Judd, Maggie Machledt, and Stephanie McCann typed the manuscript.